The ECG in Emergency Decision Making

D. MASNEY

The ECG in Emergency Decision Making

SECOND EDITION

Hein J. J. Wellens, MD, FACC, FESC, FAHA

Professor of Cardiology
University of Maastricht
The Netherlands

Mary Conover, BSN

Director of Education
Critical Care Conferences
Santa Cruz, California

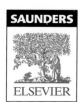
SAUNDERS

ELSEVIER

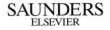

SAUNDERS
ELSEVIER

11830 Westline Industrial Drive
St. Louis, Missouri 63146

THE ECG IN EMERGENCY DECISION MAKING,
SECOND EDITION

ISBN-13 978-1-4160-0259-8
ISBN-10 1-4160-0259-6

Notice

Knowledge and best practice in this field are constantly changing. As new research and experience broaden our knowledge, changes in practice, treatment and drug therapy may become necessary or appropriate. Readers are advised to check the most current information provided (i) on procedures featured or (ii) by the manufacturer of each product to be administered, to verify the recommended dose or formula, the method and duration of administration, and contraindications. It is the responsibility of the practitioner, relying on their own experience and knowledge of the patient, to make diagnoses, to determine dosages and the best treatment for each individual patient, and to take all appropriate safety precautions. To the fullest extent of the law, neither the Publisher nor the Authors assume any liability for any injury and/or damage to persons or property arising out or related to any use of the material contained in this book.

The Publisher

ISBN-13 978-1-4160-0259-8
ISBN-10 1-4160-0259-6

Editor: Sandra Clark Brown
Senior Developmental Editor: Cindi Anderson
Publishing Services Manager: Deborah L. Vogel
Senior Project Manager: Deon Lee
Design Manager: Teresa McBryan

Printed in the United States of America

Last digit is the print number: 9 8 7 6 5 4 3 2

Preface

In cardiac emergencies, the correct diagnosis of the underlying cause is the first step to optimal treatment. With that goal in mind, the second edition of *The ECG in Emergency Decision Making* provides a systematic approach to the 12-lead ECG for accurate and effective decision making in cardiac emergencies. We offer concise and logical steps to the ECG recognition of underlying mechanisms in cardiac, pulmonary, drug-related, electrolyte, hypothermic, pacing, and defibrillator emergencies. This book is meant to be a quick and ready guide to health care professionals familiar with the basics of electrocardiography.

Chapter 1 discusses the *early* recognition of myocardial infarction (MI) in order to prevent irreversible myocardial damage by timely reperfusion. This chapter explains how to use the ST segment changes to rapidly estimate the location and size of the area at risk and to decide which reperfusion strategy is needed and especially when *percutaneous coronary intervention* is preferred.

Chapter 2 is devoted to the emergency response to and prognosis of patients who present with cardiac chest pain without an ST elevation MI ECG, but with other important changes indicating MI potential or real myocardial damage, depending on the troponin T level.

Chapter 3 discusses the emergency approach to sinoatrial and atrioventricular conduction abnormalities.

Chapter 4 offers a systematic approach to the ECG differential diagnosis of paroxysmal supraventricular tachycardia, and **Chapter 5** provides ECG clues to rapid recognition of ventricular tachycardia.

The remaining chapters provide step-by-step emergency approaches to drug-induced ECG changes and arrhythmias, including digitalis toxicity, potassium derangements, acute pulmonary embolism, and life-threatening hypothermia.

Monogenic diseases are covered in **Chapter 11.** During the last decade, it became possible to make a genetic diagnosis in a number of patients with certain ECG features, providing a means of risk stratification and management of carriers of monogenic diseases prone to cardiac arrhythmias and sudden death.

Chapters 12 and **13** provide guidance in emergency decision making regarding pacing, defibrillator, and prehospital emergencies.

The **appendixes** are helpful and instructive in regard to emergency drugs, electrical treatment of arrhythmias, axis determination, and mechanisms of aberrancy.

As a learning tool we have provided a brief outline and refresher of emergency management on detachable cards at the end of the book.

We strongly believe that an informed health care professional can provide correct interpretation of the ECG in an emergency situation, providing a better outcome for many patients.

Hein J. J. Wellens

Mary Conover

Acknowledgments

Almost all of the ECGs in this book were provided by colleagues from the Department of Cardiology of the Academic Hospital Maastricht. I am very grateful for their contributions.

Among them, a special word of thanks goes to Dr. Anton Gorgels for his continuous support and supply of great ECGs.

Most of the artwork was done by Adrie van den Dool. Her help is gratefully acknowledged.

M. C. would like to thank Candice Walker, Chief Librarian, and her assistant, Catherine Mountjoy, at Dominican Hospital in Santa Cruz, who once again cheerfully responded to requests for references, diligently seeking out articles not at hand. I would also like to acknowledge and thank John R. Buysman, PhD, of Medtronic for his support over the years.

Hein J. J. Wellens

Mary Conover

Abbreviations

The abbreviations listed here are well known and in common usage. They will therefore not be expanded again in the text.

APB	atrial premature beat
AV	atrioventricular
CX	circumflex (coronary artery)
ECG	electrocardiogram
LAD	left anterior descending (coronary artery)
LBBB	left bundle branch block
LV	left ventricle
MI	myocardial infarction
PSVT	paroxysmal supraventricular tachycardia
QTc	QT interval corrected for heart rate
RBBB	right bundle branch block
RCA	right coronary artery
RV	right ventricle
SA	sinoatrial
SVT	supraventricular tachycardia
VPB	ventricular premature beat
VT	ventricular tachycardia

Contents

CHAPTER 4
Narrow QRS Tachycardia, 91

CHAPTER 6
Digitalis-Induced Emergencies, 158

C H A P T E R

1

The ECG in Acute ST Segment Elevation MI

EMERGENCY DECISIONS
1. Ascertain the time from onset of pain.
2. Determine the size and severity of cardiac ischemia and the location of the occlusion in the coronary artery by analyzing the amount and direction of the ST segment deviation vector.
3. Look for conduction disturbances, especially bundle branch block.
4. Decide on the necessity and type of reperfusion attempt (fibrinolysis or a primary percutaneous coronary intervention).

The earliest change in the ECG in acute cardiac ischemia after a coronary occlusion is a deviation of the ST segment from the isoelectric line. The location and severity of ischemia are indicated by the amount and direction of ST segment deviation. This stage is when reperfusion can salvage or limit the damage to the jeopardized area. Failure to restore blood flow will be followed by loss (necrosis) of myocardial tissue (MI) with changes in the QRS and T wave.

ST SEGMENT ELEVATION MI

ST segment elevation MI (STEMI) is a condition in which a patient has chest pain along with ST elevation in two or more ECG leads. In recent years, the emphasis has been placed on *early* recognition of MI because in the early phase of MI, damage can be prevented by timely reperfu-

sion of the ischemic area. Therefore the terms *ST segment elevation MI (STEMI)* and *non–ST segment elevation MI (non-STEMI)* are now being used. The differentiation between STEMI and non-STEMI is suggested because in the acute stage, STEMI must be managed differently from non-STEMI. However, it is important to understand that in patients with left main or CX occlusion, ST depression may be present in most ECG leads, and those patients should not be classified as having non-STEMI. The knowledge of how to use the ST segment changes to estimate rapidly the location and size of the area at risk and decide what reperfusion strategy is needed is therefore essential in cases of acute cardiac ischemia. Obviously, if the area at risk is large, a *percutaneous coronary intervention* is preferred and the patient should be referred to an institution where this can be performed.

THE IMPORTANCE OF ST SEGMENT DEVIATION

It is common knowledge that localized, acute, severe cardiac ischemia leads to ST segment elevation in the ECG leads representing the involved myocardial region, with reciprocal ST segment depression in leads opposite that area.

ST SEGMENT DEVIATION SCORE

The ST segment deviation score is calculated by adding the number of millimeters that the ST segment deviates (elevation or depression) from the isoelectric line in all 12 ECG leads. Examples of how to determine the ST segment deviation score in STEMI are shown in Figure 1-1. *A score of more than 12 mm* indicates an ischemic area of such a size that timely reperfusion will result in salvage of a substantial amount of myocardial tissue.

As early as 1986, when thrombolytic therapy was beginning to be used as a treatment for acute MI, an ST segment deviation score was used to determine the site and size of the area at risk. At that time, the benefit from thrombolytic therapy was shown to be related to the height of the ST segment deviation score.[1-4]

Limitations

The ST deviation score has the following two important limitations:

1. ST segment deviation fluctuates with the degree of ischemia present at a certain point in time. Those fluctuations may underestimate the area at risk when the ECG is recorded at a moment of moderate ST segment deviation. Thus a better determinant of the size of the area at risk would be the *ST segment deviation vector.*

2. The extremity leads give more global information—and the precordial leads more local information—about location and extent of ischemia.

ST SEGMENT DEVIATION VECTOR

More recently, the concept of the *ST segment deviation vector*, also called the *vector of ischemia*, was introduced to predict the site of occlusion in the coronary artery and thus the approximate size of the area at risk; the more proximal the location of the occlusion in the coronary artery, the greater the area at risk.[5-8]

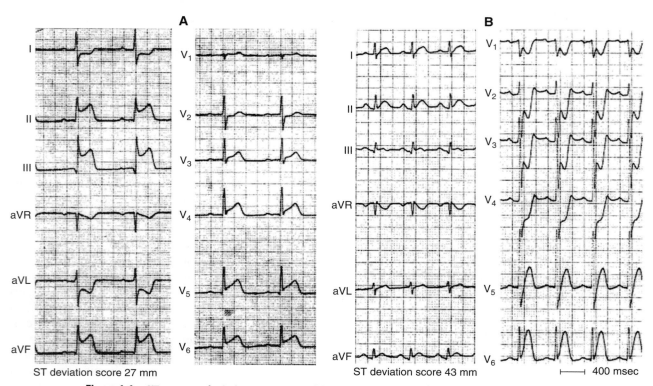

A

ST deviation score 27 mm

B

ST deviation score 43 mm

⊢——⊣ 400 msec

Figure 1-1 ST segment deviation score. **A,** In this patient with an acute inferolateral MI, by using all 12 leads, the total amount of ST segment deviation measures 27 mm. **B,** This patient with an acute inferoposterolateral MI has an ST segment deviation score of 43 mm.

The ST segment deviation vector is determined by the same method as is the QRS vector, described in Appendix A:

1. Look for the isoelectric ST segment in the limb leads to determine the lead axis perpendicular to the ST segment vector.
2. Find the most positive or most negative ST segment deviation to determine the direction of the ST segment vector.

Determining the Site of Occlusion in the Coronary Artery

INFEROPOSTERIOR ST SEGMENT ELEVATION MI

As indicated in Figure 1-2, inferoposterior ischemia can be caused by an occlusion in the RCA or the CX coronary artery.

ECG changes in response to RCA or CX occlusion are summarized in Box 1-1 and described below. The limb leads and lead V_4R provide information about RCA and CX occlusion, whereas the precordial leads provide information about the presence of ischemia of the RV and the posterior wall of the LV.

RCA Occlusion

The RCA usually perfuses the inferior and posteromedial parts of the LV as well as the RV and the AV node. Figure 1-2 shows that with an RCA occlusion the ST deviation vector in the frontal plane points to lead III, resulting in more ST elevation in lead III than in lead II (Figure 1-3).

Also, the ST vector is away from the negative electrode in lead I, causing ST depression in that lead. These facts are summarized in Box 1-1.

BOX 1-1

ECG Findings Indicating the Location of ST Elevation MI and Site of Occlusion in the Culprit Vessel in Inferoposterior MI (RCA or CX Occlusion)

RCA Occlusion
- ST depression in lead I
- ST elevation lead III greater than in lead II

Proximal
- ST elevation more than 1 mm with positive T wave in lead V_4R

Distal
- ST isoelectric with a positive T wave in lead V_4R

CX Coronary Artery Occlusion
- ST elevation in lead II greater than lead III
- ST isoelectric or elevated in lead I
- ST isoelectric or depressed with negative T wave in lead V_4R

Extension to Posterior Wall
- ST depression in precordial leads

Extension to Lateral Wall
- ST elevation in leads I, aVL, V_5, and V_6

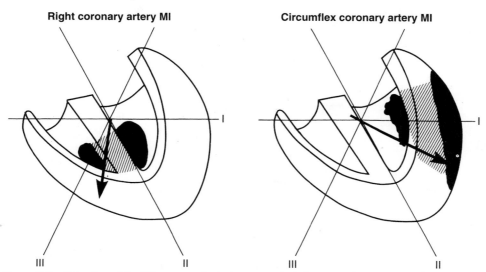

Figure 1-2 Behavior of the ST segment deviation vector in inferoposterior MI. As explained in the text, in RCA occlusion, the vector points inferiorly, to the right, and is closer to the lead III axis than to the lead II axis. In CX occlusion, the vector points to the left and is closer to the lead II axis than to lead III.

CX Coronary Artery Occlusion

The CX coronary artery perfuses the posterolateral area of the LV. In contrast to an RCA occlusion, the ST deviation vector in CX occlusion points to lead II, leading to more ST elevation in lead II than in lead III and an isoelectric or elevated ST segment in lead I (see Figure 1-3 and Box 1-1). Lead V_4R is extremely helpful in diagnosing CX occlusion when there is no difference in height of ST elevation between leads II and III (Figure 1-10).

RV Involvement

Proximal RCA occlusion. When inferoposterior cardiac ischemia is complicated by RV involvement, ST segment elevation is present with a positive T wave in the right precordial lead, V_4R (Figure 1-4).[9,10] That finding indicates an occlusion in the RCA *proximal* to the RV branch. Additionally it identifies patients at significant risk for developing advanced AV nodal block.[10-16]

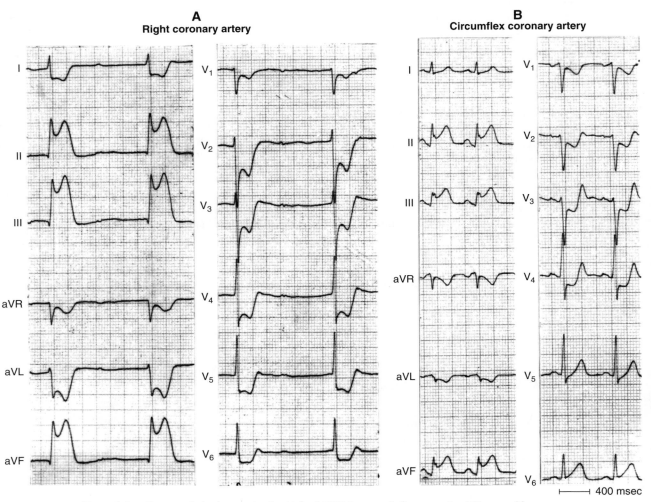

A
Right coronary artery

B
Circumflex coronary artery

├──────┤ 400 msec

Figure 1-3   Characteristic changes in the 12-lead ECG in acute inferoposterior MI, caused by either an RCA occlusion (**A**) or CX occlusion (**B**). **A,** In RCA occlusion ST depression is shown in lead I and ST elevation in the inferior leads but is more marked in lead III than in lead II. Leads V_2 to V_6 show ST depression because of posterior wall involvement. The patient also has complete AV block. **B,** In CX occlusion, ST elevation in lead II is higher than in lead III. Lead I shows an isoelectric ST segment with a positive T wave. ST depression in the precordial leads indicates posterior wall involvement; ST elevation in V_6 suggests lateral ischemia.

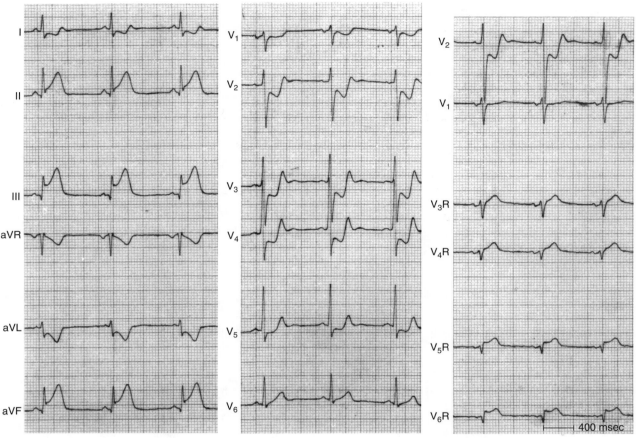

Figure 1-4 Inferoposterior ST segment elevation in MI with RV involvement caused by occlusion of the proximal RCA. RCA occlusion is diagnosed by ST depression in lead I and ST elevation in the inferior leads (more ST elevation in lead III than in lead II). The diagnosis that occlusion is proximal in the RCA is based on ST elevation with a positive T wave in lead V_4R.

Distal RCA occlusion. When the occlusion in the RCA is *distal* to the RV branch, the RV is not involved. Thus a positive T wave will be present in V_4R but without ST elevation (Figure 1-5).

Posterior LV Wall Involvement

When, in inferoposterior STEMI, ischemia of the posterior LV wall is present, the ST deviation vector in the horizontal plane will point to the posterior wall. The anterior precordial leads will therefore show ST segment depression; this is the case in CX occlusion. Lead V_4R will then show ST segment depression and a negative T wave (Figure 1-6).

Posterior wall MI secondary to an occluded branch of the CX may be erroneously diagnosed as non-STEMI because of the ST depression in the precordial leads. However, those patients will show ST elevation when more posteriorly located precordial leads (V_7-V_9) are recorded.

Lateral Wall Involvement

When inferoposterior cardiac ischemia is complicated by lateral wall involvement, the ST deviation vector in the horizontal plane will point to the lateral wall, reflected by ST segment elevation in leads V_5 and V_6, as well as in leads I and aVL. Lateral wall ischemia may occur because of a dominant RCA or CX occlusion, with the CX being the most common site of occlusion. Figure 1-7 is an example of acute inferoposterolateral MI caused by CX occlusion.

Value of Lead V_4R

Lead V_4R is quite helpful in localizing the site of coronary occlusion in inferoposterior MI (Figure 1-8). However, because the RV is thin walled, ST segment changes last a shorter length of time than the ST changes in leads recording LV events (Figure 1-9).

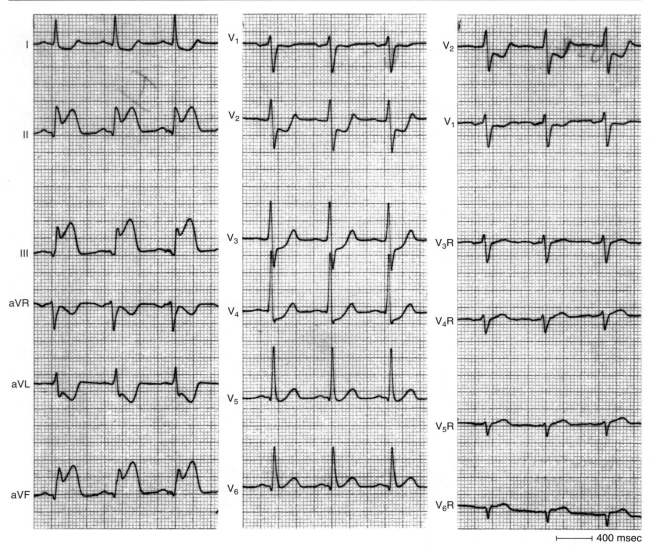

├──────────┤ 400 msec

Figure 1-5 ■ Inferoposterior ST segment elevation MI with no RV involvement. Note that leads I, II, and III indicate occlusion of the RCA (ST depression in lead I and elevation in II, III, and aVF, with more ST elevation in III than in II). Lead V_4R shows no ST elevation because the occlusion is distal to the RV branch.

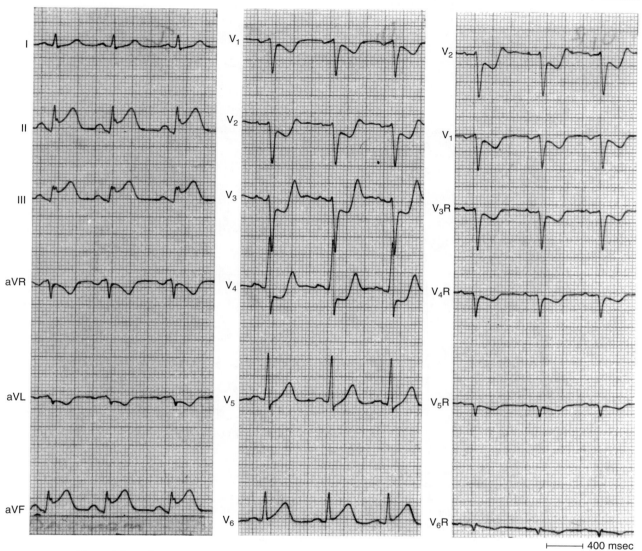

├────────────┤ 400 msec

Figure 1-6 Inferoposterior ST segment elevation MI caused by CX coronary artery occlusion, reflected in the facts that ST elevation is more marked in lead II than in lead III, and ST segment depression and a negative T wave are shown in lead V_4R. Lead I also shows a positive T wave. Of interest is the notch at the end of the QRS in leads II, III, and aVF, indicating delayed activation of the basolateral area, a typical finding in CX coronary artery occlusion.

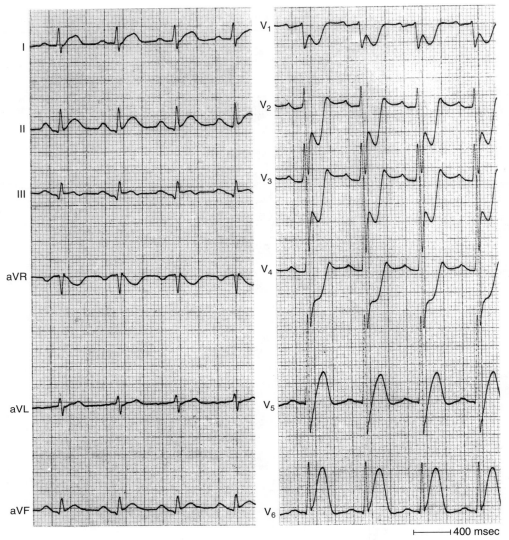

Figure 1-7 Inferoposterior ST segment elevation MI with lateral wall involvement. Note the ST elevation in leads reflecting the lateral wall (I, aVL, V$_5$, and V$_6$). As indicated by the ST depression in V$_1$ to V$_4$, this is an occlusion of a dominant CX coronary artery.

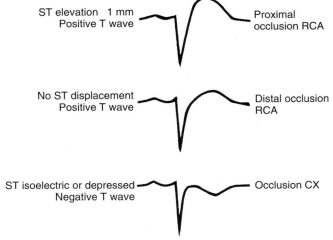

Figure 1-8 Value of ST-T segment changes in lead V$_4$R in acute inferoposterior MI.

Onset of chest pain 9:30 AM

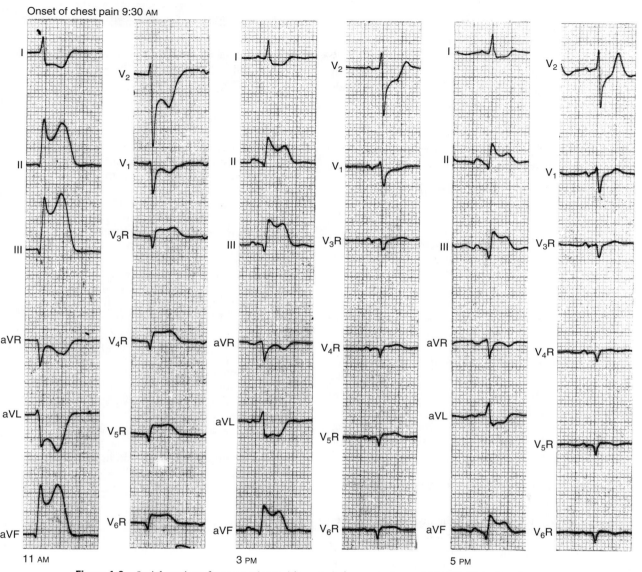

11 AM   3 PM   5 PM

Figure 1-9 Serial tracings from a patient with acute inferoposterior and RV MI. Note that the diagnostic changes for an RV infarction seen in lead V_4R have disappeared 7.5 hours after the onset of pain.

When lead V_4R is not recorded, differentiating between an RCA or CX occlusion may be difficult when the ST segment in lead I is isoelectric with equal ST elevation in leads II and III (Figure 1-10).

As pointed out by Fiol et al,[17] when V_4R is not recorded, the ratio of the sum of ST depression in leads V_1 to V_3 divided by the sum of ST elevation in leads II, III, and aVF should be determined. If this ratio is greater than 1, the occluded artery is the CX; if it is equal to or less than 1, the RCA is the culprit artery, and lateral wall involvement may occur when the RCA is dominant.

ISOLATED RV ST SEGMENT ELEVATION MI

Figure 1-11 shows the ST segment changes in acute isolated RV infarction.

Note that ST elevation is present in the right and even in the left precordial leads because of the anterior location of the RV.[18,19] This pattern may at first be confused with anterior wall STEMI, but as explained later, such confusion should not be the case when the different ECG patterns in anterior wall STEMI are known.

ANTERIOR ST SEGMENT ELEVATION MI

In acute anterior wall MI, ST elevation is present in the precordial leads. Interestingly, the location of the site of occlusion in the culprit coronary artery, the LAD branch, is diagnosed by determining the direction of the ST segment vector in *the frontal plane leads*, as explained below and outlined in Box 1-2.[6-8]

Occlusion Proximal to the First Septal and First Diagonal Branch

When, as shown in Figure 1-12, the occlusion is located *very proximal in the LAD*, that is, proximal to the first septal and first diagonal branches, the dominant ischemic area is in the basal part of the LV and therefore the ST elevation vector points *to the base of the heart* (toward leads aVR and aVL) and away from the apex (away from leads II, III, and aVF).

Also, because the first septal branch perfuses the subnodal AV conduction system, conduction disturbances may occur in the bundle of His and in the right bundle branch with or without delay or block in the fascicles of the left bundle branch.

Occlusion Between the First Septal and the First Diagonal Branch

When the LAD occlusion is between the first septal and the first diagonal branch, the dominant ischemic area is located high in the anterolateral area of the LV and the

ST segment deviation vector therefore points *toward aVL and away from lead III* (Figure 1-13).

Occlusion Between the First Diagonal and the First Septal Branch

Occasionally, the diagonal branch or an intermediate branch takes off from the LAD before the first septal branch. The ST segment deviation vector then points *toward leads aVR and III and away from lead aVL* (Figure 1-14).

Occlusion Distal to the Diagonal Branch(es)

When the LAD is occluded distal to the diagonal branch(es), the ST segment vector points *toward the apical area* (Figure 1-15). This results in ST elevation in the inferior leads, with more in lead II than in lead III.

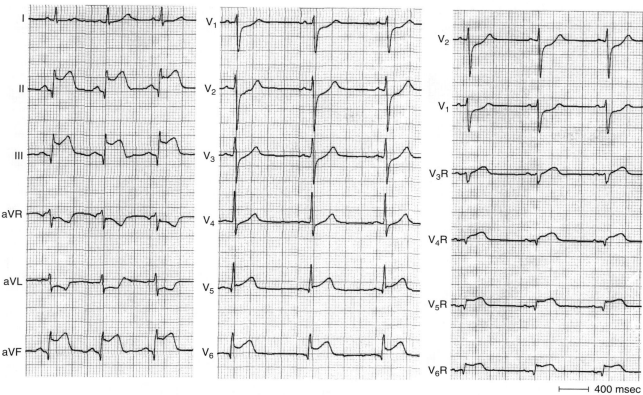

← 400 msec

Figure 1-10 A patient with acute inferior MI with the same amount of ST segment elevation in leads II and III and an isoelectric ST segment with a positive T wave in lead I. Lead V_4R indicates a proximal RCA occlusion. If no RV leads had been available, the diagnosis of RCA occlusion would have been suggested by the ratio of the sum of ST depression in leads V_1 to V_3, divided by the sum of ST elevation in the inferior leads.

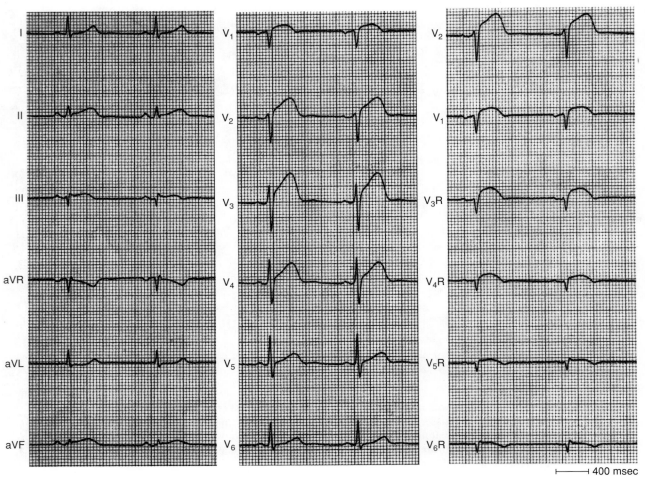

├─────┤ 400 msec

Figure 1-11 Acute isolated RV MI. Note that ST elevation is present in right and left precordial leads. This pattern should not be confused with that of anterior wall STEMI.

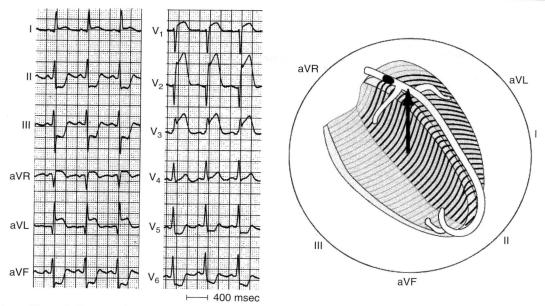

⊢——⊣ 400 msec

Figure 1-12 Acute anterior MI caused by an LAD occlusion proximal to the first septal and the first diagonal branch. Global ischemia of the whole anterior and septal aspects of the LV leads to a superiorly directed ST deviation vector because the anterobasal segment is the dominant ischemic area. This vector leads to ST elevation in leads aVR, aVL, and V_1, with reciprocal ST depression in the inferior leads and leads V_5 and V_6.

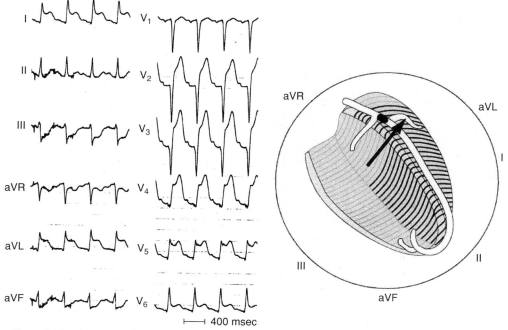

⊢——⊣ 400 msec

Figure 1-13 Acute anterior MI caused by an occlusion site in the LAD distal to the first septal branch but proximal to the first diagonal branch. The dominant ischemic area is located anterolaterally, leading to an ST deviation vector pointing in that direction. This results in ST elevation in leads I and aVL and ST depression in lead III. Lead II is isoelectric because of the perpendicular orientation of the ST vector in that lead.

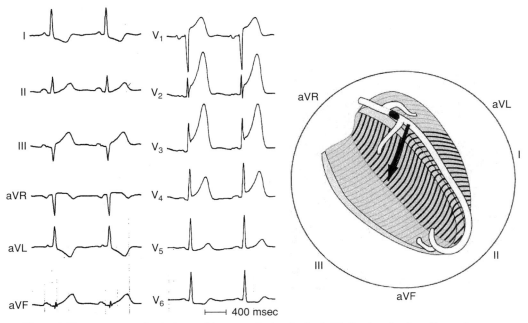

Figure 1-14   Acute anterior MI caused by an occlusion in the LAD distal to the first diagonal or intermediate branch but proximal to the first septal branch. This occlusion results in dominant ischemia in the anteroseptal area leading to a rightward and inferiorly directed ST deviation vector, which in turn results in ST elevation in leads V_1, aVR, and III and ST depression in leads I and aVL.

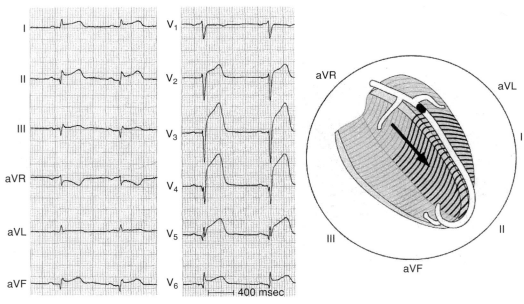

Figure 1-15   Acute anterior MI caused by a distal LAD occlusion. Because the ischemic area is located inferoapically, the ST deviation vector in the frontal plane points in an apical direction, resulting in ST elevation in the inferior leads (lead II greater than lead III), V_5, and V_6.

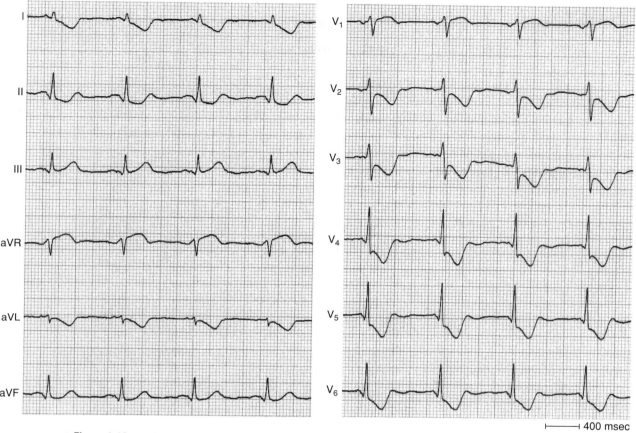

Figure 1-16 Left main occlusion. Apart from signs of an occlusion proximal to the first septal branch (ST elevation in leads aVR, aVL, and V$_1$), the ECG also shows evidence of posterobasal ischemia (ST depression in leads II, aVF, V$_4$, and V$_5$). Note that ST elevation in lead aVR is greater than that in V$_1$ and that the amount of ST depression in lead V$_6$ is more than the ST elevation in lead V$_1$.

ST elev aVR / V1
ST dep V2 - V6

Left Main Coronary Artery Occlusion

When the left main coronary artery is occluded acutely, ischemia will occur both in the territory supplied by the LAD and the CX, resulting in an ST deviation vector pointing *toward lead aVR*. In addition to ST elevation in lead aVR, ST elevation in lead V$_1$ is also present (Figure 1-16).

As reported by Yamaji et al,[20] the ST elevation in lead aVR is usually higher than the ST elevation in lead V$_1$. The ST depression in the inferior leads reflects basal ischemia. The ST depression in the precordial leads to the left of V$_2$ reflects posterior wall ischemia. Marked ST depression in the precordial leads is usually present, mostly in lead V$_4$. Often ST depression in V$_6$ is more

than ST elevation in lead V$_1$. Often RBBB is present (Figure 1-17) because of the interruption of blood supply to the sub-AV nodal conduction system.

In summary, the following ST deviations are present in the acute phase of left main coronary artery occlusion:
- ST elevation in lead aVR (ST deviation vector points to this lead)
- ST elevation in lead V$_1$ (lower than that of lead aVR)
- ST depression in leads II and aVF (basal ischemia)
- ST depression in the precordial leads to the left of V$_2$ (posterior wall ischemia)

In addition, conduction disturbances are often present in the right bundle branch with or without hemiblock.

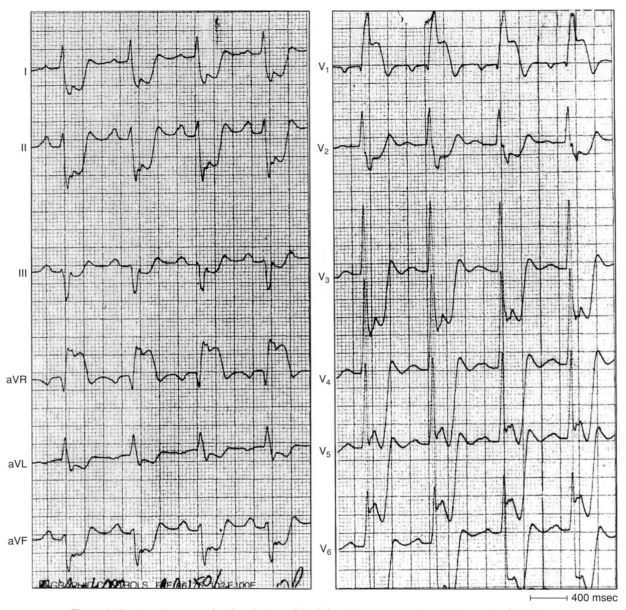

Figure 1-17   Another example of occlusion of the left main coronary artery. Note acquired RBBB with ST elevation in leads aVR and V_1 and extensive ST segment depression in the other leads.

LIMITATIONS OF THE ST DEVIATION VECTOR APPROACH IN MI DIAGNOSIS

As pointed out elsewhere,[8] the behavior of the ST segment vector in the different locations of MI is made on the basis of observations in patients with single coronary artery occlusions. The specificity and positive predictive accuracy are high, but the sensitivity is rather low. Additionally, the ST segment deviation vector concept is of limited or no value in a number of situations, such as:

- Presence of an old infarction(s)
- Preexisting ST segment abnormalities
- Altered ventricular activation (LBBB, ventricular pacing, ventricular preexcitation)
- Multivessel disease
- Dominance or underdevelopment of coronary arteries
- Abnormal site of origin of a coronary artery

Risk Stratification

PRIMARY PERCUTANEOUS CORONARY INTERVENTION VERSUS THROMBOLYTIC THERAPY

Primary coronary intervention has been shown to be superior to intravenous thrombolysis, not only because it reduces the risk of intracranial bleeding and the need for blood transfusions associated with thrombolysis, but also because it reduces short- and long-term mortality rates, the incidence of recurrent ischemia, and infarct vessel reocclusion.[21-28]

Because of the scarcity of experienced operators and centers equipped to manage acute coronary syndromes, Topol et al[29] have suggested the establishment of regional "centers of excellence" capable of handling high volumes and staffed with skilled operators and teams for the care of patients with acute ischemic heart disease. Patients with chest pain initially admitted to smaller hospitals would be categorized according to risk on the basis of the admission ECG, clinical findings, protein markers, and imaging results.

Unfortunately, referral for a percutaneous coronary intervention is not possible in many areas, and therefore knowledge of how to identify patients most likely to profit from thrombolytic therapy remains an essential skill in the risk stratification of patients with acute MI. Reperfusion therapy is most beneficial in patients with acute MI seen or admitted soon after the onset of chest pain and with signs of a large infarction or extensive cardiac ischemia. That diagnosis can in most patients be made on the basis of the ST segment behavior, as previously outlined.

RECOGNITION OF THE HIGH-RISK PATIENT

Decision making regarding which patients with STEMI should be transferred to a center where a primary percutaneous intervention can be performed should be made on the basis of the following four observations:

1. Size and severity of the ischemic area
2. Presence of conduction disturbances
3. Vital signs
4. Time interval between onset of chest pain and presentation

Size of the Ischemic Area

As already discussed, the ECG gives immediate information about the size of the ischemic area in the patient with STEMI.

Anterior wall MI. The direction of the ST deviation vector reveals the location of the occlusion in the LAD.

The closer the occlusion to the origin of the LAD, the larger the jeopardized area.

Inferoposterior MI. A proximal RCA occlusion (recognized in lead V_4R) means RV involvement and a high chance of advanced AV nodal conduction disturbances.

Posterior wall MI. The *extent of posterior wall ischemia* is known by the number of precordial leads showing ST segment depression and the depth of that depression.

Posterolateral MI. The presence of *posterolateral ischemia* is indicated by ST elevation in leads I, aVL, V_5, and V_6.

Severity of Ischemia

Sclarovsky and Birnbaum[30,31] pointed out that typical ECG changes can indicate the severity of cardiac ischemia during STEMI. They divided the ischemic changes after occlusion of the coronary artery into the following three grades from mild to severe (Figures 1-18 to 1-20):

Grade 1: Peaked symmetrical T waves without ST elevation

Grade 2: ST elevation without distortion of the terminal portion of the QRS complex

Grade 3: Distortion of the terminal portion of the QRS, ST elevation, and a junction point/R-wave ratio greater than 0.5

They also looked at the prognostic significance of the three grades of ischemia on presentation and found them to be correlated with inhospital mortality rate, final infarct size, severity of LV dysfunction, and late mortality.

Early reperfusion therapy (within 2 hours after onset of symptoms) was also found to result in similar beneficial results in grade II and grade III ischemia. Beneficial results were less when reperfusion therapy was applied later, grade III ischemia then having a significantly higher inhospital mortality rate. That finding suggests that ischemia grading in relation to time interval after onset of symptoms can also give an indication of reversibility of ischemia. Grade III ischemia was accompanied by a higher incidence of complications such as high-degree AV block and reinfarction. These data suggest that an early *percutaneous coronary intervention* should be considered in patients with grade III ischemia.[32]

Risk Index

Apart from the ECG, determining risk in the patient with STEMI can be done in other ways. Recently, Wiviott

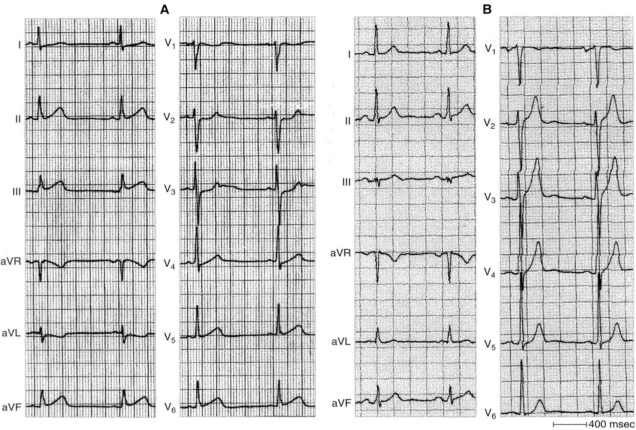

Figure 1-18   Grade I ischemia in inferior and anterior MI. **A,** Acute inferoposterolateral MI. Note the peaked symmetrical T waves without ST elevation in leads II, III, aVF, V_5, and V_6. **B,** Acute anterior wall MI. In leads V_2 to V_5, note the peaked symmetrical T waves without ST elevation.

et al[33] reported the simple *risk index* noted here, based on age and vital signs that accurately predicted inhospital death in a large number of patients involved in clinical trials of fibrinolysis (Table 1-1).

TABLE 1-1	Inhospital Death in Patients with ST Elevation MI in Relation to Risk Index
Risk Index	**Inhospital Mortality Rate**
<30	<5%
60	5%-30%
≥60	>30%

Patients with heart rates <50 and >150 beats/min are excluded.

$$\text{Risk index} = \frac{\text{Heart rate} \times (\text{Age}/10) \times 2}{\text{Systolic blood pressure}}$$

Time Interval Between Onset of Chest Pain and Presentation

The availability of reperfusion strategies for patients with a coronary occlusion places the emphasis on *ST segment changes during acute cardiac ischemia*. The purpose of this emphasis is to recognize those patients who would benefit from reopening of the culprit coronary artery to prevent or reduce cardiac damage with loss of muscle cells. Unfortunately, the interval between onset of chest pain and ECG diagnosis may be such that the phase of ischemia is over and cell necrosis is ongoing. In these cases the patient presents with pathologic Q waves. What then are the time limits for reperfusion therapy?

Transient Q waves. First, the fact that *Q waves do not necessarily indicate myocardial necrosis* is important knowledge. Extensive ischemia can result in the appearance of transient Q waves caused by conduction delay in

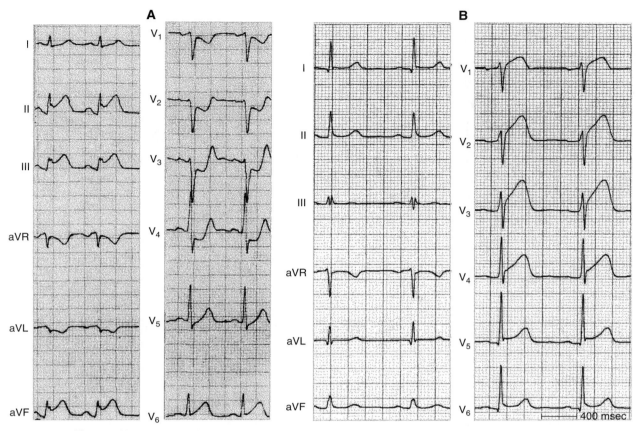

Figure 1-19   Grade II ischemia in inferior and anterior MI. **A,** Acute inferoposterior MI. In the inferior leads, note the ST elevation without distortion of the terminal portion of the QRS complex. **B,** Acute anterior wall MI. Note the precordial ST elevation without distortion of the terminal portion of the QRS complex.

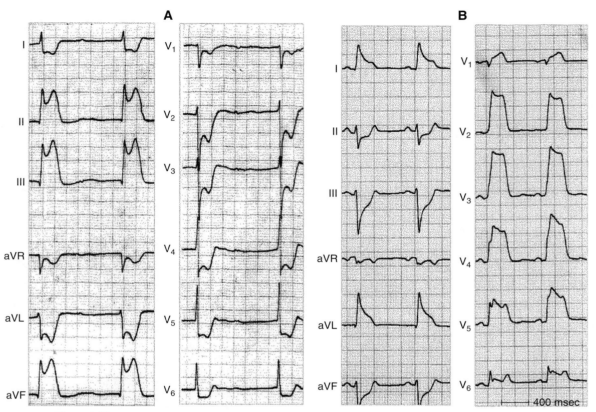

Figure 1-20   Grade III ischemia in inferior and anterior MI. **A,** Acute inferoposterior MI. In the inferior leads, note the distortion of the terminal portion of the QRS, ST elevation, and a junction point/R-wave ratio more than 0.5. **B,** Acute anterior wall MI. In leads V_2 to V_5 note the distortion of the terminal portion of the QRS, ST elevation, and loss of S waves.

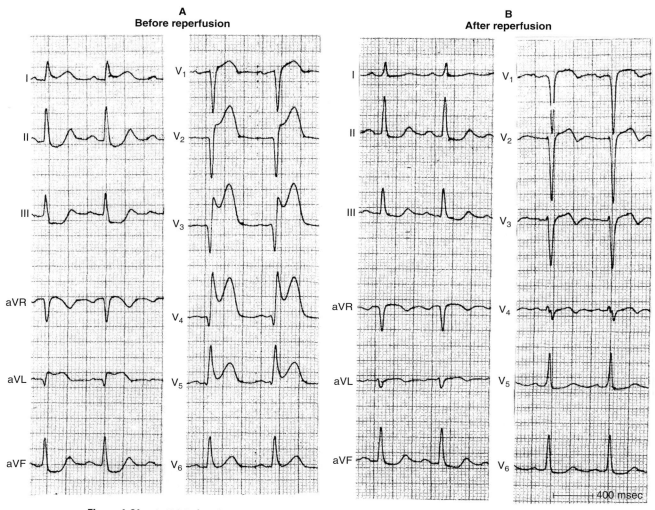

Figure 1-21 **A,** ECG showing an acute anteroseptal MI. Q waves are present in leads aVL and V_2 to V_5. **B,** After successful fibrinolytic therapy, the Q waves have disappeared, indicating that the myocardial tissue was still salvageable.

the zone under that electrode.[34] Thus significant myocardial salvage by reperfusion can be accomplished in patients with new pathologic Q waves. This situation is especially true with qR complexes, when ST segment elevation infarct size can be limited by reperfusion therapy (Figure 1-21). It can also be demonstrated when the patient presents with acquired RBBB in the setting of a large anterior wall MI (Figure 1-22).

Time frame. Time from the onset of symptoms to myocardial necrosis is also influenced by factors such as the presence of collateral circulation to the ischemic area and "intermittent" coronary occlusion. Although the golden rule is to start reperfusion therapy as soon as possible after coronary occlusion, definite time limits cannot be given.

The ability to produce a patent infarct artery (and reduce myocardial cell loss) depends less on the duration

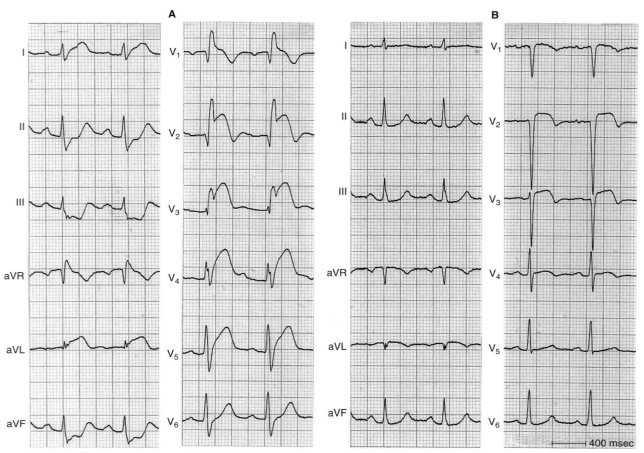

Figure 1-22   Q waves during severe ischemia in a patient with acquired RBBB in the setting of a large anterior wall MI. **A,** An acute anterior wall MI on admission is shown with acquired RBBB showing a QR complex in lead V$_1$ because of an LAD occlusion proximal to the first septal branch. An ECG recorded 3 minutes after primary percutaneous transluminal coronary angioplasty, shows disappearance of RBBB and the development of terminal T-wave inversion in leads V$_1$ to V$_4$ **(B).** Shortening of the PR interval from 0.24 seconds **(A)** to 0.16 seconds **(B)** is also shown. These changes indicate successful reperfusion of the anteroseptal area and normalization of sub-AV nodal conduction.

of symptoms in patients undergoing percutaneous coronary intervention than on treatment with fibrinolytic therapy. For patients in whom symptoms started more than 3 hours before presentation, percutaneous coronary intervention is therefore preferred because it will probably save more myocardial tissue than fibrinolytic therapy, especially when a large area is threatened.

CONDUCTION DISTURBANCES IN ACUTE MI

The emergence of conduction disturbances between the sinus node and the right atrium, and between the atrium and ventricles, in the acute phase of MI is of prognostic and therapeutic significance and should therefore be immediately recognized. The site of block is related to the particular occluded coronary artery.

Blood Supply to the Conduction System

Sinus node and SA region.   The sinus node and the SA region are, in 55% of cases, perfused by an atrial branch from the proximal part of the RCA and, in 45% of cases, by a proximal branch of the CX coronary artery.[35] A proximal occlusion of the RCA or CX coronary artery

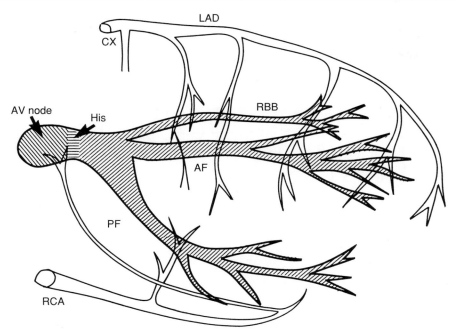

Figure 1-23   Scheme of the blood supply to the AV conduction system. *AF,* anterior fascicle; *PF,* posterior fascicle; *His,* His bundle; *RBB,* right bundle branch.

may therefore lead to ischemia of the sinus node and the surrounding atrium.

The AV conduction system. The AV conduction system consists of the AV node, the bundle of His, and the bundle branches (Figure 1-23). The RCA perfuses the AV node and the proximal part of the bundle of His. The distal part of the His bundle, the right bundle branch, and the anterior fascicle of the left bundle branch are supplied by the septal branches of the LAD coronary artery. The posterior fascicle of the left bundle branch is supplied by septal branches from both the LAD and the RCA.[35]

Sinus Bradycardia

Sinus bradycardia is shown in Figure 1-24. It is three times more common in inferoposterior than in anterior MI.[36] Possible mechanisms for sinus bradycardia are listed in Box 1-3. In general, sinus bradycardia

indicates a smaller infarct because it is usually vagally induced.

BOX 1-3

Possible Mechanisms for Sinus Bradycardia After an Acute MI[8]

- Neurologic reflexes (Bezold-Jarisch reflex)
- Coronary chemoreflexes (vagally mediated)
- Humoral (nonneural) reflexes (e.g., pH, enzymes, adenosine, potassium)
- Oxygen conserving ("diving") reflex
- Infarction or ischemia of the sinus node or surrounding atrium

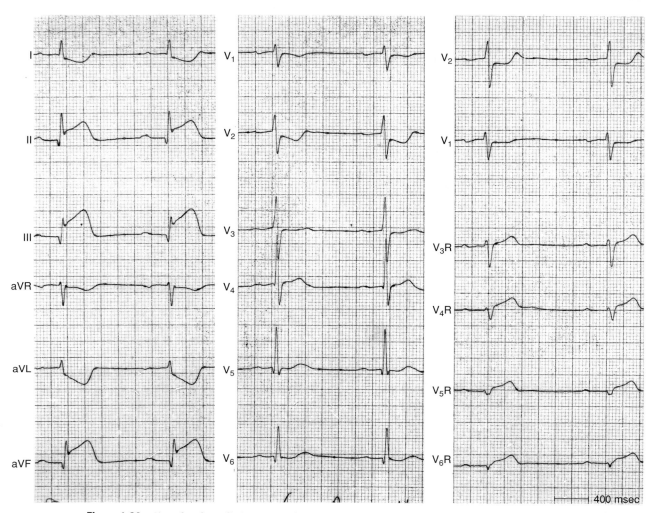

Figure 1-24 Sinus bradycardia in acute inferior MI with RV involvement because of a proximal occlusion of the RCA. The patient also has a prolonged PR interval.

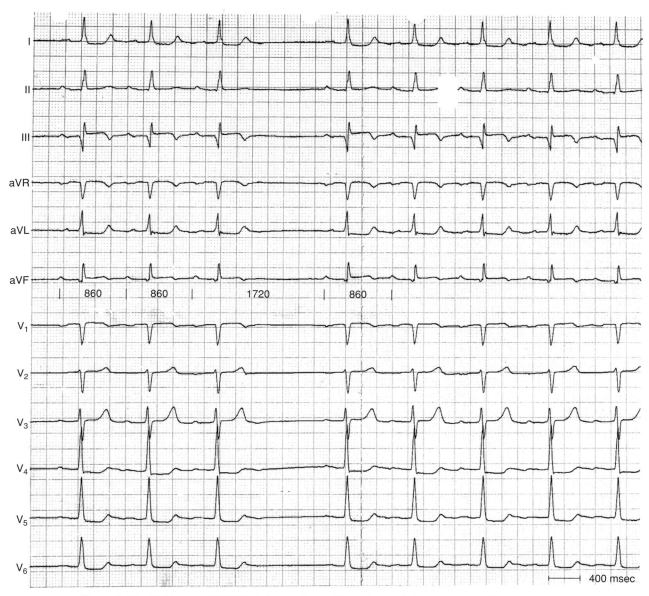

Figure 1-25   Mobitz type II SA block in a patient with a subacute inferior MI. This finding suggests a coronary occlusion proximal to the SA branch.

SA Block and Sinus Arrest

Figure 1-25 shows Mobitz II second-degree SA block. Figure 1-26 shows complete SA block or absence of impulse formation in the sinus node. Grade 2 or complete SA block suggests a proximal occlusion in the RCA or CX and is often accompanied by *atrial infarction*. This type of occlusion is a sign of a large infarction, suggesting that a *percutaneous coronary intervention* should be performed.

Pacing is indicated when the slow heart rate leads to a low cardiac output or increased ventricular ectopic impulse formation.

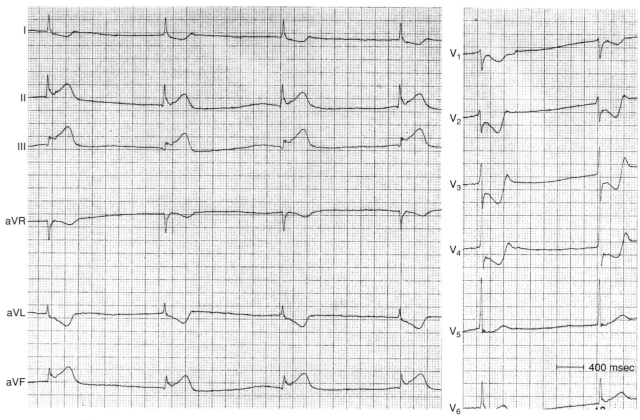

Figure 1-26   Complete SA block or sinus arrest in a patient with acute inferior MI after an occlusion of the RCA. The junctional escape rhythm is followed by retrograde conduction to the atrium.

Conduction Abnormalities at the AV Nodal Level

Conduction abnormalities at the level of the AV node are usually seen in cases of an occlusion of the *RCA proximal to the RV branch*.[10] They may present as one of the following:

- A prolonged PR interval of more than 200 msec
- Second-degree AV block (of the Wenckebach type, or two-to-one block)
- Complete AV nodal block

Examples are given in Figures 1-27 to 1-29. In all three examples a proximal RCA occlusion was responsible for inferoposterior MI. Typical for two-to-one AV nodal block is the markedly prolonged PR interval of the conducted P wave, in contrast to two-to-one conduction in the sub-AV nodal conduction system, where the PR interval of the conducted P wave is usually normal.

The occurrence of high-degree (second degree or more) AV nodal block in the setting of acute MI has important prognostic implications.[37-40] This situation is still true in the reperfusion era, with an excess mortality rate of two to three times the mortality rate when no AV nodal conduction disturbances are present. Second-degree or worse AV conduction disturbances in acute MI are summarized in Table 1-2. These disturbances stress the necessity of early reperfusion, preferably by primary percutaneous coronary intervention.

AV nodal block after inferior MI is rarely permanent.[41] *Long-term pacing* is only indicated when symptomatic second-degree or complete AV nodal block persists more than 2 weeks after inferior MI.

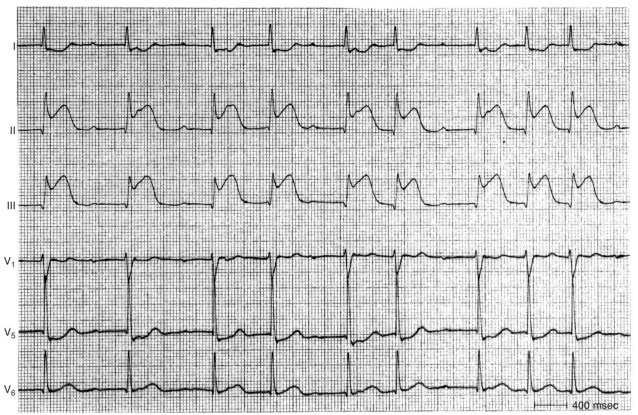

Figure 1-27   An example of variable (two to one, three to two, and four to three) AV Wenckebach block in a patient with an acute inferior MI from an RCA occlusion.

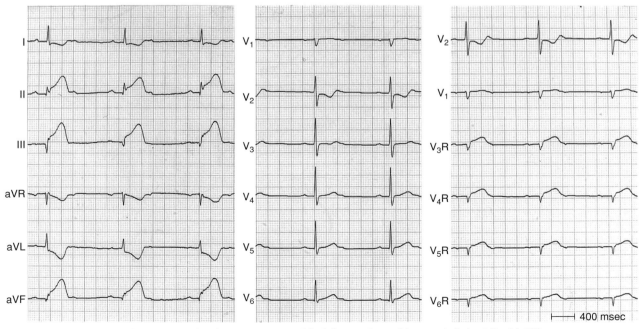

Figure 1-28   An example of a two-to-one AV block in a patient with acute inferior MI with RV involvement caused by an occlusion in the RCA.

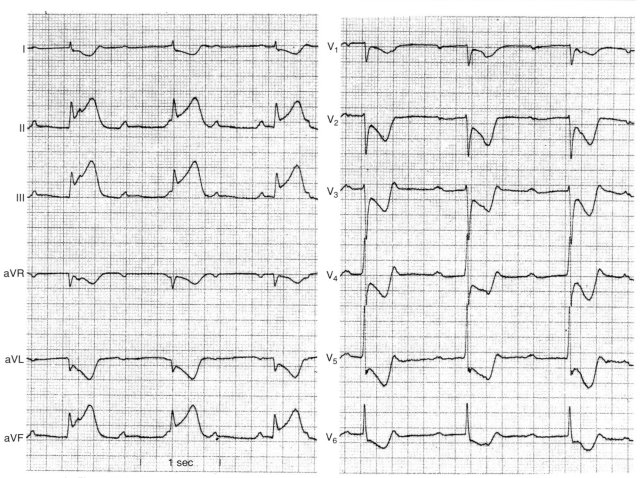

Figure 1-29   Complete AV nodal block in a patient with an RCA occlusion. Also note the signs of atrial infarction (Pta elevation in leads II, III, and aVF).

TABLE 1-2	AV Conduction Disturbances in Acute MI (Second Degree or Worse)	
Infarct Location	**Inferoposterior**	**Anterior**
Culprit coronary artery	Proximal RCA	Proximal LAD
Escape rhythm	Narrow or wide QRS	Wide QRS
		Rate: <40 beats/min
	Rate: 40-60 beats/min	
Incidence	12%-20%	5%
Duration	Usually transient	Usually transient
Excess inhospital mortality rate compared with no conduction disturbance	2-3 times	4 times

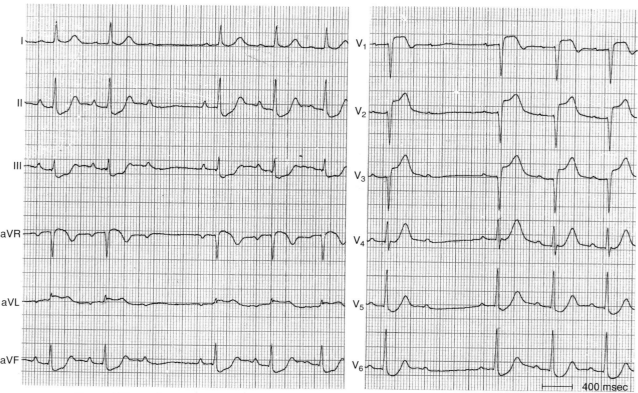

Figure 1-30   Mobitz type II block in the bundle of His in acute anterior MI caused by an LAD occlusion proximal to the first septal branch. Note the ST deviation vector, indicating a very proximal LAD occlusion.

Conduction Disturbances Below the AV Node

The development of conduction disturbances in or below the bundle of His associated with acute MI is a specific marker for a very proximal occlusion of the LAD and therefore indicates a large area of the LV in jeopardy. The poor prognosis of these patients (see Table 1-2) makes emergency coronary intervention the preferred treatment. The conduction disturbances take the form of Mobitz II second-degree AV block (Figure 1-30), two-to-one block (Figure 1-31), and RBBB, with or without left anterior or left posterior fascicular block. Often the conducted QRS complexes are preceded by a PR interval of normal length because of a normal or abbreviated AV nodal conduction time.

The most common type of sub-AV nodal conduction disturbance in an LAD occlusion proximal to the first septal branch is RBBB with or without left fascicular block (Figure 1-32). This disturbance is much more common than the development of complete LBBB.

When RBBB is the result of the MI, the prognosis is ominous, especially when accompanied by left fascicular block.[40,42-47] Early death may occur within a few days because of pump failure. The patient surviving the critical early days has a 30% chance that sustained VT or ventricular fibrillation will develop 1 to 2 weeks later in the remodeled, scarred LV.[43,44]

Acquired Versus Preexisting RBBB

When the patient presenting with MI also has RBBB, discerning whether the block was already present before the MI (preexisting) or was caused by the MI (acquired) is important relative to the prognosis. As shown by Lie et al,[42] when RBBB was preexisting, hospital mortality rate was no different from patients without RBBB. In contrast acquired RBBB, which typically occurs in a very proximal LAD occlusion, indicates a poor prognosis.[43] The ECG can help differentiate acquired and preexisting RBBB.

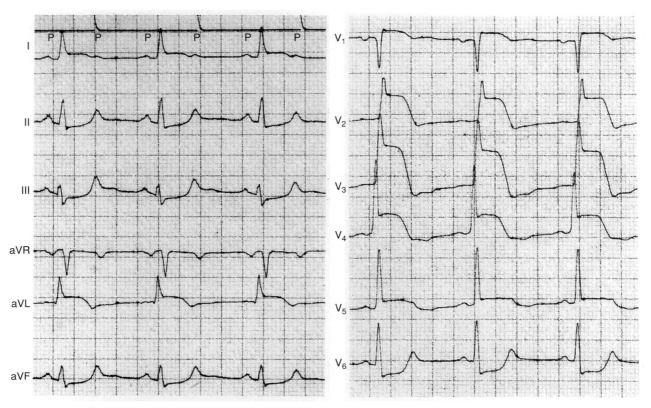

Figure 1-31 An example of two-to-one intra-Hissal block in acute anterior MI caused by an LAD occlusion proximal to the first septal branch. Note the normal PR interval of the conducted P wave. This finding in two-to-one AV block is typical for a conduction disturbance below the AV node.

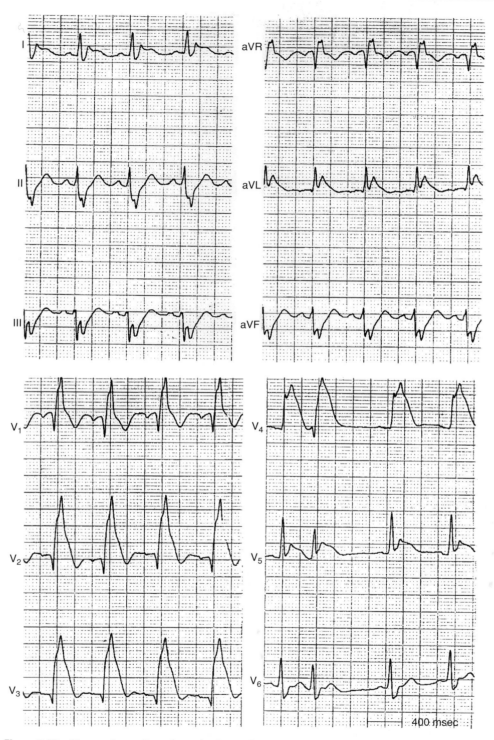

Figure 1-32   Sinus tachycardia and acquired complete RBBB with left anterior hemiblock in a patient with an acute anterior MI.

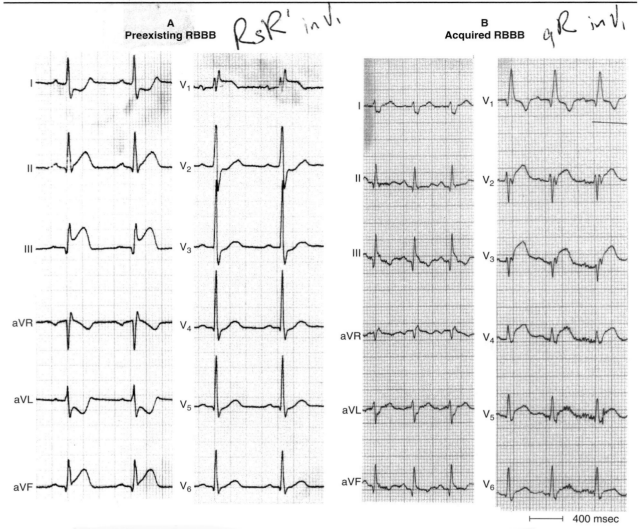

Figure 1-33   Preexisting RBBB versus acquired RBBB after MI. **A,** The ECG of a patient with preexisting RBBB admitted with an inferior MI from an RCA occlusion. The QRS during RBBB shows an RsR′ configuration in lead V_1. The ST elevation in lead V_1 indicates RV involvement. **B,** The ECG of a patient with an acute anterior wall MI with acquired RBBB and left posterior hemiblock. The QRS during RBBB shows a qR configuration in lead V_1.

As shown in Figure 1-33, acquired RBBB is characterized by a QR or qR complex, whereas preexisting RBBB shows an RsR′ configuration in lead V_1. Preexisting RBBB is more commonly found in elderly patients.

LBBB and MI

Complete LBBB secondary to acute anterior wall MI is rare (Figure 1-34). As previously stated, acquired bundle branch block in anterior MI is typically located in the right bundle branch with or without left hemiblock.

As shown in Figure 1-35, LBBB may occur in infero-posterior MI during second-degree AV nodal block and slow heart rates.[48] These LBBB complexes are either conducted sinus beats or AV junctional escape beats. The fact that LBBB occurs only after a long interval indicates that the mechanism is phase 4 (bradycardia dependent) block (see Chapter 3).

DIAGNOSIS OF MI DURING ABNORMAL VENTRICULAR ACTIVATION

The ECG diagnosis of MI, the area at risk, and the culprit coronary artery are determined on the basis of changes in the pattern of normal depolarization and repolarization during AV conduction over an intact bundle branch

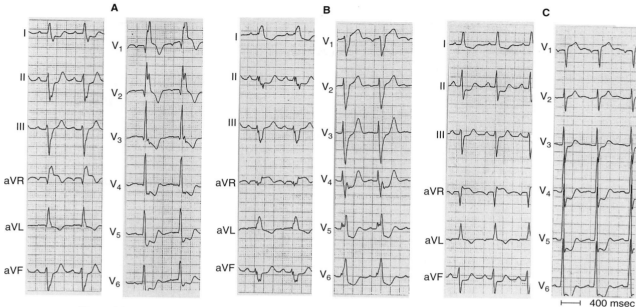

Figure 1-34 Patient with an LAD occlusion proximal to the first septal branch. **A,** Acquired RBBB and left anterior hemiblock. **B,** Complete LBBB recorded 5 minutes later. Note the disappearance of changes diagnostic for anterior wall MI. **C,** Normalization of intraventricular conduction after reperfusion by fibrinolytic therapy. ST segment changes are still present.

TABLE 1-3	Three ECG Criteria to Diagnose MI in the Presence of LBBB[50]		
Criteria		**Odds Ratio (95% CI)**	**Score**
1. ST segment elevation >1 mm concordant with the QRS with positive T waves in leads I, aVL, V$_5$, and V$_6$		25.2 (11.6-54.7)	5
2. ST segment depression >1 mm in leads V$_1$, V$_2$, or V$_3$		6.0 (1.9-19.3)	3
3. ST segment elevation >5 mm discordant with the QRS in leads V$_2$ to V$_4$		4.3 (1.8-10.6)	2

To obtain a sensitivity of 78% and a specificity of 90%, the minimal total score should be 3.
CI, Confidence interval.

system during sinus rhythm. Those changes allow the clinician to locate the ischemic or infarcted area.

RBBB does not affect activation of the LV and therefore has little effect on the ECG diagnosis of LV ischemia or infarction.[8] However, LV activation is markedly different during LBBB, RV pacing, and some types of ventricular preexcitation.

ECG Diagnosis of LBBB in MI

In LBBB the LV is activated by radial spread from the exit of the right bundle branch. This means that areas of the LV normally activated early (e.g., the exit sites of the anterior fascicle, the posterior fascicle, and septal fibers) are now activated much later in the QRS complex, making it difficult to impossible to recognize ischemia or infarction in those areas. Unfortunately, the difficulties in making the diagnosis of MI in LBBB leads to marked

underuse of reperfusion therapy in these patients. Not surprisingly, several investigators have tried during the past 3 decades to identify ECG findings that could be of help in suspecting MI in LBBB.[49]

The current most commonly used ECG findings for MI in LBBB come from a study by Sgarbossa et al.[50] In that retrospective study, ECGs from patients with LBBB and MI were compared with asymptomatic patients with LBBB. Table 1-3 lists the three ECG criteria to diagnose MI in the presence of LBBB according to these authors (Figure 1-36). Table 1-3 also indicates that some criteria are more valuable than others.

Subsequently Shlipak et al[51] and Gula et al[52] determined that these criteria have a low prevalence and poor sensitivity. When present they are helpful, but approximately half of the patients with LBBB and MI do not have them.

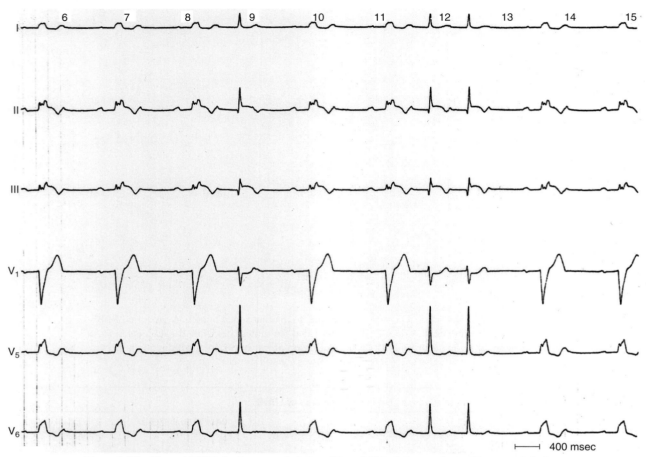

Figure 1-35 Phase 4 LBBB during second-degree AV nodal block in a patient with recent inferior MI. Phase 4 LBBB is only present during the longest RR intervals. During Wenckebach conduction the shorter RR intervals show a narrow QRS complex. Also note that during LBBB notching of the QRS and ST segment elevation are shown in leads II and III.

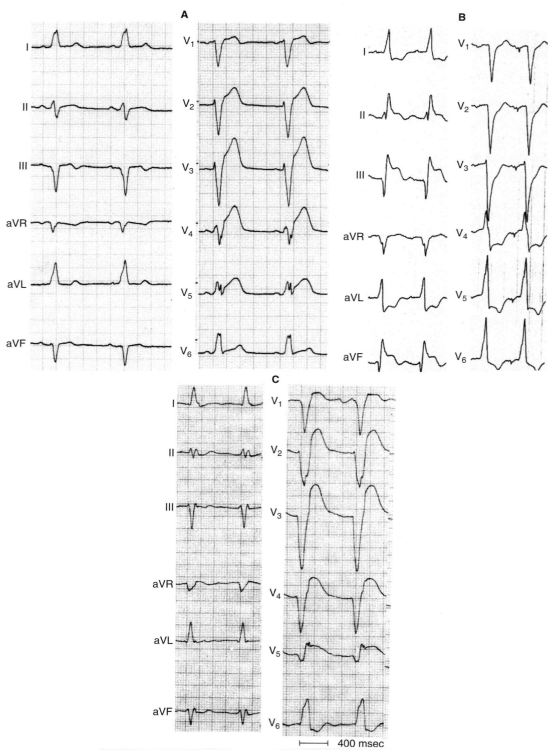

Figure 1-36 Three findings in LBBB that have been advanced as helpful in diagnosing the presence of MI. **A,** ST segment elevation more than 1 mm, concordant with the QRS complex in leads I, V_5, and V_6. **B,** ST segment depression more than 1 mm in leads V_1 to V_3. **C,** ST segment elevation more than 5 mm discordant with QRS in leads V_2 to V_4. Also see Table 1-3.

400 msec

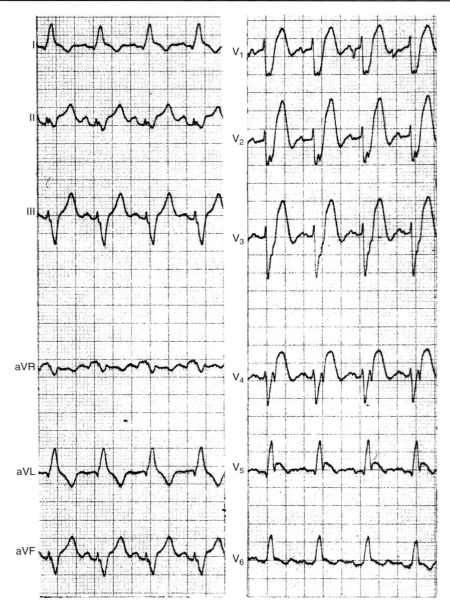

Figure 1-37   Anterior wall MI in a patient with LBBB. Q waves are present in leads I, aVL, and V_5. Also present are an initial R in lead V_1, notching of the QRS complex, and marked ST elevation in leads V_1 to V_5.

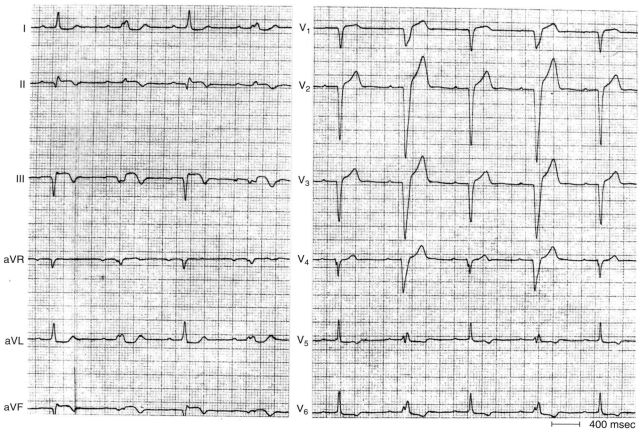

Figure 1-38   Two-to-one LBBB in inferior MI. Note persistence of ST elevation and terminal T-wave inversion in the inferior leads during LBBB.

Other criteria have been reported,[8] such as the presence of q waves in leads I, aVL, and V_5 or V_6 in anteroseptal MI (Figure 1-37), and persistence of ST segment elevation during LBBB in leads II, III, and aVF in inferoposterior MI (Figure 1-38), but their sensitivity and specificity have not been analyzed.

Conclusion. The conclusion, therefore, should be that the ECG is not a reliable source of information in patients with LBBB and chest pain to make the diagnosis of ischemia or MI.

The authors believe that reperfusion therapy should be given to the patient with LBBB when the clinical presentation suggests MI.[53] This belief is opposed to the guidelines of the American College of Cardiology and the American Heart Association,[54] which suggest that reperfusion therapy should only be given to patients with new or presumably new bundle branch block. As discussed earlier, LBBB is seldom caused by acute ischemia; most people with LBBB and chest pain have preexisting LBBB!

During chest pain

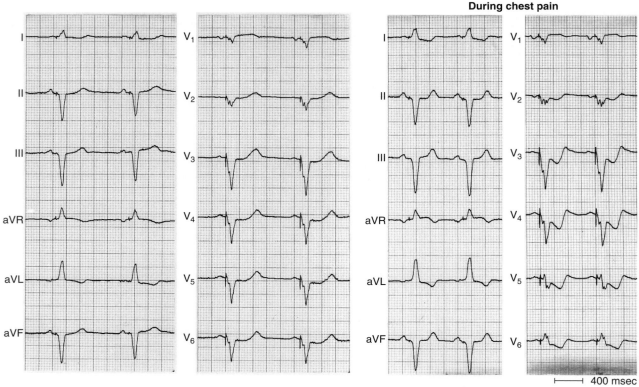

Figure 1-39 Ventricular paced complexes before (**A**) and after (**B**) CX coronary artery occlusion. Note that after occlusion the ST segment is depressed in the precordial leads V_2 to V_5. Widening and notching of the QRS are also present in the precordial leads.

Paced Ventricular Rhythm

Currently most ventricular pacing is performed from the RV, resulting in sequential activation of first the RV and then the LV similar to ventricular activation in cases of LBBB. Thus the same type of QRS and ST segment changes are seen as in LBBB (Figure 1-39).[55-57] Occasionally, *electrical alternans* of the paced QRS complexes may be present in severe and extensive cardiac ischemia, such as in the patient whose ECG is shown in Figure 1-40. In this case coronary angiography revealed an occlusion of the left main coronary artery.

Ventricular Preexcitation

During ventricular preexcitation the ventricles are not activated in a normal sequence. The ability to mask MI by ventricular preexcitation depends on the location of the accessory AV pathway. In general, if the location of the MI is contralateral to the accessory pathway, the resulting ECG pattern will mask infarction, as shown in Figure 1-41, whereas an ipsilateral location will allow recognition of ischemia or infarction, as shown in Figure 1-42.

Ventricular preexcitation may also produce pseudo-infarct patterns because of early activation of a part of

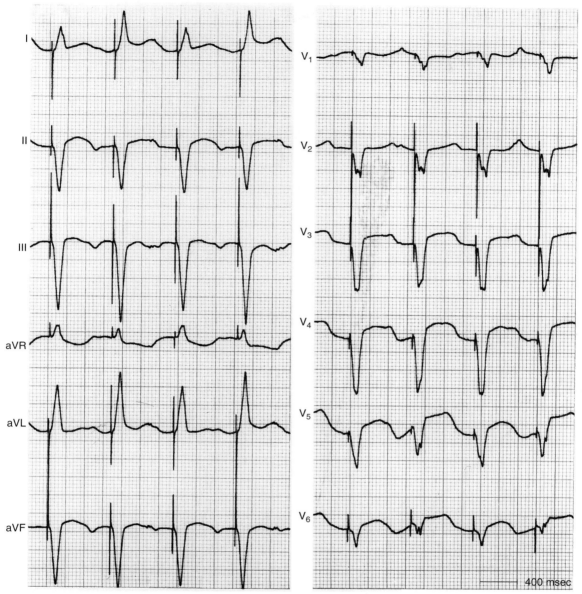

Figure 1-40   QRS electrical alternans during a paced rhythm in a patient with an occlusion of the left main coronary artery.

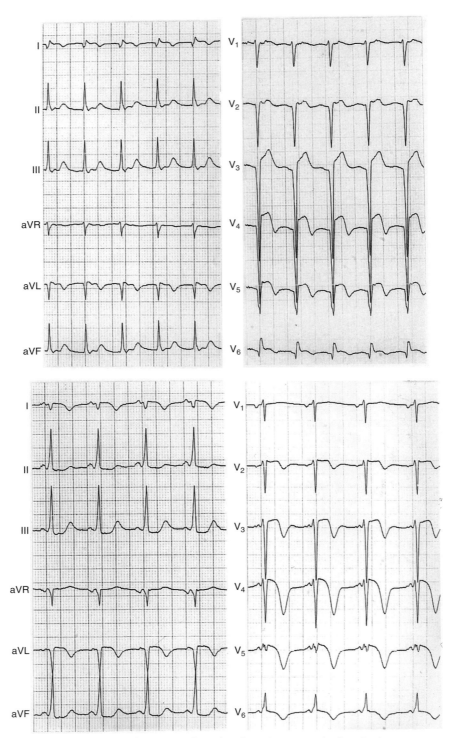

Figure 1-41 Accessory pathway contralateral to the MI. **A,** An orthodromic circus movement tachycardia in a patient with Wolff-Parkinson-White syndrome. The QRS and ST segment changes indicate a subacute anterior wall MI. **B,** Ventricular preexcitation over a left-sided accessory AV pathway in the same patient, recorded 6 hours later. During preexcitation initial QRS positivity (delta wave) is shown in the precordial leads because ventricular activation starts in the left posterior wall. Also note QRS notching in lead V_5 and the ST-T segment changes.

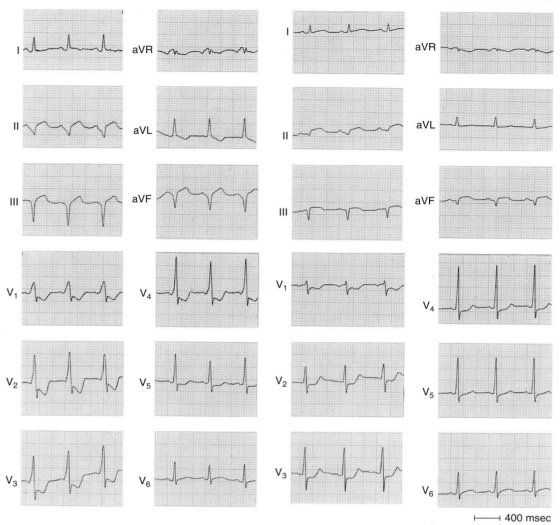

├────────┤ 400 msec

Figure 1-42 Accessory pathway ipsilateral to the MI. **A,** Preexcitation over a left posteroseptal accessory pathway with ST segment elevation in leads II, III, and aVF. ST segment depression is present in leads V_1 to V_5. Positive delta waves are prominent in leads II, aVR, and V_1 to V_4. **B,** AV conduction over the AV node only in the same patient 12 hours later. The same signs of inferoposterior MI caused by a CX occlusion are visible.

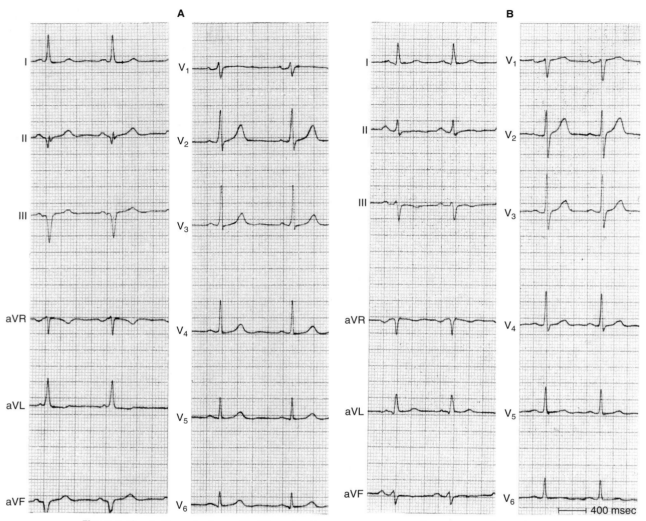

Figure 1-43 **A,** Sinus rhythm with AV conduction over a posteroseptal accessory pathway. A pseudo inferior MI pattern caused by the negative delta waves is present in leads II, III, and aVF. **B,** Same patient during AV conduction over the AV node only.

the heart. As shown in Figure 1-43, a pseudo-infarct pattern is created because of conduction over an inferoposterior septal accessory pathway, leading to initial QRS negativity (the delta wave) in the inferior leads.

ECG Signs of Reperfusion

ST SEGMENT CHANGES

The 12-lead ECG is an inexpensive tool to monitor coronary vessel patency and myocardial perfusion during treatment. In the absence of reperfusion, only minor changes in the amount of ST segment deviation occur during the first hours after occlusion of the coronary artery.

Resolution of ST segment deviation of more than 70% within 1 hour after fibrinolytic therapy strongly suggests patency of the infarct-related coronary artery.[58-62] The absence of ST resolution after reperfusion does not accurately predict an occluded coronary artery but does suggest impaired myocardial perfusion (no myocardial reflow). This situation can be found in approximately 50% of patients with no (<30%) ST resolution.

After fibrinolytic therapy, half of the patients show an *increase in ST segment elevation* at the time of reperfusion, followed by a significant decrease in ST segment elevation.[60,61] This situation is less often seen on reperfusion in patients undergoing a percutaneous cardiac intervention (10% versus 50%).[62]

Important differences may exist between anterior and inferior MI regarding ST segment resolution. Restoration of epicardial blood flow frequently shows significantly less ST resolution in anterior than in inferior MI.[63] De Lemos et al[64] therefore suggest that resolution of ST deviation by more than 70% is the optimal threshold for patients with inferior MI, but more than 50% may be optimal for anterior MI.

Normalization of the ST segment has important prognostic significance. As shown by van't Hof et al,[65] the relative risk of death among patients with no resolution compared with that of patients with a normalized ST segment was 8.7, and the relative risk of death among patients with partial resolution compared with that of patients with normalized ST segment was 3.6.

The best way to evaluate the effect of the reperfusion procedure is continuous *ST segment monitoring.* As shown by Johanson et al,[66] small variations in ST segment shift during the first 4 hours after acute MI predict a worse outcome. Continuous ST segment monitoring also allows early recognition of reocclusion, making optimal management possible.

T-WAVE CHANGES

After reperfusion, when the decrease in ST segment deviation occurs, *terminal T-wave inversion* is also usually present in the leads showing decreasing ST segment elevation (Figure 1-44). In anterior wall MI this terminal T-wave inversion can be seen in the precordial leads, and in inferior MI it can be seen in leads II, III, and aVF. In posterior MI, with ST segment depression in the precordial leads, the reverse pattern can be found; that is, the terminal part of the T wave becomes positive. *Late T-wave inversion (>4 hours)* is not an indicator of reperfusion but a feature of the ST segment behavior after myocardial necrosis.

VENTRICULAR ARRHYTHMIAS

Restoration of patency of an occluded coronary vessel is frequently accompanied by arrhythmias. They may occur at the ventricular and atrial level (Box 1-4), but following reperfusion, arrhythmias at the ventricular level are more common. The reperfusion ventricular arrhythmias are the accelerated idioventricular rhythm (AIVR), VPBs, and nonsustained VT.

BOX 1-4

Reperfusion Arrhythmias

Accelerated idioventricular rhythm: Run of more than three ventricular complexes with a rate between 60 and 120 beats/min starting late in diastole
Nonsustained VT: Ventricular rhythm more than 120 beats/min lasting less than 30 seconds
Increase in VPBs: Twofold increase in the number per 5-minute interval
Ventricular fibrillation
Atrial tachycardia/atrial fibrillation: Run of more than three regular or irregular rapid atrial complexes

---

Accelerated Idioventricular Rhythm

AIVR is a very specific reperfusion arrhythmia with a specificity of more than 80% and a positive predictive value of more than 90% (Figures 1-45 and 1-46).[67-69] AIVR is probably caused by reperfusion damage.[68] Although it is a transient, self-terminating arrhythmia that does not need treatment, has no major hemodynamic consequences, and is not a precursor to more malignant ventricular arrhythmias, it is, however, a predictor of worsening of LV function after the acute phase. Engelen et al[70] showed a relation between the incidence and severity of AIVR and LV wall motion abnormalities several weeks after MI. Importantly, AIVR is less common *after percutaneous cardiac intervention* than after reperfusion by fibrinolytic treatment.[62,70]

Sustained Monomorphic VT

Sustained monomorphic VT is not a reperfusion arrhythmia. When it occurs in the setting of an acute MI, a scar from a previous MI is usually present.[71]

Nonsustained VT

Nonsustained VT may occur. However, the clinical importance of this arrhythmia as an indicator of reperfusion is limited because it is frequently seen in the absence of reperfusion.

Polymorphic VT and Ventricular Fibrillation

Polymorphic VT and ventricular fibrillation were found to occur more often in patients receiving thrombolytics compared with placebo in a large randomized trial assessing the safety of thrombolytic therapy at home.[72] Discussion is ongoing about the significance of primary ventricular fibrillation on the long-term prognosis of patients with MI.[73-79]

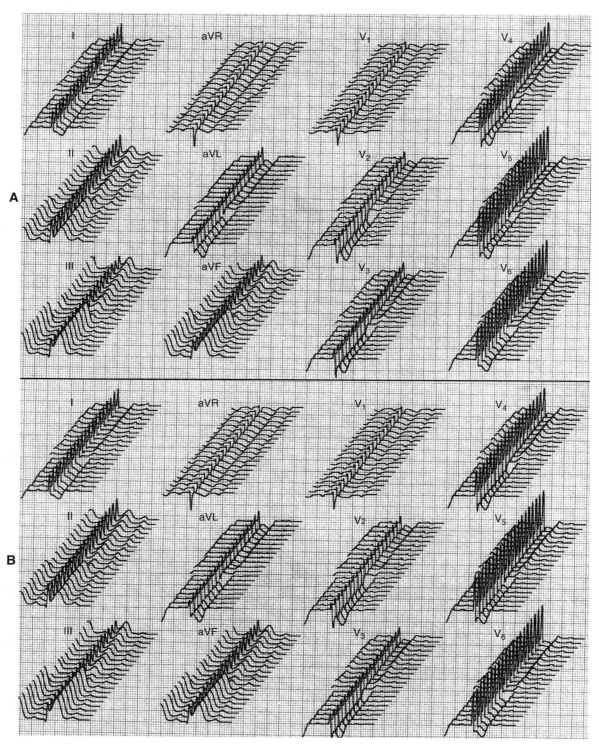

Figure 1-44 Sequential recording of the 12-lead ECG at 45-second intervals in acute inferior MI. **A,** Loss of ST segment deviation on RCA reperfusion. **B,** Short-lasting ST segment elevation at the time of RCA reperfusion.

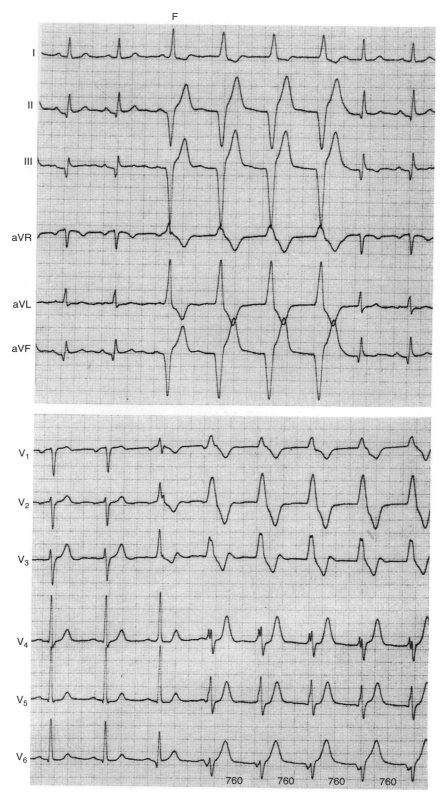

Figure 1-45 Accelerated idioventricular rhythm in the setting of inferior wall MI. The rhythm begins with a fusion beat *(F)* and has an RBBB configuration with left axis deviation.

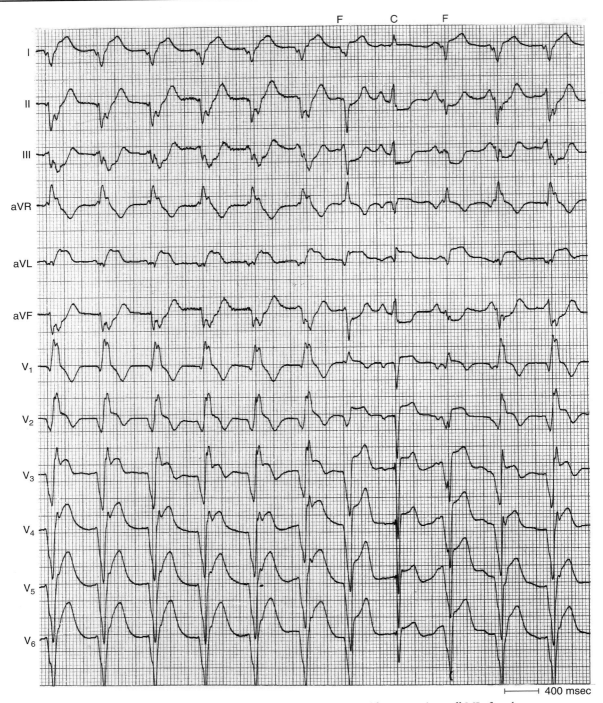

├────────┤ 400 msec

Figure 1-46 Accelerated idioventricular rhythm in a patient with an anterior wall MI after the reopening of an LAD occlusion proximal to the first septal branch. Note that beats 7 to 9 are fusion *(F)* and capture *(C)* beats.

35

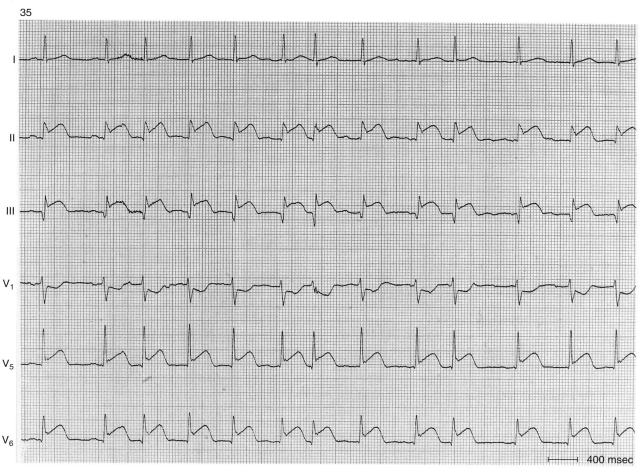

Figure 1-47 Atrial fibrillation occurring 37 minutes after the start of thrombolytic therapy in a patient with inferior MI.

SUPRAVENTRICULAR ARRHYTHMIAS

Atrial tachycardia and atrial fibrillation, shown in Figure 1-47, may occur in the setting of reperfusion. The significance of these arrhythmias is not clear. Of course, they must be differentiated from atrial fibrillation occurring later after MI as an expression of pump failure.

Bradycardia, usually sinus bradycardia, may also occur, especially in inferior wall MI and occasionally because of complete SA block (see Figure 1-23). A transient bradycardia occurring during vessel reopening does not influence the short- or long-term prognosis.

Differential Diagnosis

The clinical presentation of acute MI may be mimicked by the following five relatively common clinical conditions, which should always be considered in the differential diagnosis of acute MI:

1. Acute pulmonary embolism
2. Acute pericarditis
3. Aortic dissection
4. Pancreatitis
5. Cholecystitis

In addition, the newly described tako-tsubo syndrome (transient LV apical ballooning without coronary artery stenosis) mimics acute MI and is also discussed.

ACUTE PULMONARY EMBOLISM

Acute massive pulmonary embolism (see Chapter 9) involving the main pulmonary arteries may simulate acute MI, especially because both conditions may present with chest pain, shortness of breath, and hypotension and may be associated with a fall in cardiac output, abnormal Q waves, ST segment elevation, T-wave changes, and modest troponin elevation. For example, right axis deviation with Q waves and T-wave changes in the inferior leads mimics inferior MI. Although the RBBB pattern and ST segment elevation in lead V_1 raise the suspicion of pulmonary embolism, especially if a positive T wave is present in that lead, this pattern is also seen when RBBB is associated with acute anteroseptal infarction, acute pericarditis, and the early repolarization pattern.

The ECG signs of acute pulmonary embolism are not 100% diagnostic, and prior cardiac disease may make these ECG signs even less specific and less obvious. However, certain ECG findings can cause the informed examiner to have a high degree of suspicion, in which case the diagnosis can be confirmed by an emergency echocardiogram, which sensitively reflects the RV pressure and volume overload of acute pulmonary embolism.

Additionally, cases of acute pulmonary embolism are associated with physical symptoms, ECG, and chest x-ray that, although nonspecific, may help in the differential diagnosis.

In acute pulmonary embolism the following statements can be made:

- Acute respiratory distress is more pronounced than would be expected in MI, unless the acute MI is accompanied by pulmonary edema.
- The abnormal ECG is inconsistent with that usually seen in MI. For example, in one 12-lead ECG both inferior and anterior MI may be suggested, in that Q waves may be seen in leads III and aVF, but not in lead II, and may be associated with a QR pattern in lead V_1.
- The chest radiograph does not show pulmonary congestion, although severe dyspnea and hypoxemia are present.

ACUTE PERICARDITIS

The signs and symptoms of pericarditis can mimic those of acute MI in that there is ST segment elevation and there may be chest pain. The diagnosis of pericarditis is based on the following:

- Characteristic chest pain that is sharp, pleuritic, worse on inspiration or with recumbency, and relieved by leaning forward

- No response to nitroglycerin
- Pericardial friction rub heard along the left lower sternal border or the left precordium
- ECG changes; classically, ECG changes occur in four stages, with some cases that do not include all four stages:
    Stage I: Diffuse concave ST segment elevation present during the first few days of pericardial inflammation, lasting up to 2 weeks. The concave appearance of the ST segment elevation of pericarditis differs from the usually convex appearance of acute MI.
    Stage II: The ST segments return to baseline and the T wave flattens. This stage lasts from days to several weeks.
    Stage III: T-wave inversion begins at the end of the second or third week.
    Stage IV: The T wave gradually resolves, which may take up to 3 months.

Other helpful clues include the following:

- Q waves are absent.
- Reciprocal changes are absent.
- ST segment elevation does not localize into right or left coronary artery distribution.
- The *echocardiogram* is helpful in making the differential diagnosis because pericardial effusion is frequently present as a result of pericarditis.

AORTIC DISSECTION

In aortic dissection the character of the pain may differ from that of acute MI in the following ways:

- Posterior transmission is frequently seen.
- Pain may be pulsatile, rhythmic, and synchronized with systole.
- Nitroglycerin does not provide a response.
- The ECG may be normal or ST segment changes may be present, especially if the patient has hypertension and LV hypertrophy.
- ECG changes may be present and associated with pericarditis if the dissection involves the aortic root and pericardial hemorrhage has occurred.

The diagnosis is suspected on *chest radiographs* and confirmed either by *computed tomographic scan*, *transesophageal echocardiography,* or *magnetic resonance imaging.* Aortography is rarely needed for diagnosis.

MYOCARDITIS

The clinical presentation of myocarditis can mimic that of acute MI. Sarda et al[80] showed that among 45 patients who presented with symptoms of acute MI but a normal coronary angiogram, 40% had myocarditis.

The diagnosis is made by:

- Exclusion of acute MI
- The clinical course of the patient, and if needed
- Endomyocardial biopsy

PANCREATITIS AND CHOLECYSTITIS

Pancreatitis and cholecystitis can present a clinical picture mimicking acute MI with chest pain. The differential diagnosis between these two disorders and MI is made with *abdominal ultrasound* and determination of appropriate *blood tests*.[81]

TRANSIENT LV APICAL BALLOONING (TAKO-TSUBO CARDIOMYOPATHY)

Tako-tsubo cardiomyopathy is the acute onset of transient LV apical ballooning without significant coronary stenosis that mimics acute MI in symptoms and ECG findings. Most patients who survive recover completely and relatively quickly, although the possibility of recurrence exists.[82]

Satoh et al[83] in 1990 and Dote et al[84] in 1991 described this syndrome and named it "tako-tsubo type cardiomyopathy" because on ventriculogram its unique apical ballooning resembled the ampulla-shaped "tako-tsubo" fishing pot used for trapping octopus in Japan.

In 2001, a series of 88 patients was presented by Tsuchihashi et al.[85] This and other studies have demonstrated that the syndrome is seen predominantly in women,[86-89] and in some patients it is possibly triggered by emotional or physical stress.[90,91]

These patients present with dyspnea, chest pain, or pulmonary edema. Progression to cardiogenic shock or ventricular fibrillation has been reported.[92] Cardiac markers rise only minimally, which is especially notable when compared with the dramatic extent of the akinetic zone.[93]

Typical ECG Features

Acute phase
- ST elevation in chest leads (especially V_3 to V_6) and lead I
- Q waves in chest leads in 15% of cases

Subacute phase
- Disappearance of Q waves
- Deep T-wave inversion in precordial leads and leads I, II, and aVL
- QT prolongation maximal on day 3

Conclusion

The ECG pattern shows transient Q waves, ST segment elevation evolving to deep negative T waves, and QT prolongation peaking by day 3.

ST segment elevation. The ECG on admission may be normal, but subsequent changes, although rarely typical, are compelling mimics of acute anterior MI with ST segment elevation in leads V_1 to V_6.

Negative T waves. Additionally, in all 88 patients of the study by Tsuchihashi et al,[85] negative T waves developed in the anterior leads.

Prolonged QTc intervals. Abe et al[94] reported prolonged QTc intervals during the acute phase, returning to normal during the chronic phase.

Visual Findings

Echocardiogram. In all patients, echocardiography revealed akinesia of the apical and mid portions of the LV.

Ventriculogram. Left ventriculogram revealed unique LV apical ballooning with hypercontraction at the basal segment.

Angiogram. Coronary angiography demonstrated no significant obstruction in the coronary arteries.

Clinical Implications

- Tako-tsubo LV dysfunction mimics anterior MI and may needlessly expose the patient to fibrinolytic agents.
- Optimal treatment for one patient may harm other patients, emphasizing the need for a better understanding of the pathophysiologic characteristics and treatment options.
- The possibility of recurrence exists.

Treatment of ST Segment Elevation MI

The golden rule in the treatment of acute coronary syndromes is to make the time interval between onset of ischemia and restoration of myocardial blood flow as short as possible. Many factors play a role, including:

- Length of time from the onset of chest pain until medical attention is sought
- Rapidity with which emergency medical services are provided to the patient
- Accuracy of the diagnosis in the acute phase
- Availability of prehospital treatment facilities, including thrombolytic therapy
- Availability of inhospital facilities, such as percutaneous cardiac intervention

- Optimal management of acute chest pain at each step from home to hospital
- A written chest pain protocol, indicating what to do with patients with suspected or confirmed STEMI in both the prehospital and hospital phases

The goal is rapid recognition and treatment of patients with STEMI, with, depending on the selected reperfusion strategy, a medical contact to fibrinolytic treatment within 30 minutes and a medical contact to *percutaneous cardiac intervention* in fewer than 90 minutes. Of great help are the American College of Cardiology/American Heart Association guidelines for the management of patients with STEMI found in Antman et al[54] and at *www.acc.org/clinical/guidelines/stemi/index.htm.*

Important in the early phase is the knowledge required to provide a correct ECG diagnosis, which is essential for decision making. When needed in the prehospital setting, the ECG interpretation can be helped by using computerized algorithms or advice from a hospital physician.

MANAGEMENT RELATIVE TO TIME INTERVAL FROM PAIN TO MEDICAL ATTENTION

The management of MI depends on the time interval between the onset of chest pain and the availability of prehospital and inhospital facilities. Three situations are given below along with the course of action to be taken.

Decision making is significantly influenced by the presence or absence of a *percutaneous cardiac intervention* center nearby. Suggestions on how to proceed in different situations, with the emphasis on ECG findings, are also provided.

Situation A: A Percutaneous Cardiac Intervention Center Can Be Reached Within 30 Minutes

1. Record a 12-lead ECG, along with lead V_4R in case of inferoposterior MI.
2. Determine the time interval from the onset of pain to the ECG recording.
3. Give, unless contraindicated or already used by the patient, nitroglycerine, aspirin, a beta-blocking agent, and pain medication.
4. Transmit the ECG of patients with STEMI to a *percutaneous cardiac intervention* center.
5. Transmit the ECG of patients with chest pain and conduction disturbances, including LBBB and paced rhythms, to a *percutaneous cardiac intervention center,* followed by transport to the center.

6. Transmit the ECG in patients with non-STEMI to a *percutaneous cardiac intervention* center for advice about transport to that center in relation to the extent and degree of ST depression.

Situation B: A Percutaneous Cardiac Intervention Center Can Be Reached Within 30 to 60 Minutes

1. Record a 12-lead ECG, along with lead V_4R in case of inferoposterior MI.
2. Determine the time interval from the onset of pain to the ECG recording.
3. Give, unless contraindicated or already used by the patient, nitroglycerine, aspirin, a beta-blocking agent, and pain medication.
4. Make a risk profile (ST deviation score, location of the coronary occlusion, degree of ischemia, conduction disturbances).
5. Start intravenous fibrinolytic therapy in all patients with STEMI not having contraindications to fibrinolysis.
6. Send high-risk patients with STEMI to a percutaneous cardiac intervention center. High-risk patients with STEMI include those with the following:
   - Shock or heart failure
   - ST deviation score more than 15 mm
   - LAD occlusion proximal to first septal or first diagonal branch
   - Proximal RCA occlusion
   - Dominant CX occlusion
   - Conduction disturbances at the SA, AV, and bundle branch level
   - Recurrent MI
   - Contraindications for fibrinolytic therapy
7. Admit other patients with STEMI and non-STEMI to the local hospital.

Situation C: A Percutaneous Cardiac Intervention Center Cannot Be Reached in 60 Minutes

1. Record a 12-lead ECG, along with lead V_4R in case of inferoposterior MI.
2. Determine the time interval from the onset of pain to the ECG recording.
3. Give, unless contraindicated or already used by the patient, nitroglycerine, aspirin, a beta-blocking agent, and pain medication.
4. Treat all patients with STEMI and symptom onset within the previous 4 hours with fibrinolytic therapy unless contraindications are present.
5. Consider transfer of high-risk patients with STEMI to a percutaneous cardiac intervention center, especially when fibrinolytic therapy fails or is contraindicated.

SUMMARY

The ECG is of great value in STEMI to risk stratify the patient and select optimal management. For risk stratification, the following five ECG parameters are important:

1. ST segment deviation score
2. Severity of ischemia as indicated by the ST-T segment behavior
3. ST segment deviation vector in the frontal plane to detect the site of occlusion in the culprit coronary artery and estimate the size of the area at risk
4. ST segment deviation vector in the horizontal plane (lead V_4R) to detect RV involvement and risk for the development of high-degree AV nodal block and the extent and severity of posterior wall ischemia
5. Presence of AV and intraventricular conduction disturbances

REFERENCES

1. Vermeer F, Simoons ML, Bar FW, et al: Which patient benefits most from early thrombolytic therapy with intracoronary streptokinase? *Circulation* 74:1379-89, 1986.
2. Bar FW, Vermeer F, De Zwaan C, et al: Value of admission electrocardiogram in predicting outcome of thrombolytic therapy in acute myocardial infarction, *Am J Cardiol* 59:6-13, 1987.
3. Long-term effects of intravenous thrombolysis in acute myocardial infarction: final report of the GISSI study. Gruppo Italiano per lo Studio della Streptochi-nasi nell'Infarto Miocardico (GISSI), *Lancet* 2(8564):871-4, 1987.
4. Aldrich HR, Wagner NB, Boswick J, et al: Use of the ST segment deviation for prediction of final electrocardiographic size of acute myocardial infarction, *Am J Cardiol* 61:749-53, 1988.
5. Foerster JM, Vera Z, Janzen DA, et al: Evaluation of precordial orthogonal vector cardiographic lead ST segment magnitude in the assessment of myocardial ischemia injury, *Circulation* 55:728-35, 1977.
6. Engelen DJ, Gorgels AP, Cheriex EC, et al: Value of the electrocardiogram in localizing the occlusion site in the left anterior descending coronary artery in acute anterior myocardial infarction, *J Am Cardiol* 34:389-95, 1999.
7. Hurst JW: Methods used to interpret the 12-lead electrocardiogram: pattern memorization vs. the use of the vector concept, *Clin Cardiol* 24:4-13, 2004.
8. Wellens HJJ, Gorgels APM, Doevendans PA: *The ECG in acute myocardial infarction and unstable angina: diagnosis and risk stratification*, Boston, 2003, Kluwer Academic Publishers.
9. Braat SH, Brugada P, De Zwaan C, et al: Value of the electrocardiogram in diagnosing right ventricular involvement in patients with an acute inferior wall myocardial infarction, *Br Heart J* 49:368-72, 1983.
10. Braat SH, De Zwaan C, Brugada P, et al: Right ventricular involvement with acute myocardial infarction identifies high risk of developing atrioventricular nodal conduction disturbances, *Am Heart J* 107:1183-7, 1984.
11. Braat SH, Gorgels APM, Bar FW, et al: Value of the ST-T segment in lead V_4R in inferior wall acute myocardial infarction to predict the site of coronary artery occlusion, *Am J Cardiol* 62:146-52, 1988.
12. Berger PB, Ryan TJ: Inferior myocardial infarction: high risk subgroups, *Circulation* 81:401-11, 1990.
13. Berger PB, Ruocco NA Jr, Ryan TJ, et al: Frequency and significance of right ventricular dysfunction during inferior wall left ventricular myocardial infarction treated with thrombolytic therapy (results from the thrombolysis in myocardial infarction [TIMI] II trial). The TIMI Research Group, *Am J Cardiol* 71:1148-52, 1993.
14. Zehender M, Kaperc W, Kauder E, et al: Right ventricular infarction as independent predictor of prognosis after acute myocardial infarction, *N Engl J Med* 328:981-8, 1993.
15. Zeymer U, Neuhaus KL, Wegscheider K, et al: Effects of thrombolytic therapy in acute inferior myocardial infarction with or without right ventricular involvement. HIT-4 Trial Group. Hirudin for Improvement of Thrombolysis, *J Am Coll Cardiol* 32:876-81, 1998.
16. Mehta SR, Eikelboom JW, Natarajan MK, et al: Impact of right ventricular involvement on mortality and morbidity in patients with inferior myocardial infarction, *J Am Coll Cardiol* 37:37-43, 2001.
17. Fiol M, Cygankiewicz I, Carrillo A, et al: Value of electrocardiographic algorithm based on "ups and downs" of ST in assessment of a culprit artery in evolving inferior wall acute myocardial infarction, *Am J Cardiol* 94:709-14, 2004.
18. Mittal SR: Isolated right ventricular infarction, *Int J Cardiol* 46:53-60, 1994.
19. Van der Bolt CLB, Vermeersch PHMJ, Plokker HWM: Isolated acute occlusion of a large right ventricular branch of the right coronary artery following coronary balloon angioplasty, *Eur Heart J* 17:247-50, 1996.
20. Yamaji H, Iwasachi S, Kusachi S, et al: Prediction of acute left main coronary obstruction by 12-lead electrocardiogram: aVR ST-segment elevation with less V_1 ST-segment elevation, *J Am Coll Cardiol* 38:1348-54, 2001.
21. Indications for fibrinolytic therapy in suspected acute myocardial infarction: collaborative overview of early mortality and major morbidity results from all randomised trials of more than 1000 patients. Fibrinolytic Therapy Trialists' (FTT) Collaborative Group, *Lancet* 343:311-22, 1994.
22. Hartzler GO, Rutterford BD, McConahay DR, et al: Percutaneous transluminal coronary angioplasty with and without thrombolytic therapy for treatment of acute myocardial infarction, *Am Heart J* 106:965-70, 1983.
23. Grines CL, Browne KF, Marco J, et al: A comparison of immediate angioplasty with thrombolytic therapy for acute myocardial infarction. The Primary Angioplasty in Myocardial Infarction Study Group, *N Engl J Med* 328:673-9, 1993.
24. Zijlstra F, De Boer MJ, Hoorntje JCA, et al: A comparison of immediate coronary angioplasty with intravenous streptokinase in acute myocardial infarction, *N Engl J Med* 328:680-4, 1993.
25. Gibbons RJ, Holmes DR, Reeder GS, et al: Immediate angioplasty compared with the administration of a thrombolytic agent followed by conservative treatment for myocardial infarction, *N Engl J Med* 328:685-9, 1993.
26. Weaver WD, Simes RJ, Betriu A, et al: Comparison of primary coronary angioplasty and intravenous thrombolytic therapy for acute myocardial infarction: a quantitative review, *JAMA* 278:2093-9, 1997.
27. Zijlstra F, Hoorntje JC, De Boer MJ, et al: Long term benefit of primary angioplasty as compared with thrombolytic therapy for acute myocardial infarction, *N Engl J Med* 341:1413-8, 1999.

28. Keeley EC, Boura JA, Grines CL: Primary angioplasty versus intravenous thrombolytic therapy for acute myocardial infarction: a quantitative review of 23 randomised trials, *Lancet* 361:13-20, 2003.

29. Topol EJ, Kereiakes DJ: Regionalization of care for acute ischemic heart disease, *Circulation* 107:1463-6, 2003.

30. Sclarovsky S: *Electrocardiography of acute myocardial ischemic syndromes,* London, 1999, Martin Duntz.

31. Birnbaum Y, Sclarovsky S: The grades of ischemia on the presenting electrocardiogram of patients with ST elevation acute myocardial infarction, *J Electrocardiol* 34(suppl):17-26, 2001.

32. Birnbaum Y, Hertz I, Sclarovsky S, et al: Prognostic significance of the admission electrocardiogram in acute myocardial infarction, *J Am Coll Cardiol* 27:1128-33, 1996.

33. Wiviott SD, Morrow DA, Frederick PD, et al: Performance of the thrombolysis in myocardial infarction risk index in the national registry of myocardial infarction-3 and -4. A simple index that predicts mortality is ST segment elevation myocardial infarction, *J Am Coll Cardiol* 44:783-9, 2004.

34. Durrer D, Van Dam RTH, Freud GE, et al: Total excitation of the isolated human heart, *Circulation* 41:899-912, 1970.

35. James TN: The coronary circulation and conduction system in acute myocardial infarction, *Prog Cardiovasc Dis* 10:410-28, 1968.

36. Zipes DP: The clinical significance of bradycardic rhythm in acute myocardial infarction, *Am J Cardiol* 24:814-9, 1969.

37. Tans A, Lie Ki, Durrer D: Clinical setting and prognostic significance of high degree AV block in acute inferior myocardial infarction: a study of 144 patients, *Am Heart J* 99:4-8, 1980.

38. Berger P, Ruocco N, Ryan T, et al: Incidence and prognostic implications of heart block complicating acute inferior myocardial infarction treated with thrombolytic therapy: results from TIMI II, *J Am Coll Cardiol* 20:533-40, 1992.

39. Kimura K, Kosuge M, Ishikawa T, et al: Comparison of results of early reperfusion in patients with inferior wall acute myocardial infarction with and without complete atrioventricular block, *Am J Cardiol* 84:731-3, 1999.

40. Simons GR, Sgarbossa E, Wagner G, et al: Atrioventricular and intraventricular conduction disorders in acute myocardial infarction: a reappraisal in the thrombolytic era, *Pacing Clin Electrophysiol* 21:2651-63, 1998.

41. Barold SS: American College of Cardiology/American Heart Association guidelines for pacemaker implantation after acute myocardial infarction. What is persistent advanced block at the atrioventricular node? *Am J Cardiol* 80:770-4, 1997.

42. Lie KI, Wellens HJJ, Schuilenburg RM: Bundle branch block and acute myocardial infarction. In Wellens HJJ, Lie KI, Jansse MJ, editors: *The conduction system of the heart,* Philadelphia, 1976, Lea and Febiger, pp 663-72.

43. Lie KI, Wellens HJJ, Schuilenburg RM, et al: Factors influencing prognosis of bundle branch block complicating acute anteroseptal infarction: the value of His bundle recordings, *Circulation* 50:935-41, 1974.

44. Newby KH, Pisano E, Krucoff MW, et al: Incidence and clinical relevance of the occurrence of bundle branch block in patients treated with thrombolytic therapy, *Circulation* 94:2424-8, 1996.

45. Harpaz D, Behar S, Gotlieb S, et al: Complete atrioventricular block complicating acute myocardial infarction in the thrombolytic era, *J Am Coll Cardiol* 34:721-8, 1999.

46. Sgarbossa EB, Pinsky SL, Topol EJ, et al: Acute myocardial infarction and complete bundle branch block at hospital admission: clinical characteristics and outcome in the thrombolytic era.

47. Go AS, Barron HV, Rundle AC, et al: Bundle-branch block and in-hospital mortality in acute myocardial infarction. National Registry of Myocardial Infarction 2 Investigators, *Ann Intern Med* 129:690-7, 1998.

GUSTO-I Investigators. Global Utilization of Streptokinase and t-PA [tissue-type plasminogen activator] for Occluded Coronary Arteries, *J Am Coll Cardiol* 31:105-10, 1998.

48. Lie KI, Wellens HJJ, Schuilenburg RM, et al: Mechanism and significance of widened QRS complexes during complete AV block in acute inferior myocardial infarction, *Am J Cardiol* 33:833-41, 1974.

49. Wackers FJT, Lie KI, David G, et al: Assessment of the value of electrocardiographic signs for myocardial infarction in left bundle branch block. In Wellens HJJ, Kulbertus HE, editors: *What's new in electrocardiography?* The Hague, 1981, Martinus Nijhoff, pp 37-57.

50. Sgarbossa EB, Pinsky SL, Barbagelata A, et al: Electrocardiographic diagnosis of evolving acute myocardial infarction in the presence of left bundle branch block, *N Engl J Med* 334:481-7, 1996.

51. Shlipak MS, Lyons WL, Go AS, et al: Should the electrocardiogram be used to guide therapy for patients with left bundle branch block and suspected myocardial infarction, *JAMA* 281:714-9, 1999.

52. Gula LJ, Dick A, Massel D: Diagnosing acute myocardial infarction in the setting of the left bundle branch block: prevalence and observer variability from a large community study, *Coron Artery Dis* 14:387-93, 2003.

53. Wellens HJJ: Acute myocardial infarction and left bundle branch block, can we lift the veil? *N Engl J Med* 334:528-9, 1996.

54. Antman EM, Anbe DT, Armstrong PW, et al: ACC/AHA guidelines for the management of patients with ST-elevation myocardial infarction—executive summary: a report of the American College of Cardiology/American Heart Association Task Force on Practice Guidelines (Writing Committee to Revise the 1999 Guidelines for the Management of Patients With Acute Myocardial Infarction), *Circulation* 110:588-636, 2004.

55. Barold SS, Ong LS, Heinle RA: Electrocardiographic diagnosis of myocardial infarction in patients with transvenous pacemakers, *J Electrocardiol* 9:99-111, 1996.

56. Dodinot B, Kubler L, Godemir JP: Electrocardiographic diagnosis of myocardial infarction in pacemaker patients. In Wellens HJJ, Kulbertus HE, editors: *What's new in electrocardiography?* The Hague, 1981, Martinus Nijhoff, pp 79-90.

57. Sgarbossa E, Pinski S, Gates K, et al: Early ECG diagnosis of acute myocardial infarction in the presence of ventricular paced rhythm, *Am J Cardiol* 77:423-24, 1996.

58. De Lemos JA, Braunwald E: ST segment resolution as a tool for assessing the efficacy of reperfusion therapy, *J Am Coll Cardiol* 38:1283-94, 2001.

59. Zeymer U, Schroder R, Tebbe U, et al: Non-invasive detection of early infarct vessel patency by resolution of ST segment elevation in patients with thrombolysis for acute myocardial infarction, *Eur Heart J* 22:769-75, 2001.

60. Arstall MA, Stewart S, Haste MA, et al: Streptokinase-induced transient aggravation of myocardial injury, *Int J Cardiol* 50:107-16, 1995.

61. Doevendans PA, Gorgels AP, van der Zee R, et al: Electrocardiographic diagnosis of reperfusion during thrombolytic therapy in acute myocardial infarction, *Am J Cardiol* 75:1206-10, 1995.

62. Wehrens XH, Doevendans PA, Oude Ophuis TJ, et al: A comparison of electrocardiographic changes during reperfusion of acute myocardial infarction by thrombolysis or PTCA, *Am Heart J* 139:430-6, 2000.

63. Buszman P, Szafranek A, Kalarus Z, et al: Use of changes in ST segment elevation for prediction of infarct artery recanalization in acute myocardial infarction, *Eur Heart J* 16:1207-14, 1995.

64. De Lemos JA, Antman EM, McCabe CH, et al: ST segment resolution and infarct related artery patency and flow after thrombolytic therapy, *Am J Cardiol* 85:299-304, 2000.

65. van't Hof AW, Liem A, De Boer MJ, et al: Clinical value of the 12-lead electrocardiogram after successful reperfusion therapy for acute myocardial infarction, *Lancet* 350:615-9, 1997.

66. Johanson P, Svensson AM, Dellborg M: Clinical implications of early ST segment variability. A report from the ASSENT 2 ST-monitoring sub-study, *Coron Artery Dis* 12:277-83, 2001.

67. Goldberg S, Greenspon AJ, Urban PL, et al: Reperfusion arrhythmia: a marker of restoration of antegrade flow during intracoronary thrombolysis for acute myocardial infarction, *Am Heart J* 105:26-32, 1983.

68. Gorgels AP, Vos MA, Letsch IS, et al: Usefulness of the accelerated idioventricular rhythm as a marker for myocardial necrosis and reperfusion during thrombolytic therapy in acute myocardial infarction, *Am J Cardiol* 61:231-5, 1988.

69. Gressin V, Louvard Y, Pezzano M, et al: Holter recording of ventricular arrhythmias during intravenous thrombolysis for acute myocardial infarction, *Am J Cardiol* 69:152-9, 1992.

70. Engelen DJ, Gressin V, Krucoff MW, et al: Reperfusion arrhythmias in acute anterior myocardial infarction are related to the mode of reperfusion and predict worsening of left ventricular function, *Am J Cardiol* 92:1143-9, 2003.

71. Wellens HJ, Lie KI, Durrer D: Further observations on ventricular tachycardia as studied by electrical stimulation of the heart. Chronic recurrent ventricular tachycardia and ventricular tachycardia during acute myocardial infarction, *Circulation* 49:647-53, 1974.

72. Boissel JP, Castaigne A, Mercier C, et al: Ventricular fibrillation following administration of thrombolytic treatment. The EMIP experience, *Eur Heart J* 17:213-21, 1996.

73. Volpi A, Maggioni A, Franzosi MJ, et al: In-hospital prognosis of patients with acute myocardial infarction complicated by primary ventricular fibrillation, *N Engl J Med* 317:257-61, 1987.

74. Behar S, Goldbourt U, Reicher-Reiss H: Prognosis of acute myocardial infarction complicated by primary ventricular fibrillation. Principal Investigators of the SPRINT Study, *Am J Cardiol* 66:1208-11, 1990.

75. Tofler GH, Stone PH, Muller JE, et al: Prognosis after cardiac arrest due to ventricular tachycardia or ventricular fibrillation associated with acute myocardial infarction (the MILIS Study). Multicenter Investigation of the Limitation of Infarct Size, *Am J Cardiol* 60:755-61, 1987.

76. Chiriboga D, Yarzebski J, Goldberg RJ, et al: Temporal trends (1975 through 1990) in the incidence and case fatality rates of primary ventricular fibrillation complicating acute myocardial infarction, *Circulation* 89:998-1003, 1994.

77. Berger PB, Ruocco NA, Ryan TJ, et al: Incidence and significance of ventricular tachycardia and fibrillation in the absence of hypotension or heart failure in acute myocardial infarction treated with recombinant tissue-type plasminogen activator: results from the Thrombolysis in Myocardial Infarction (TIMI) Phase II trial, *J Am Coll Cardiol* 22:1773-9, 1993.

78. Brezins M, Elyassov S, Elimelech I, et al: Comparison of patients with acute myocardial infarction with and without ventricular fibrillation, *Am J Cardiol* 78:948-50, 1996.

79. Doevendans PA, Cheriex E, Van der Zee R, et al: Risk stratification in the thrombolytic era: results of a prospective study, *Cardiologie* 3:319-23, 1996.

80. Sarda L, Colin P, Boccara F, et al: Myocarditis in patients with clinical presentation of myocardial infarction and normal coronary angiograms, *J Am Coll Cardiol* 37:786-92, 2002.

81. Hung SC, Chiang CE, Chen JD, et al: Pseudo-myocardial infarction, *Circulation* 101:2989-90, 2000.

82. Tsuchihashi K, Ueshima K, Uchida T, et al: Transient left ventricular apical ballooning without coronary artery stenosis: a novel heart syndrome mimicking acute myocardial infarction, *J Am Coll Cardiol* 38:11-18, 2001.

83. Satoh H, Tateishi H, Uchida T, et al: Takotsubo type cardiomyopathy due to multivessel spasm. In Dodama K, Haze K, Hon M, editors: *Clinical aspect of myocardial injury: from ischemia to heart failure* [in Japanese], Tokyo, 1990, Kagakuhyouronsya, pp 56-64.

84. Dote K, Satoh H, Tateishi H, et al: Myocardial stunning due to simultaneous multivessel spasm: a review of five cases, *J Cardiol* 21:201-14, 1991.

85. Tsuchihashi K, Ueshima K, Uchida T, et al: Transient left ventricular apical ballooning without coronary artery stenosis: a novel heart syndrome mimicking acute myocardial infarction, *J Am Coll Cardiol* 38:11-18, 2001.

86. Desmet WJR, Adriaenssens BFM, Dens JAY: Apical ballooning of the left ventricle: first series in white patients, *Heart* 89:1027-31, 2003.

87. Abe Y, Kondo M: Apical ballooning of the left ventricle: a distinct entity? *Heart* 89:974-6, 2003.

88. Abe Y, Kondo M, Matsuoka R, et al: Assessment of clinical features in transient left ventricular apical ballooning, *J Am Coll Cardiol* 41:737-42, 2003.

89. Ibanez B, Navarro F, Farre J, et al: Tako-Tsubo syndrome associated with a long course of the left anterior descending coronary artery along the apical diafragmatic surface of the left ventricles, *Rev Esp Cardio* 57:209-16, 2004.

90. Ueyama T: Emotional stress-induced Tako-tsubo cardiomyopathy: animal model and molecular mechanism, *Ann N Y Acad Sci* 1018:437-44, 2004.

91. Ibanez B, Navarro F, Farre J, et al: Tako-tsubo syndrome associated with a long course of the left anterior descending coronary artery along the apical diaphragmatic surface of the left ventricle [in Spanish], *Rev Esp Cardiol* 57:209-16, 2004.

92. Ferrer Garcia MC, Ortas Nadal MR, Daga Calejero B: Chest pain and ventricular fibrillation in transient left ventricular apical ballooning [in Spanish], *Med Clin (Barc)* 123:38, 2004.

93. Glockner D, Dissmann M, Behrens S: Atypical acute myocardial ischemia syndrome with reversible left ventricular wall motion abnormalities ("apical ballooning") without significant coronary artery disease, *Z Kardiol* 93:156-61, 2004.

94. Abe Y, Kondo M, Matsuoka R, et al: Assessment of clinical features in transient left ventricular apical ballooning, *J Am Coll Cardiol* 41:737-42, 2003.

2

ECG Recognition of Non–ST Elevation MI and Unstable Angina

EMERGENCY RESPONSE

Recognition of Extent and Severity of Coronary Artery Disease During Chest Pain

1. Count the number of leads with ST segment deviation and determine the total ST deviation score.
2. Look for ST segment elevation in leads aVR and V_1.
3. Exclude other causes of ST segment deviation such as digitalis administration.
4. Determine the troponin value.
5. Decide on early invasive versus noninvasive management.

Recognition of a Critical Narrowing in the LAD

1. Determine the troponin level. In such cases, little or no elevation is present.
2. Look for terminal T-wave negativity progressing to symmetrical T-wave inversion in the precordial leads after the chest pain has subsided.
3. If 12-lead monitoring is not available, obtain a 12-lead ECG every 4 hours to watch for terminal T-wave negativity in the precordial leads (usually most prominent in leads V_2 and V_3), progressing to deep symmetrical T-wave inversion.

NOTE: When the above ECG changes are present, an early invasive diagnostic (and possible therapeutic) approach is suggested.

Chapter 1 discussed ECG findings in patients with chest pain and ST segment elevation in two or more ECG leads, a condition known as ST elevation MI (STEMI).

It is important to examine the ECG carefully, paying attention to all ECG leads including lead aVR, which may show ST elevation, while several other leads show ST depression. A patient with these ECG findings could have left main occlusion and should not be classified as non-STEMI.

Patients may also have cardiac chest pain without a STEMI ECG. However, they may show ST-T segment changes, either ST segment depression or negative T waves in a varying number of ECG leads. In recent years, those patients have been classified as having either *non-STEMI*, when an enzyme rise is present, or unstable angina, when an enzyme rise is not present. The presence of an enzyme rise, usually *troponin T*, has been recognized as an important prognostic marker for myocardial damage and death.[1-4]

AN EARLY INVASIVE VERSUS A CONSERVATIVE (SELECTIVE INVASIVE) APPROACH IN UNSTABLE CORONARY ARTERY DISEASE

Discussion has risen in recent years regarding how to stratify these patients according to their risk of MI and death and how to select the best strategy (invasive versus noninvasive) to reduce that risk.[5-10] The TACTICS,[10] FRISC II,[8,11] and RITA-3[12] investigators argue in favor of an early invasive approach in patients with chest pain and non-STEMI (elevated troponin value).

Although these investigators found a higher infarct risk following percutaneous coronary intervention, early revascularization resulted in a lower mortality rate and fewer rehospitalizations during follow-up. The results of these studies have prompted the advice that, in patients with non-STEMI who have a positive troponin value, cardiac catheterization should be performed and followed by, when needed, revascularization within 48 hours by percutaneous coronary intervention or coronary artery bypass grafting.

More recently, however, the ICTUS investigators[13] came to a different conclusion. That study showed no differences in mortality rate after 1 year between the early invasive group and the selective invasive group.

Those findings could have been affected by the treatment of patients who were initially managed noninvasively with clopidogrel (Plavix) and high-dose statins, in addition to aspirin and enoxaparin. The differences in outcome of the studies on invasive versus noninvasive strategies in patients with non-STEMI may also be caused by the heterogeneity of these patients regarding underlying pathologic conditions and prognosis.

An important question, therefore, is: Do we have better ways of selecting patients with non-STEMI who require an early invasive approach? This chapter covers the value of the ECG in this regard.

THE VALUE OF THE ECG IN NON–ST SEGMENT ELEVATION MI AND UNSTABLE ANGINA

The 12-lead ECG is valuable for risk stratification in patients with non-STEMI and unstable angina because with it the clinician is able to compute the ST segment deviation score (see p. 2) and determine the signs of critical narrowing of the proximal LAD coronary artery.

The Importance of the Degree of ST Segment Depression in the Admission ECG

Several studies have shown the prognostic importance of ST depression on the admission ECG in patients with non-STEMI and unstable angina.[14-18] Recently, Holmvang

et al[15] demonstrated, by analyzing the ECG data from the FRISC II study, that a quantitative assessment of the sum of ST depression in the different ECG leads is valuable in risk stratification and treatment decisions. They found that when the ST segment deviation score fell in the intermediate (2.5-5.5 mm) or major (>5.5 mm) range, a 50% reduction in death or MI could be obtained with an early invasive strategy.

ST segment monitoring. A practical point is whether the ECG is recorded during chest pain. As shown in Figure 2-1, important variations may occur in ST segment behavior in relation to the presence or absence of chest pain. This fact underscores the value of continuous ST segment monitoring after the patient has been admitted.

The Value of the Number of Leads Showing ST Segment Deviation

A correlation exists between the number of ECG leads showing ST-T segment deviation and the extent and severity of coronary artery disease. In 1993 Gorgels et al[19] found that, in patients with unstable angina, the chance of having severe left main stem or three-vessel disease was quite high (71%) when ST segment elevation in leads V_1 and aVR was accompanied by ST segment depression in eight or more of the 12 ECG leads.

Additionally, the FRISC II study findings demonstrated a correlation between the severity of coronary artery disease and the number of leads showing ST segment depression. An early invasive strategy reduced MI and mortality rates by 50% when ST segment depression was seen in five to seven leads ($P < 0.005$) or eight to 11 leads ($P < 0.001$). In this study, the findings on the ST segment depression score and the number of leads with ST segment deviation were of prognostic significance independent of age, sex, or troponin T status.[15]

Value of lead aVR. Most studies reporting on ECG changes in non-STEMI and unstable angina exclude lead aVR from their measurements. This exclusion is unfortunate because that lead is of great value in diagnosing global LV ischemia. Lead aVR often shows ST segment elevation in both left main and three-vessel disease. This situation may also be the case in lead V_1, as demonstrated in Figures 2-1 and 2-2. Figure 2-2 also shows another feature, described by Atie et al,[20] of left main disease—that ST segment depression is most prominent in lead V_4.

Other factors leading to ST segment deviation. As shown in Figure 6-3 (p. 160), during digitalis intoxication the ST segment may deviate in a way similar to that seen in left main stem or three-vessel disease. However,

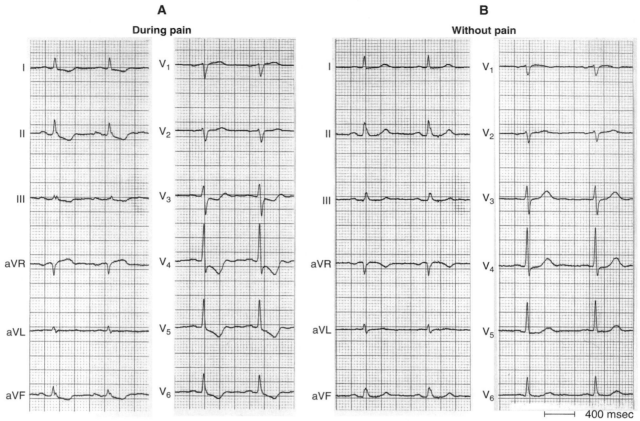

Figure 2-1   A, ECG recorded during chest pain showing ST segment deviation in many leads, including leads aVR and V_1. This pattern suggests three-vessel or left main stem disease. B, Normalization of the ST segment after the pain had subsided.

T-wave behavior and the duration of the QT interval should lead to the correct diagnosis.

Confounding factors. Another important observation resulted from the FRISC II study. The investigators found that in patients in whom ST segment analysis could not be performed because of confounding factors such as bundle branch block, LV or RV hypertrophy, or a paced ventricular rhythm, the prognosis was poor irrespective of an invasive or noninvasive treatment strategy. These confounding factors were found in approximately 25% of their patients.

The Value of T-Wave Changes After Chest Pain Has Subsided

In the 1980s de Zwaan et al[21,22] described an ECG pattern in patients admitted with a history of cardiac chest pain in whom characteristic ECG changes developed *after* the pain had subsided (Figures 2-3 and 2-4). That ECG pattern was found to indicate a critical narrowing in the LAD, usually proximally located.

In patients with unstable angina and critical LAD narrowing, the typical ECG consists of progressive symmetrical T-wave inversion in the precordial leads (after the chest pain is gone), starting in the terminal part of the T wave. This pattern is commonly seen in leads V_2 and V_3 but may also develop in the other precordial leads.

In addition to the T-wave inversion in V_2 and V_3, these patients also must show the following:

■ Little or no ST elevation
■ No loss of R-wave progression in precordial leads
■ Little or no troponin elevation

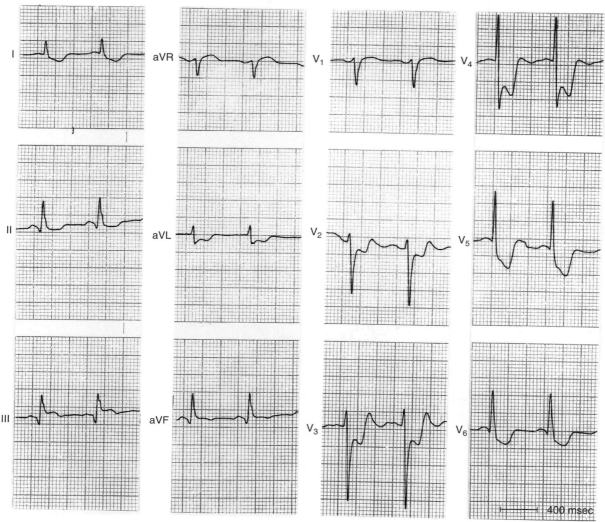

Figure 2-2 Extensive ST segment deviation in a patient with left main stem disease. Apart from marked ST depression in leads I, II, aVL, and V_2 to V_6, ST elevation in aVR and V_1 is also present. The patient had an old inferior MI. Note that lead V_4 shows the greatest amount of ST depression, which is a feature of left main stem disease.[20]

Recognition of this pattern is important because LAD occlusion leads to a large anterior wall MI, and early death may occur from pump failure or high-degree sub-AV nodal block. Early percutaneous or surgical revascularization may prevent this situation from happening.[23]

CONCLUSION

In patients with non-STEMI and unstable angina, the ECG is valuable for risk stratification. In those patients an ST segment deviation score and a count of the number of ECG leads showing ST segment deviation should be performed. The ECG should also be closely monitored

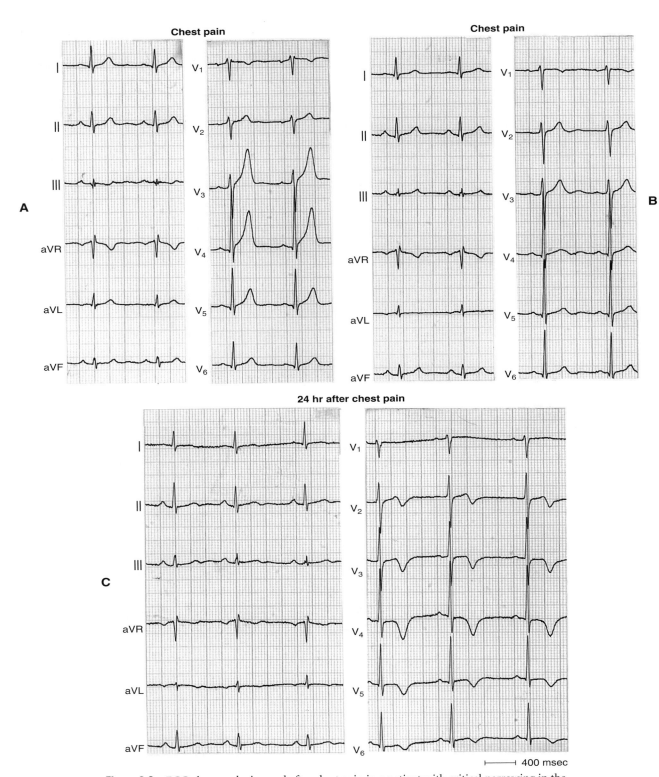

Figure 2-3 ECG changes during and after chest pain in a patient with critical narrowing in the LAD. Peaked T waves (on admission) are present in the precordial leads with slight ST elevation (**A**). When the chest pain decreased, normalization of the ST-T segment occurred (**B**). T-wave negativity in leads V_2 to V_6 (24 hours later without chest pain) indicate reperfusion of the anterior wall in the presence of a severe lesion in the LAD (**C**).

A   **B**

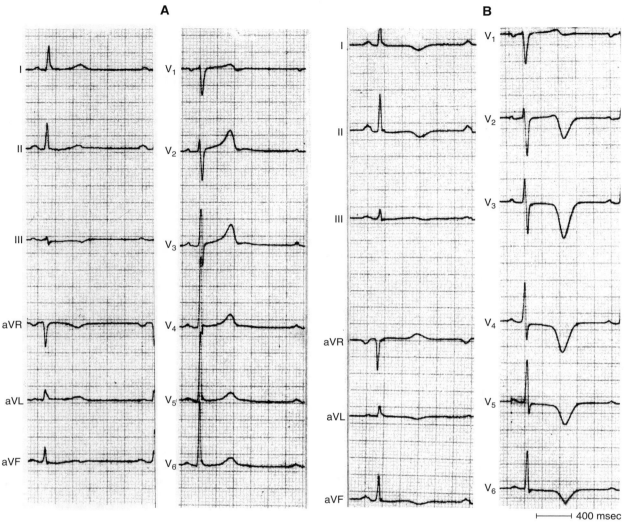

Figure 2-4   ECG changes reflecting critical proximal LAD stenosis. ECG when the patient is admitted for anginal pain (**A**). Only slight negativity is present at the end of the T waves in leads V_1 to V_3. Twelve hours later (**B**), when the pain subsided, the ST segment shows symmetrical deep T-wave inversion in leads V_2 to V_6.

after the chest pain has subsided to recognize patients with critical narrowing in the LAD.

REFERENCES

1. Ohman EM, Armstrong PW, Christenson RH, et al: Cardiac troponin T levels for risk stratification in acute myocardial ischemia. GUSTO IIA Investigators, *N Engl J Med* 335:1333-41, 1996.
2. Lindahl B, Venge P, Wallentin L: Troponin T identifies patients with unstable coronary artery disease who benefit from long-term antithrombotic protection. Fragmin in Unstable Coronary Artery Disease (FRISC) Study Group, *J Am Coll Cardiol* 29:43-8, 1997.
3. Newby LK, Christenson RH, Ohman EM, et al: Value of serial troponin T measures for early and late risk stratification in patients with acute coronary syndromes. The GUSTO-IIa Investigators, *Circulation* 98:1853-9, 1998.
4. Heeschen C, Hamm CW, Goldmann B, et al: Troponin concentrations for stratification of patients with acute coronary syndromes in relation to therapeutic efficacy of tirofiban. PRISM Study Investigators. Platelet Receptor Inhibition in Ischemic Syndrome Management, *Lancet* 354:1757-62, 1999.

5. Effects of tissue plasminogen activator and a comparison of early invasive and conservative strategies in unstable angina and non-Q-wave myocardial infarction. Results of the TIMI IIIB Trial. Thrombolysis in Myocardial Ischemia, *Circulation* 89:1545-56, 1994.

6. Anderson HV, Cannon CP, Stone PH, et al: One-year results of the Thrombolysis in Myocardial Infarction (TIMI) IIIB clinical trial. A randomized comparison of tissue-type plasminogen activator versus placebo and early invasive versus early conservative strategies in unstable angina and non-Q wave myocardial infarction, *J Am Coll Cardiol* 26:1643-50, 1995.

7. Boden WE, O'Rourke RA, Crawford MH, et al: Outcomes in patients with acute non-Q-wave myocardial infarction randomly assigned to an invasive as compared with a conservative management strategy. Veterans Affairs Non-Q-Wave Infarction Strategies in Hospital (VANQWISH) Trial Investigators, *N Engl J Med* 338:1785-92, 1998.

8. Fragmin and Fast Revascularization During Instability in Coronary Artery Disease Investigators: Invasive compared with non-invasive treatment in unstable coronary-artery disease, FRISC II prospective randomized multicentre study, *Lancet* 354:708-15, 1999.

9. Wallentin L, Lagerqvist B, Husted S, et al: Outcome at 1 year after invasive compared with a non-invasive strategy in unstable coronary artery disease: The FRISC II invasive randomized trial, *Lancet* 356:9-16, 2000.

10. Cannon CP, Weintraub WS, Demopoulos LA, et al: Comparison of early invasive end conservative strategies in patients with unstable coronary syndromes treated with the glycoprotein IIb/IIIa inhibitor tirofiban, *N Engl J Med* 344:1879-87, 2001.

11. Lagerqvist B, Husted S, Kontny F, et al: A long term perspective on the protective effects of an early invasive strategy in unstable coronary artery disease. Two year follow-up of the FRISC II invasive study, *J Am Coll Cardiol* 40:1902-14, 2002.

12. Fox KA, Poole-Wilson PA, Henderson RA, et al: Interventional versus conservative treatment for patients with unstable angina or non-ST-elevation myocardial infarction: the British Heart Foundation RITA 3 randomised trial. Randomized Intervention Trial of unstable Angina, *Lancet* 360:743-51, 2002.

13. De Winter R, for the ICTUS investigators: Presented at the European Congress of Cardiology, Munchen, August 29, 2004.

14. Diderholm E, Andren B, Frostveldt G, et al: ST depression in ECG at entry indicates severe coronary lesions end large benefits of an early invasive treatment strategy in unstable coronary artery disease: The FRISC II ECG sub study, *Eur Heart J* 23:41-9, 2002.

15. Holmvang L, Clemmensen P, Lindahl B, et al: Quantitative analysis of the admission electrocardiogram identifies patients with unstable coronary artery disease who benefit the most from early invasive treatment, *J Am Coll Cardiol* 41:905-15, 2003.

16. Holmvang L, Luscher MS, Clemmensen P, et al: Very early risk stratification using combined ECG and biochemical assessment in patients with unstable coronary artery disease, *Circulation* 98:2004-9, 1998.

17. Hyde TA, French JK, Wong CK, et al: Four years survival of patients with acute coronary syndromes without ST segment elevation and prognostic significance of 0.5 mm ST segment depression, *Am J Cardiol* 84:379-85, 1999.

18. Kaul P, Vu Y, Chang WC, et al: Prognostic value of ST segment depression in acute coronary syndromes: insights from PARAGON-A applied to GUSTO-IIb. PARAGON-A and GUSTO IIb Investigators. Platelet IIb/IIIa Antagonism for the Reduction of Acute Global Organization Network, *J Am Coll Cardiol* 38:64-71, 2001.

19. Gorgels AP, Vos MA, Mulleneers R, et al: Value of the electrocardiogram in diagnosing the number of severely narrowed coronary arteries in rest angina pectoris, *Am J Cardiol* 72:999-1003, 1993.

20. Atie J, Brugada P, Smeets JL, et al: Clinical presentation and prognosis of left main coronary artery disease in the 1980s, *Eur Heart J* 12:495-501, 1991.

21. De Zwaan C, Bar F, Wellens HJJ: Characteristic electrocardiographic pattern indicating a critical stenosis high in left anterior descending coronary artery in patients admitted because of impending myocardial infarction, *Am Heart J* 103:730-5, 1982.

22. De Zwaan C, Bar FW, Janssen JHA, et al: Angiographic and clinical characteristics of patients with unstable angina showing an ECG pattern indicating critical narrowing of the proximal LAD coronary artery, *Am Heart J* 117:657-66, 1989.

23. Wellens HJJ, Gorgels APM, Doevendans PA: *The ECG in acute myocardial infarction and unstable angina. Diagnosis and risk stratification,* Boston, 2003, Kluwer Academic Publishers, pp 117-26.

3

Bradyarrhythmias

SA Conduction Abnormalities

EMERGENCY APPROACH
1. Record a 12-lead ECG.
2. If hypotension, dizziness, and presyncope are absent, no immediate treatment is required.
3. Evaluate the ECG for the following:
   - MI
   - Mechanism of bradycardia. Look for the following:
     - P-wave regularity (indicates a regular sinus or atrial rhythm)
     - Abrupt pauses or group beating in the sinus rhythm (suggests SA block)
     - Abrupt pauses or group beating in the ventricular rhythm (suggests AV block)
     - QRS axis and width for coexistent bundle branch block
4. In case of sinus bradycardia, give no treatment unless hypotension is present, then give intravenous atropine, 0.04 mg/kg of body weight.
5. In case of SA block or sinus arrest, give no treatment unless hypotension is present or the rhythm is digitalis induced (stop the drug).
6. If the diagnosis is sick sinus syndrome, treatment depends on symptoms (dizziness, presyncope, congestive heart failure).
7. In cases of acute inferoposterior MI with SA block, coronary reperfusion is indicated.

SA block is a conduction disorder in which impulses generated in the sinus node are intermittently conducted or not conducted to the atrial myocardium (transmission failure).

Sinus arrest is a disorder of automaticity in which no impulses are generated within the sinus node (generator failure).

Sick sinus syndrome (SSS) is a dysfunction of the sinus node or SA conduction in which no adequate escape mechanism is present and the patient becomes symptomatic because of the bradycardia.

SA conduction abnormalities can be manifest as second-degree SA block or complete SA block. Second-degree

SA block may be type I (SA Wenckebach), type II (Mobitz II), or two-to-one SA block, which looks like sinus bradycardia. SA Wenckebach and Mobitz II SA block can be recognized on the ECG and differentiated from each other because of the pattern of the PP intervals before the dropped P wave.

MECHANISM

Determining the mechanisms of SA block and sinus arrest is possible only by recording a sinus node electrogram.[1,2] To do so, a catheter is placed in the right atrium close to the sinus node. Without such a recording it is impossible to determine if atrial bradycardia or the absence of sinus P waves is caused by abnormalities of sinus node impulse formation, impulse conduction, or both.

CAUSES

Sinus node dysfunction, SA conduction disturbances, and SSS can be based on intrinsic changes in the sinus node and surrounding atrium or extrinsic causes.

Intrinsic

The intrinsic causes of SA conduction abnormalities include the following:
- Aging (fibrotic degeneration of the sinus node and surrounding atrium)
- Ischemic disease
- Infiltrative disorders such as amyloidosis, hemachromatosis, and tumors
- Inflammatory damage (myocarditis, pericarditis)
- Musculoskeletal skeletal disease (myotonic dystrophy, Friedreich's ataxia)
- Collagen diseases (lupus erythematosus, scleroderma)

The most important intrinsic cause of SA conduction abnormalities is fibrotic degeneration of the sinus node area and surrounding atrium from aging. After the age of 50 years, 1% of heart muscle each year is replaced by fibrous tissue in the atrium, the conduction system, and the ventricle. These changes play an important role in the development of SSS, atrial fibrillation, AV conduction disturbances, and diastolic dysfunction of the ventricles.

The sinus node area may also be damaged during cardiac surgery (e.g., congenital heart disease, cardiac transplant). Or there may be familial (inborn) abnormalities in impulse formation in the sinus node.

Extrinsic

The extrinsic causes of SA conduction abnormalities include the following:
- Drugs (Table 3-1)

TABLE 3-1	Drugs Affecting Sinus Node Function	
Drug Types	**Examples**
Antiarrhythmics	Class IA (quinidine, procainamide, disopyramide)
	Class IC (flecainide, propafenone)
	Class III (sotalol)
	Amiodarone
Beta-blocking agents	
Calcium channel blockers	Verapamil
	Diltiazem
Cardiac glycosides	
Miscellaneous	Lithium
	Cimetidine
	Diphenylhydantoin

- Electrolyte abnormalities (hyperkalemia)
- Endocrine disorders (hypothyroidism)
- Neurally mediated conditions (vasovagal syncope, carotid sinus syndrome, postmicturition syncope, cough-sneeze syncope, Bezold-Jarisch reflex in inferior MI)
- Intracranial hypertension
- Obstructive jaundice

DIAGNOSIS

SA conduction disturbances can lead to intermittent SA conduction or complete SA block.

Intermittent conduction can be divided into type I (SA Wenckebach), type II (SA Mobitz II), and high-degree SA block.

SA Wenckebach is the progressive lengthening of SA conduction until no P-wave appears for one beat and the sequence begins again.

ECG Recognition
- Group beating
- Shortening PP intervals
- Pauses less than twice the shortest cycle

Figure 3-1, A, shows two instances of SA Wenckebach with a four-to-three conduction ratio. Four discharges occur from the sinus node, with three conducted to produce three P waves. This pattern of SA conduction is illustrated in the laddergram. Note that SA conduction time lengthens until one sinus impulse is not conducted.

TYPE II SECOND-DEGREE SA BLOCK (SA MOBITZ II)

In type II SA block, regular firing of the sinus node occurs, but periodic failure of conduction to the atrium

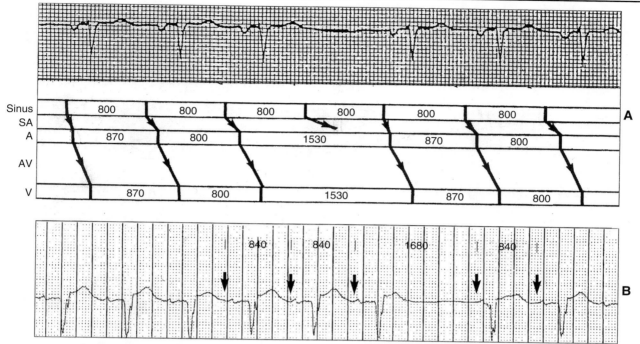

Figure 3-1   A, SA Wenckebach. In the ECG the firing of the sinus node and AV conduction are, of course, not seen. However, they can be deduced from the typical Wenckebach pattern noted in the ECG and described here. As indicated in the laddergram, regular impulse formation in the sinus node but four-to-three conduction to the atrium are present, that is, each Wenckebach period shows three P waves for every four generated. Because the greatest increment in SA lengthening is in the second SA conduction time of each sequence, the PP interval decreases before the blocked beat. **B,** Mobitz II SA block. No change in PP interval occurs until a P wave is dropped and a sudden doubling of the PP intervals occurs. This is characteristic for this type of SA conduction disturbance.

is present. Unlike SA Wenckebach, the failure of conduction associated with type II SA block is not preceded by increments in SA conduction time.

ECG Recognition

- PP intervals are fixed before and after the pauses (because of no increments in SA conduction time)
- The pause itself is twice the PP interval

Figures 3-1 and 3-2 are examples of type II second-degree SA block. Figure 3-2 is from a patient with a subacute inferior MI. The combination of inferior wall MI and type II second-degree SA block suggests an occlusion of the RCA or CX before the SA branch.

TWO-TO-ONE SA BLOCK

Two-to-one SA block is characterized by regular firing of the sinus node, with every other sinus impulse being blocked from entering atrial tissue. Figure 3-3 shows episodes of two-to-one SA block. Typically, the prolonged PP interval is twice the normal PP interval.

Differential Diagnosis

Two-to-one SA block can be simulated when bigeminal nonconducted APBs hide in T waves, especially if they are followed by overdrive suppression of the sinus node. In such a case, the differential diagnosis can usually be made by carefully examining and comparing the shape of the T waves before the pauses. If a P wave is hiding within, it will distort the T wave because it is not part of the repolarization mechanism. Thus the T waves of the bradycardia will be a different shape from the T waves that do not precede a pause and will also be different from each other.

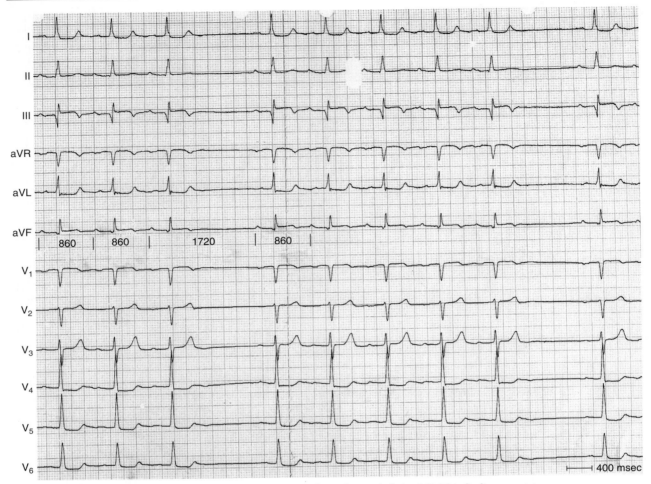

Figure 3-2 Mobitz II SA block in a patient with a subacute inferior MI. This finding suggests an occlusion of the right or CX coronary artery before the SA branch.

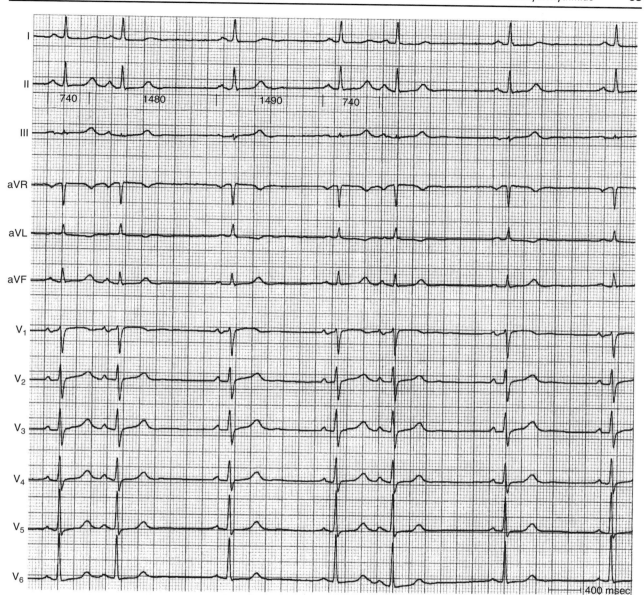

Figure 3-3 Episodes of two-to-one SA block. Note that the PP of the cycle with the missing P wave is often twice that of the normal PP interval.

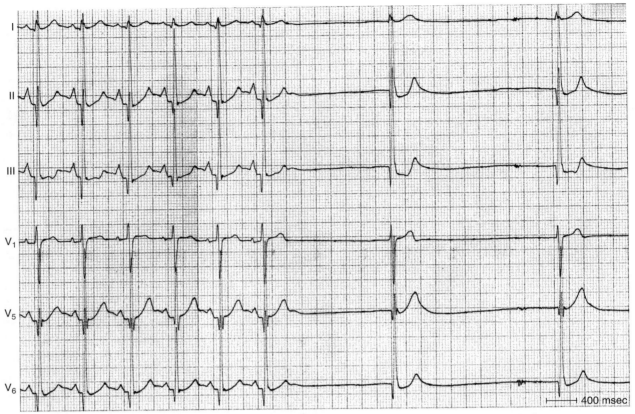

Figure 3-4   Sudden cessation of P waves after sinus rhythm at a rate of 100 per minute. Note that the pause is terminated by AV junctional escape beats. This is either complete SA block or sudden cessation of impulse formation in the sinus node.

COMPLETE SA BLOCK AND SINUS ARREST

In complete SA block conduction between the sinus node and atrial tissue fails completely (Figure 3-4).

In sinus arrest impulses are not generated in the sinus node, and differentiating between complete SA block and sinus arrest from the surface ECG is not possible.

Figure 3-5 is from a patient with acute inferior MI. Sinus P waves are completely absent. The AV junctional escape rhythm is followed by retrograde activation of the atrium (negative P waves in the inferior leads).

In cases of digitalis toxicity, complete SA block may be masked by coexisting impulse formation elsewhere in the atria and/or AV junction (atrial tachycardia and/or junctional tachycardia). The mechanism and arrhythmias of digitalis toxicity are discussed in detail in Chapter 6.

SICK SINUS SYNDROME

SSS is a condition associated with abnormalities in sinus node automaticity and SA conduction, together with failure of an adequate escape mechanism; it is often associated with AV nodal disease. SSS is frequently intermittent and unpredictable and may occur in the absence of other cardiac disease. For reasons previously outlined, the occurrence of SSS increases with age.

ECG Recognition

In SSS the heart rate is episodically much too slow. This pattern may alternate with a rapid heart rhythm, usually atrial fibrillation (the bradycardia-tachycardia syndrome).

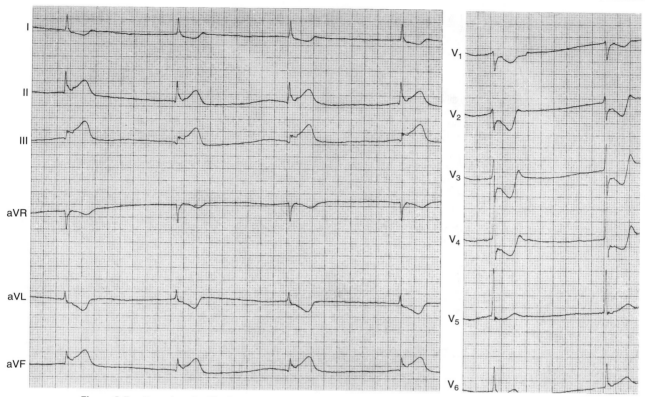

Figure 3-5 Complete SA block or sinus arrest in a patient with acute inferior wall MI. A junctional escape rhythm with retrograde P waves is present at the end of the QRS complex. The P waves are best seen in the inferior leads.

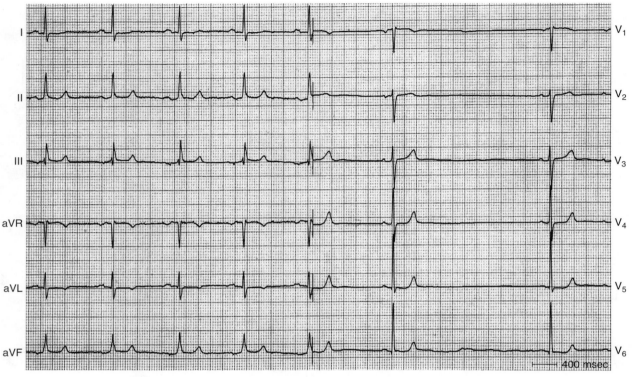

Figure 3-6 Inappropriate sinus arrhythmia with a pause of 2.5 seconds.

The diagnosis is made when cerebral perfusion is inadequate because of any of the following, singly or alternating with each other:

- Marked or inappropriate sinus bradycardia. Sinus bradycardia is marked when it is persistent at fewer than 40 beats/min; it is inappropriate when the heart rate fails to accelerate during exercise or fever.
- Marked or inappropriate sinus arrhythmia (Figure 3-6). The slowing of the sinus node to fewer than 40 beats/min that produces pauses of more than 2 seconds is rare among normal individuals, with the exception of endurance athletes, and suggests SSS.
- Sinus arrest or SA block.

- Slow atrial rhythm with an unreliable junctional escape rhythm.
- Bradycardia-tachycardia syndrome.
- Sudden prolonged sinus pauses, especially after premature atrial beats or after an episode of atrial tachycardia.

Bradycardia-Tachycardia Syndrome

The tachycardia phase of SSS is frequently paroxysmal atrial fibrillation but may be any other type of SVT (Figure 3-7). Often, in the transition between the tachycardia and the bradycardia, long pauses caused by inappropriate overdrive suppression of the sinus node are present. The bradycardia-tachycardia syndrome often

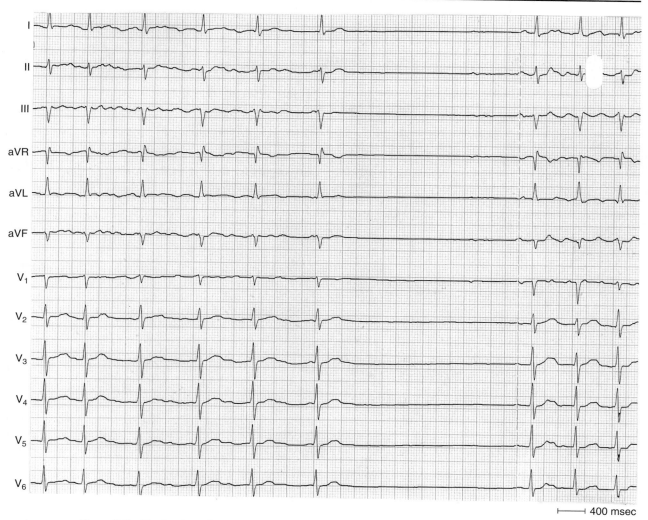

┝━━━┥ 400 msec

Figure 3-7   The bradycardia-tachycardia syndrome. The tachycardia is atrial fibrillation. When atrial fibrillation stops, a long pause occurs before a single sinus P wave appears. Thereafter, atrial fibrillation starts again.

precedes the development of chronic atrial fibrillation and is a common manifestation of SSS.

Causes

The causes of SSS are discussed above under the causes of abnormalities in impulse generation and conduction in the sinus node area.

Diagnosis and Mechanisms

The invasive tests to evaluate sinus node conduction and function, introduced in the 1970s and 1980s, such as sinus node recovery time and SA conduction time, are no longer used because of their unreliability. Even non-invasive testing, such as the evaluation of the amount of sinus node acceleration after atropine, isoproterenol, or exercise, is now rarely used.

Therefore, because of the intermittent character of sinus node disease, the best information comes from long-lasting rhythm recordings either by a Holter monitor or by an implantable device. Event recorders with the capability to transmit cardiac analysis are also very helpful.

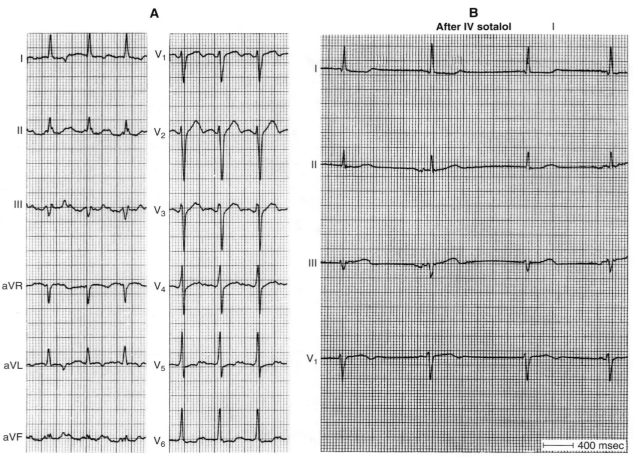

Figure 3-8   Atrial tachycardia with two-to-one AV conduction (**A**). After intravenous sotalol, complete SA block occurs with an escape rhythm alternating between the AV junction and a low atrial focus (**B**).

Latent Sick Sinus Syndrome

Latent SSS may become manifest because of extrinsic causes, such as after the termination of an atrial arrhythmia by intravenous sotalol (Figure 3-8).

Management

■ Careful history-taking to discover possible causes.

■ If a 12-lead ECG does not show the typical findings discussed, a 24-hour Holter recording or an event recorder gives important information because most patients with SSS have intermittent symptoms.

■ The correction of all possible causes, including the discontinuation of possible offending drugs. If this step is unsuccessful, a pacemaker is indicated in symptomatic patients. An AAI pacemaker is recommended, but additional AV nodal conduction disturbances have to be excluded before pacemaker implant.

AV Conduction Disturbances

EMERGENCY APPROACH

1. Record a 12-lead ECG.
2. Determine by noninvasive methods the site of AV block.

In Acute Inferior Wall MI

- The site of block is in the AV node.
- Early reperfusion is indicated for high-grade AV nodal block; resolution of the block indicates successful reperfusion.
- AV nodal conduction problems are transient and usually do not require a pacemaker. The patient should be observed.
- If complete AV nodal block develops, the escape pacemaker is usually a dependable AV junctional rhythm not requiring a pacemaker. The patient should be observed.
- Insert a temporary or dual-chamber pacemaker in cases of pump failure, cardiogenic shock, or when both frequent ventricular ectopic activity and high-degree AV nodal block are present.
- The need for permanent pacing is quite rare and is only indicated when symptomatic second- or third-degree AV nodal block is present and persists for more than 2 weeks after MI.

Type II AV Block (Mobitz II AV Block)

- Determine the likely site of AV block by measuring the PR interval and the effect of exercise, carotid sinus pressure, and atropine on AV conduction.
- A temporary pacemaker is required when type II AV block is associated with syncope.
- In patients with chronic fibrotic disease of the conduction system, a permanent pacemaker is necessary.

Two-to-One AV Block

- Determine the level of AV block by measuring the PR interval.
- Although the block may become complete in acute inferior wall MI, a pacemaker is usually not necessary because of a dependable junctional escape mechanism.
- A temporary pacemaker may be indicated in acute anterior wall MI if the QRS is broad and the patient is symptomatic (syncope or hemodynamic deterioration).

Complete AV Block (Third-Degree AV Block)

- The insertion of a pacemaker is usually required when associated with a broad QRS.
- No immediate treatment is necessary when the QRS is narrow. Determine the cause of the block and then make a judgment regarding the necessity of pacemaker insertion.
- Complete AV block in acute anterior MI requires temporary pacing. A permanent pacemaker is usually not needed if the patient survives the acute stage of MI.

Paroxysmal AV Block

- A pacemaker is indicated because of the unreliability of the escape mechanism and risk of sudden death.

CLASSIFICATION OF AV BLOCK

AV block is traditionally divided into first-, second-, and third-degree block.

- The term *first-degree AV block* is a misnomer in that every P wave is, in fact, conducted to the ventricles, albeit with a prolonged PR interval.
- *Second-degree AV block* manifests with P waves not conducted to the ventricles. This category is divided into type I (Wenckebach), type II (Mobitz II), and second-degree block with two-to-one conduction.
- *Third-degree AV block* is characterized by no conduction between the atrium and ventricles.

AV nodal conduction disturbances are seen in acute inferior wall and RV MI when the occlusion is of the RCA above the RV branch and takes the form of prolonged PR interval, AV Wenckebach, two-to-one block, and complete AV nodal block.

Intra-Hisian conduction disturbances are seen in acute anterior wall MI when the occlusion is of the proximal LAD coronary artery and takes the form of two-to-one, Mobitz II, and complete block, which are signs of the critical involvement of a large area of LV myocardium.

NONINVASIVE METHODS FOR DETERMINING SITE OF AV BLOCK

In AV block the conduction defect may be located in the AV node, bundle of His, bundle branches, or any combination of these (Figure 3-9).[3] Because AV nodal block has a better prognosis and treatment differs from that for subnodal block, determination of the location and type of block is important. In this regard, much can be learned on the surface ECG from the PR interval, QRS duration, and the response of the block to noninvasive interventions such as atropine, exercise, or vagal maneuvers (Table 3-2).

PR interval. Generally, the longer PR intervals (≥0.28 seconds) are associated with a pathologic condition in the AV node. In fact, when the pathologic condition is subnodal, the PR interval of the conducted beat is often normal.

QRS duration. A QRS duration of 0.12 seconds or more indicates a pathologic condition in the bundle branches, whereas a narrow QRS indicates a pathologic condition in the AV node or bundle of His.

Response to noninvasive interventions. Interventions, such as vagal maneuvers, that slow AV nodal conduction worsen AV nodal block, but because the number of impulses passing through the AV node declines, they improve subnodal block. This fact is demonstrated in Figure 3-10 by the application of carotid sinus massage in a patient with two-to-one AV block. On the other hand, interventions such as atropine and exercise improve AV nodal conduction (Figure 3-11), but because of the increase in the number of impulses conducted through the AV node, they worsen subnodal conduction problems.

In summary, carotid sinus massage worsens AV nodal block and improves subnodal block; atropine and exercise improve AV nodal conduction and worsen subnodal block (see Table 3-2).

HIS BUNDLE ELECTROGRAM

The His bundle electrogram is an intracardiac recording of the electrical activity in the atrium, bundle of His, and ventricle.[3,4] These three complexes seen on a His bundle electrogram are depicted in Figure 3-9. They give the following information:

Atrial electrogram (A): Indicates the time of low right atrial activation
His bundle electrogram (His): Indicates the time of His bundle activation
Ventricular electrogram (V): Indicates the time of ventricular activation
Normal AH interval: 60 to 125 msec
Normal HV interval: 35 to 55 msec

PROLONGED PR INTERVAL

The PR interval reflects AV conduction time and is measured from the onset of the P wave to the beginning of the QRS complex. A prolonged PR interval (do not use the term "first-degree block") may be the result of conduction delay in the atrium, AV node, bundle of His, or bundle branches. Although the actual site of delay

TABLE 3-2	Noninvasive Interventions to Determine Site of AV Block: Effect on AV Conduction	
Intervention	AV Nodal Conduction	Subnodal Conduction
Atropine	Improves	Worsens
Exercise	Improves	Worsens
Carotid sinus massage	Worsens	Improves

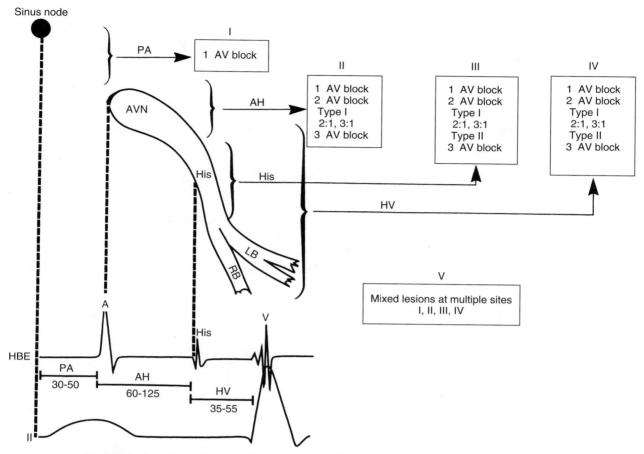

Figure 3-9 Location and types of block from the sinus node area to the ventricles and the corresponding measurements in the His bundle electrogram. Shown in the left lower portion of the figure are a His bundle electrogram and lead II tracing. The intervals noted are PA, AH, and HV; normal values are shown in milliseconds. *PA interval,* From the beginning of the P wave in the ECG to the atrial deflection in the His bundle electrogram; *AH interval,* From the atrial deflection to the first deflection of the His bundle (corresponds to AV nodal transmission time); *HV interval,* From the onset of the His bundle deflection to the onset of the ventricular deflection in the His bundle electrogram, indicating the time required to travel from the bundle of His to the ventricles over the bundle branch system; *AVN,* AV node; *LB,* left branch; *RB,* right branch. (Modified from Narula OS: *Cardiac arrhythmias: electrophysiology, diagnosis and management,* Baltimore, 1979, Lippincott, Williams & Wilkins.)

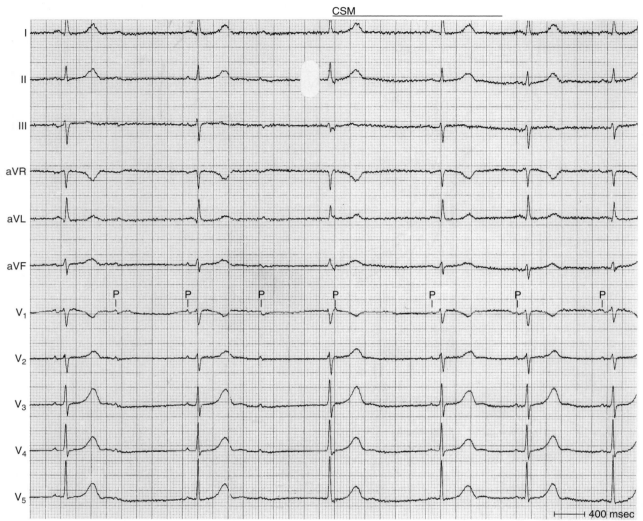

Figure 3-10 Improvement in AV conduction during slowing of the sinus rate by carotid sinus massage *(CSM)*. Two-to-one AV block *(left)* changes to one-to-one AV conduction *(right)*. This change indicates that the two-to-one block was located below the AV node in view of the narrow QRS. Thus the site of block must have been in the bundle of His.

cannot be determined on the surface ECG, a prolongation to 0.28 seconds or more usually indicates an AV nodal pathology. In fact, markedly prolonged PR intervals are typical for AV nodal Wenckebach and two-to-one AV nodal block. When pathology of these blocks is subnodal, shorter or even absent PR prolongation is seen.[5]

An accurate measure of the site of delay in a prolonged PR interval can be obtained only by recording a His bundle electrogram, which indicates whether the prolonged PR interval is based on an AV nodal conduction delay, a subnodal conduction problem (HV interval longer than 55 msec), or both.[3-5]

SECOND-DEGREE AV BLOCK

In both type I (Wenckebach) and type II (Mobitz II) second-degree AV block, some of the sinus impulses are

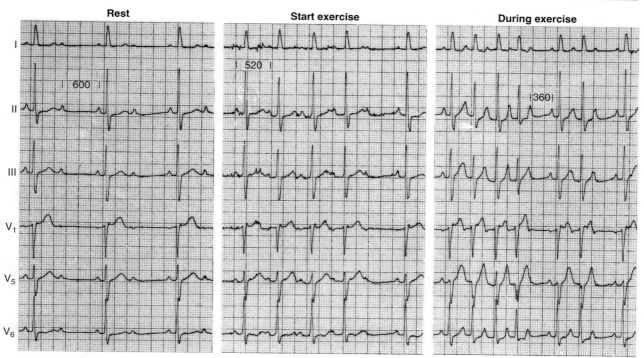

Figure 3-11 *Left,* Two-to-one AV block. AV nodal conduction improves with exercise, which indicates that the AV conduction disturbance is located in the AV node.

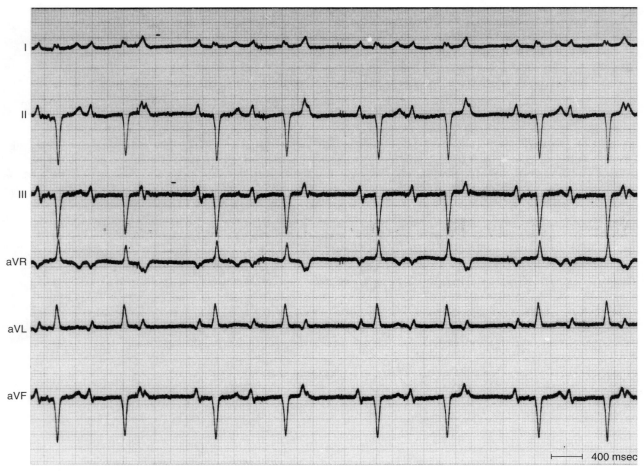

Figure 3-12 Type I second-degree AV block (AV Wenckebach). Note the lengthening PR intervals, blocked P waves, and group beating.

not conducted to the ventricles. The pathologic condition may be either in the AV node or within or below the bundle of His; each situation has different clinical implications, treatment, and prognosis. A QRS duration of less than 0.12 seconds indicates that the block is in the AV node or the bundle of His. When a QRS of 0.12 seconds or longer is present, apart from block in the bundle branch system, an additional block in the AV node or bundle of His is possible.

TYPE I AV BLOCK (AV WENCKEBACH)
ECG Recognition

P waves. P waves originate in the sinus node.

PR intervals. The PR intervals progressively lengthen before the dropped beat.

QRS. The QRS may be narrow or wide, depending on the presence or absence of bundle branch block.

Rhythm. Group beating is present.

RR intervals. RR intervals shorten because the largest increment in the PR interval is usually between the first and second PR interval; however, the pattern may be atypical. Pauses are less than twice the shortest cycle.

An example of three-to-two AV Wenckebach is given in Figure 3-12; for every three P waves, only two are conducted. Note the group beating and marked lengthening of the second PR interval of each group; the third P wave is not conducted.

Lead V₄R. In acute inferior wall MI the development of AV nodal conduction problems can frequently be anticipated when ST elevation is present in lead V_4R, indicating a proximal RCA occlusion. Approximately 45% of patients with inferior wall MI caused by a proximal RCA occlusion have second-degree or complete AV block develop, placing them at two to three times the risk of those who do not have block develop (see Chapter 1).[6-8]

Mechanism

Mechanisms of AV nodal block are the same as those for block at the SA level. As mentioned, when the pathologic condition is AV nodal, conduction improves with atropine and exercise and worsens with carotid sinus massage (see Table 3-2). If AV nodal block is caused by vagal stimulation it will resolve with atropine.

Incidence

AV nodal block is common among patients with inferior infarction (12% to 20%),[6] even in the era of reperfusion, and is associated with an increased mortality rate because it usually occurs in the setting of proximal RCA occlusion with RV involvement.[6]

During the acute phase of such a large inferoposterior and RV MI from proximal RCA occlusion, approximately 45% have advanced AV nodal block.[9] The incidence of complete AV nodal block in acute inferoposterior wall MI is approximately 10%.

Prognosis

Chronic type I second-degree AV nodal block is usually benign in patients without organic heart disease. However, when organic heart disease is present, the prognosis is related to the underlying disease.

Management

Reperfusion. When high-grade AV nodal block is associated with inferior wall MI, the posterior wall and the RV are usually also involved because of an occlusion in the proximal RCA. Early reperfusion is usually followed by a resolution of the AV nodal block, which itself is an ECG sign of reperfusion.

Temporary pacing. In acute inferior wall MI, AV conduction problems are transient and usually require only observation. Approximately half of the type I AV blocks associated with acute inferior wall MI progress to complete AV block. If complete AV block develops as a result of inferior wall MI, the escape pacemaker is usually a dependable AV junctional rhythm and the patient may only require observation.

However, when inferior wall MI is associated with pump failure, cardiogenic shock, or when both frequent ventricular ectopic activity and high-degree AV nodal block are present, temporary ventricular or dual-chamber pacing is indicated.

Permanent pacing. The need for permanent pacing in acute inferior wall MI is rare and is only indicated when second- or third-degree AV nodal block is present and persists more than 2 weeks after MI.[10]

TYPE II (MOBITZ II) AV BLOCK
ECG Recognition

P Waves. The P waves originate in the sinus node and have a regular interval.

PR Intervals. PR intervals are normal or slightly prolonged and are exactly the same length before and after the nonconducted P wave.

QRS. The QRS duration is narrow when the lesion is within the His bundle and broad (≥ 0.12 seconds) when the pathology involves the bundle branches.

Ventricular rhythm. The ventricular rhythm is irregular because of nonconducted beats.

Conduction. Some sinus P waves are not conducted to the ventricles.

Conduction worsens with atropine and exercise because of an increased sinus rate. Conduction improves when carotid sinus massage slows the sinus rate. The typical ECG of type II AV block is illustrated in Figure 3-13. Note the nonconducted sinus P waves during a regular PP interval with a fixed PR interval throughout the tracing, and the broad QRS, all hallmarks of type II AV block. The PR interval is slightly prolonged.

Mechanism

The lesion in type II AV block is located either in the His bundle (narrow QRS) or involves both bundle branches (broad QRS), one completely and the other intermittently. When both bundle branches are involved, the persistent block of one bundle causes the ventricular complexes to be broad; intermittent block of the other bundle causes nonconducted beats.

Clinical Implications

Symptomatic patients. Type II second-degree AV block is often accompanied by syncope and may progress

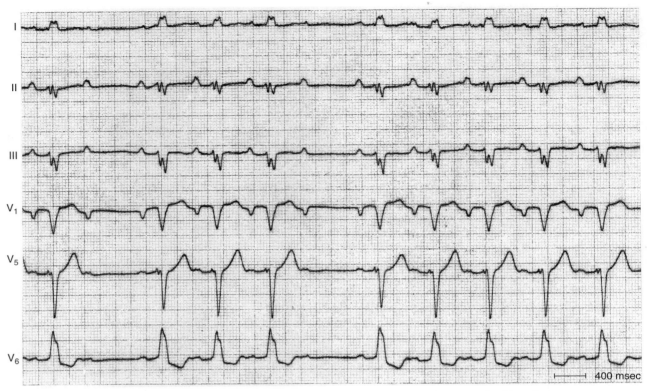

Figure 3-13   Type II second-degree AV block (Mobitz II). Note that the PR intervals, although prolonged, are identical before and after the dropped beat. The QRS is broad with a typical LBBB configuration, indicating that the Mobitz II block is located in the right bundle branch.

to complete heart block with a slow ventricular escape rhythm.

    Proximal LAD coronary artery occlusion. Subnodal conduction impairment (type II AV block, two-to-one AV block, and bundle branch block) accompanying acute anterior wall MI indicates a very proximal LAD coronary artery occlusion and identifies a high-risk patient in whom a large area of the LV is endangered.

Causes

The most common cause of type II AV block is chronic fibrotic disease of the conduction system in the elderly. Type II AV block may also occur in anteroseptal MI (see Chapter 1).

Prognosis

The prognosis of a patient with anterior MI and sub-nodal conduction impairment is determined by the degree of AV block, LV function, and whether life-threatening ventricular arrhythmias are present.[6]

Management

Type II AV block associated with syncope requires the insertion of a temporary pacemaker followed by a permanent pacemaker in patients with chronic fibrotic disease of the conduction system.

TWO-TO-ONE AV BLOCK
ECG Recognition

    P waves. The P waves originate in the sinus node.

    PR intervals. PR intervals are normal or prolonged.

    QRS. If the conduction problem is in the AV node or His bundle, the QRS is narrow. In cases of bundle branch pathology the QRS is broad.

    Rhythm. The atrial and ventricular rhythms are regular.

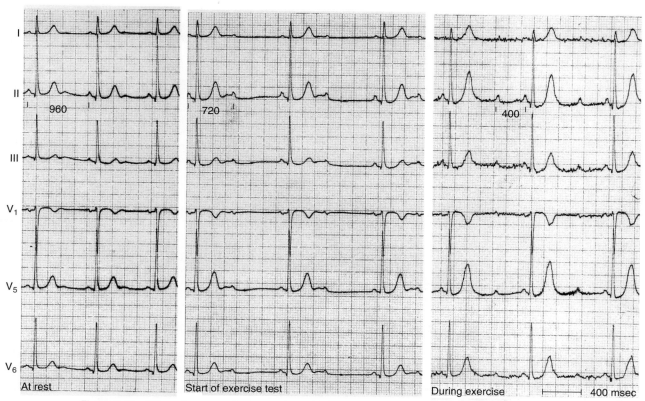

Figure 3-14 When the patient is at rest, sinus rhythm with a normal PR interval is present. However, during exercise a high-degree AV block develops in this patient with a narrow QRS complex. This sequence of events indicates the block must be in the bundle of His.

Conduction. Every other P wave is conducted to the ventricles.

Figure 3-14 shows, with the patient at rest, one-to-one AV conduction with a normal PR interval at a sinus rate of 65 beats/min. During exercise, when the sinus rate accelerates, two-to-one AV block devel-ops first, changing to three-to-one AV conduction with a further increase in sinus rate during exercise. The worsening of AV block during exercise indicates a sub-nodal lesion (see Table 3-2). The fact that the QRS is narrow indicates the block is located in the bundle of His.

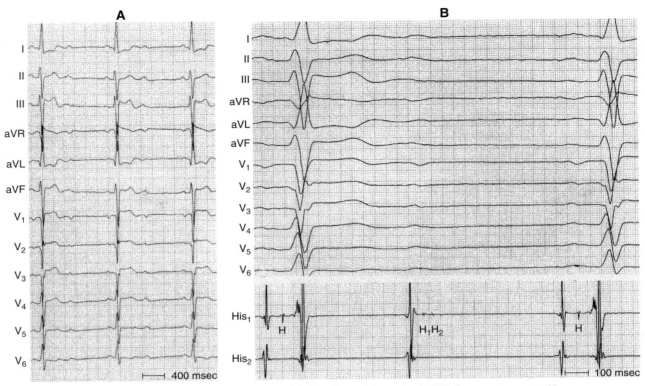

Figure 3-15   Two-to-one AV block below the AV node. **A,** The 12-lead ECG shows two-to-one AV block in a patient with an old anterior wall MI. The PR interval is 160 msec. **B,** The His bundle recording from the same patient reveals that the site of block is in the bundle of His.

Distinguishing Between Two-to-One Block in and Below the AV Node

During two-to-one AV block, the site of block can be suspected by measuring the PR interval of the conducted beat. If the PR interval is 0.18 seconds or less, the block is usually located below the AV node (Figure 3-15). However, when the PR of the conducted beat is more than 0.28 seconds the block is usually in the AV node (Figures 3-16 and 3-17).

Clinical Implications

The clinical implications of two-to-one AV block depend on the site of the pathology (either AV nodal or subnodal). The level of block can be determined by noninvasive methods (see Table 3-2) as well as by measuring the PR interval. The level of block can be invasively determined by a His bundle electrogram (see Figure 3-9).

Management

Acute inferior wall MI. Although the block may become complete in acute inferior wall MI, a pacemaker is usually not necessary because of a dependable junctional escape mechanism.

Acute anterior wall MI. A temporary pacemaker may be indicated in acute anterior wall MI if the QRS is broad and the patient is symptomatic (syncope or hemodynamic deterioration).

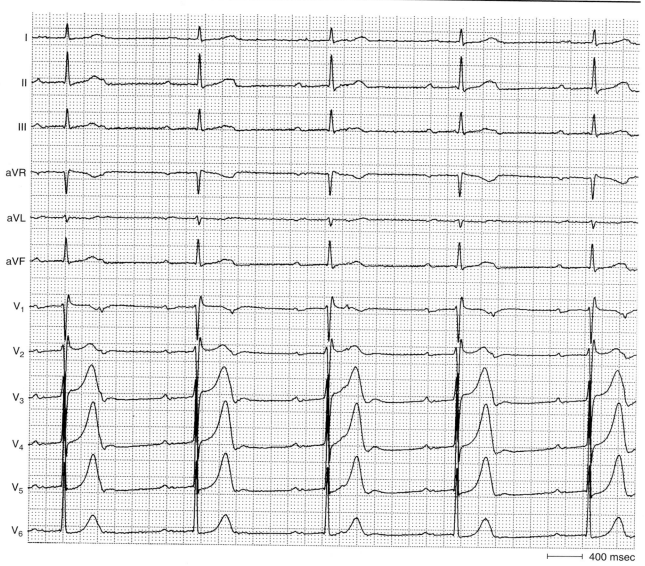

├────┤ 400 msec

Figure 3-16   Example of two-to-one block in the AV node. Note the prolonged PR interval.

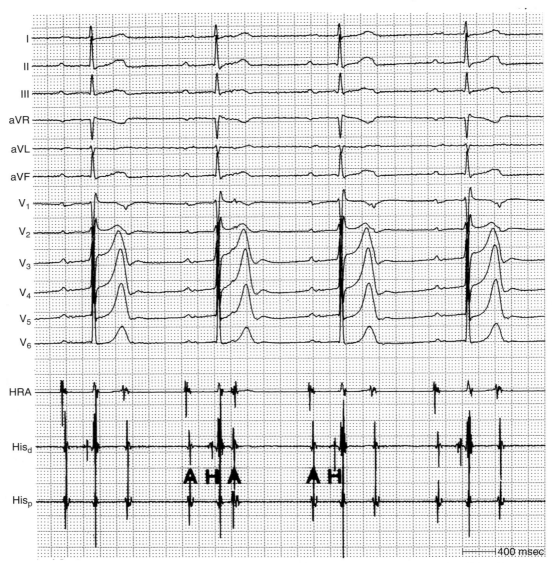

Figure 3-17   Same patient as in Figure 3-16. However, now a His bundle recording shows that the site of two-to-one block is in the AV node, as suspected by the prolonged PR interval.

COMPLETE AV BLOCK (THIRD-DEGREE AV BLOCK)

ECG Recognition

P waves. The P waves originate in the sinus node.

P/QRS relation. No P/QRS relation exists (AV dissociation).

QRS. The QRS is narrow if the site of block is in the AV node or the His bundle and the escape rhythm origi-nates in the AV junction, that is, above the branching portion of the His bundle. The QRS is broad if the escape rhythm occurs in a ventricle or in the AV junction in the presence of bundle branch block.

Rate. The ventricular rate is less than 50 beats/min, except in congenital complete AV block, which may have a higher rate.

Rhythm. AV dissociation is present.

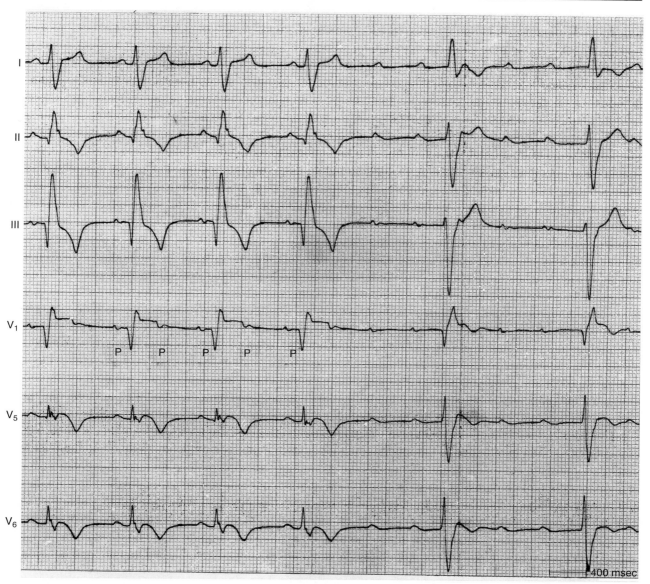

Figure 3-18   At the beginning of the tracing two-to-one AV block is present with a QRS configuration, indicating block in the posterior fascicle (right axis deviation) and the right bundle branch. This pattern suddenly changes into complete AV block with an escape rhythm arising in the left posterior fascicle (left axis deviation).

Figure 3-18 shows two-to-one AV block and the sudden onset of complete AV block in a patient with anteroseptal MI, RBBB, and left posterior hemiblock. The QRS configuration of the conducted beats at the beginning of the tracing shows RBBB with right axis deviation as the result of left posterior hemiblock. When complete AV block suddenly occurs (after the fourth

QRS complex), the morphologic characteristic of the escape ventricular rhythm is that of a focus in the left posterior fascicle. This is known because RBBB configuration of the QRS complexes in lead V_1 indicates a focus in the left bundle branch, and the left axis deviation during the complete AV block indicates impulse formation in the posterior fascicle of the left bundle branch.

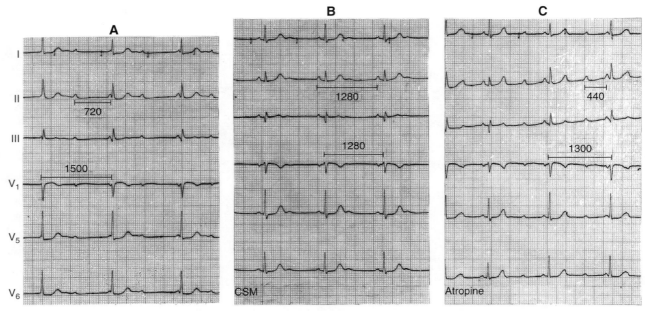

Figure 3-19 How carotid sinus massage *(CSM)* and atropine administration help in locating the site of block in a patient with complete AV block with a narrow QRS **(A).** Slowing of the sinus node by CSM improves AV nodal conduction **(B),** and atropine worsens conduction **(C).** This pattern indicates that the conduction abnormality is located in the bundle of His.

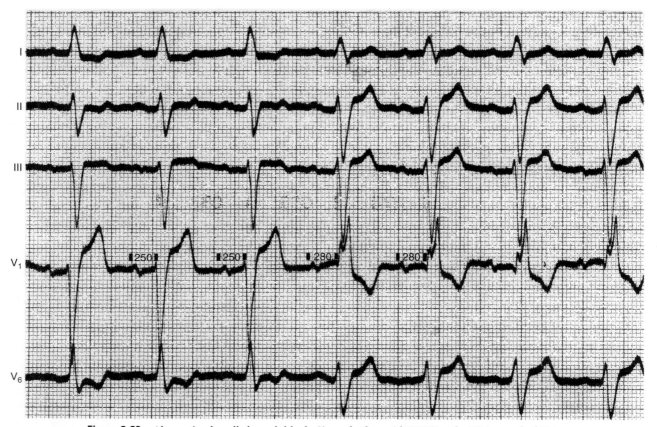

Figure 3-20 Alternating bundle branch block. Sinus rhythm with LBBB and a PR interval of 250 msec *(left)* suddenly changes to RBBB with a PR interval of 280 msec.

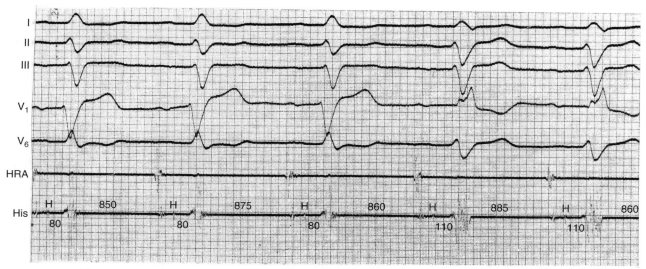

Figure 3-21   His bundle recording from the patient in Figure 3-20 showing that during LBBB an HV interval (from the onset of the His bundle deflection to the onset of the ventricular deflection in the His bundle electrogram) of 80 msec suddenly prolongs to 110 msec with the appearance of RBBB. *HRA,* High right atrium.

Figure 3-19, *A,* is an example of third-degree AV block with a narrow QRS complex. The level of block could therefore be either AV nodal or within the bundle of His.

Figure 3-19, *B,* shows that carotid sinus massage (CSM) depresses AV nodal conduction and one-to-one conduction ensues because of sinus slowing, proving that the AV node is not involved.

In Figure 3-19, *C,* when atropine is given to increase the rate of the sinus node and shorten AV nodal conduction time, high-degree AV block is seen. These observations indicate that the lesion is in the bundle of His and not in the AV node.

Clinical Implications

In complete AV block the rate and dependability of the ventricular rhythm are related to the level of the lesion and the rate of the escape rhythm. In general, the dependability of the escape rhythm is better the higher its location in the conduction system.

Alternating bundle branch block. Those at highest risk for complete AV block development are patients with alternating bundle branch block. In such cases, during sinus rhythm one bundle branch block pattern (e.g., LBBB) suddenly changes to the other pattern of bundle branch block (e.g., RBBB). As shown in Figures 3-20 and 3-21, that finding implies severe conduction abnormalities in both bundle branches and indicates

the necessity for implantation of a permanent pacemaker.

Management

Broad QRS. Complete AV block with a broad QRS usually requires the insertion of a pacemaker.

Narrow QRS. If the QRS is narrow, no immediate treatment is necessary. In such a case, the cause of the block should be determined and a judgment made regarding the necessity of pacemaker insertion.

Anteroseptal MI. Complete AV block in anterior MI requires temporary pacing. If the patient survives the acute stage of MI, implantation of a permanent pacemaker is rarely needed.

PAROXYSMAL AV BLOCK

A particular (and dangerous) type of block in the AV conduction system is paroxysmal complete AV block, in which one-to-one AV conduction suddenly changes to complete AV block.[11]

ECG Recognition

Paroxysmal AV block can be detected by a critical lengthening of the PP interval followed by complete AV block (Figure 3-22). Following a conducted APB, the sinus node is suppressed, causing a prolonged interval from the APB to the next sinus P wave (840 msec), which is then conducted through the AV node

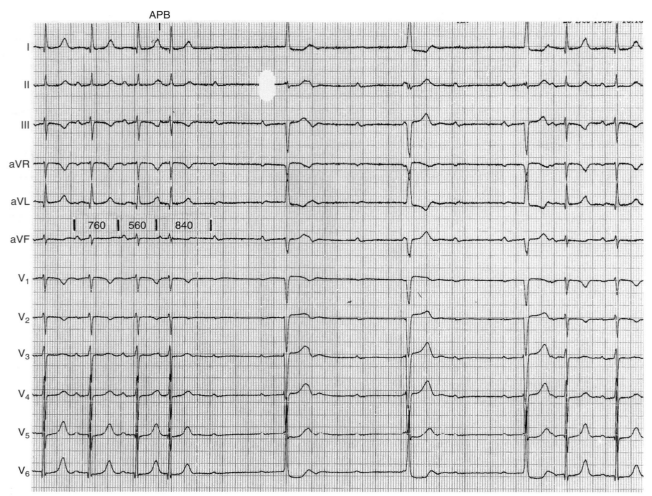

Figure 3-22 Paroxysmal complete AV block after a conducted APB. As indicated, after the APB is an interval to the next P wave that is longer than the preceding sinus PP interval. That PP lengthening creates a pause long enough to produce local phase 4 block in the bundle of His. Certainty about the location of the block in the His bundle is deducted from the narrow QRS of the conducted beats and the escape rhythm that, based on QRS width, is arising in the bundle of His distal to the site of block. One-to-one AV conduction resumes near the end of the recording.

and into the His bundle, where it encounters refractory cells because of local phase 4 depolarization (phase 4 block). In this case, an escape rhythm is present, arising more distally in the His bundle with resumption of one-to-one AV conduction at the end of the recording.

Other Possible Scenarios

After a critically prolonged PP interval (see Figure 3-22) localized phase 4 block may occur distal to the AV node, in the bundle of His, or in the bundle branches (phase 4

bundle branch block). Thus paroxysmal complete AV block can occur following:

- APBs, conducted (see Figure 3-22) or nonconducted (Figure 3-23)
- Retrogradely conducted VPBs (Figure 3-24)
- His bundle extrasystoles retrogradely conducted to the atrium but with block to the ventricle during carotid sinus massage (Figure 3-25) *or*
- During a Valsalva maneuver

As shown in Figures 3-23 and 3-25, a certain amount of time may pass before an escape mechanism becomes

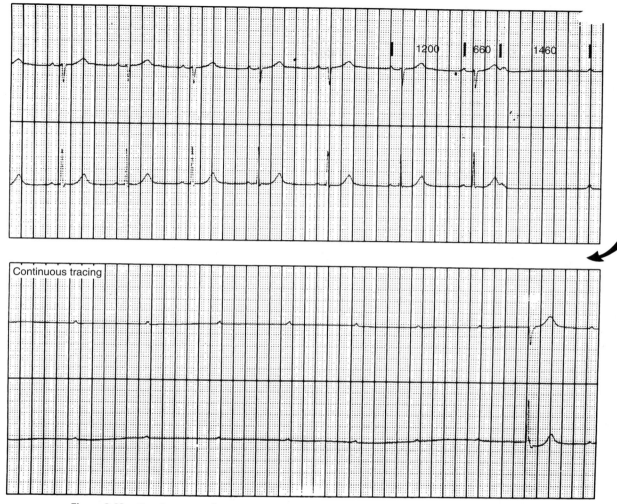

Figure 3-23 Continuous Holter recording of paroxysmal complete AV block after a nonconducted APB (toward the end of the top tracing). Note that the PR interval and QRS before paroxysmal block are perfectly normal, illustrating the difficulty of making the diagnosis outside an episode of block.

manifest, resulting in paroxysmal episodes of syncope or sudden death.

Five Characteristics of Paroxysmal AV Block

1. Occurs after a critical lengthening of the PP interval.
2. Location is sub-AV nodal.
3. Mechanism is local phase 4 block in the sub-AV nodal conduction system.
4. Dangerous, because of the unreliable escape mechanism.
5. Diagnosis is often missed because of its paroxysmal character against a background of absent AV conduction disturbances.

Mechanisms

For conduction to take place anywhere in the heart, the transmembrane potential of a given fiber must have achieved a certain negativity (usually more than −65 mV) to give it excitability and responsiveness. During electrical diastole, cells with the capability of pacing slowly reduce their transmembrane potential (phase 4 depolarization). When the time of diastole is prolonged, a given location in the sub-AV nodal conduction system may have reduced its potential to a level that will not allow conduction. However, phase 4 block is not a usual or a normal condition because, in addition to a

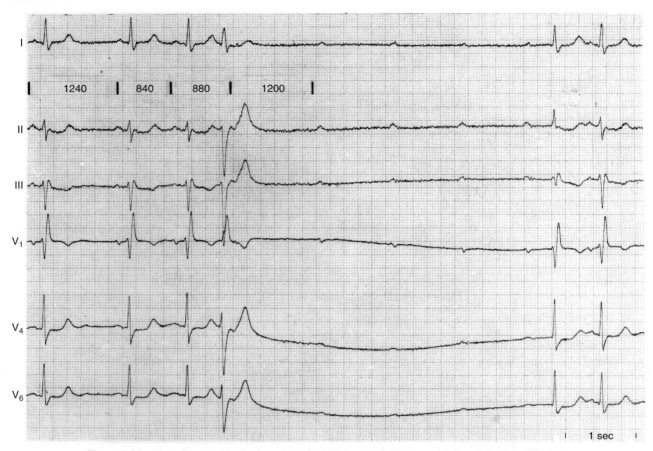

Figure 3-24 Complete AV block after a VPB in a patient with RBBB and left anterior hemiblock, leaving only the posterior fascicle for conduction. Note the retrograde conduction to the atrium after the VPB (retrograde P wave immediately after the VPB). The most likely mechanism is induction of phase 4 block in the posterior fascicle. *Numbers* above lead II indicate the length of the PP intervals.

prolonged interval of inactivation within the sub-AV nodal conduction system, it also requires one or more of the following conditions:

- Phase 4 depolarization
- A shift in the membrane threshold potential toward zero (decrease in excitability) so that time is available for the local tissue in question to reach a potential at which conduction is impaired
- Deterioration in membrane responsiveness so that significant conduction impairment develops at −75 mV instead of at −65 mV[12]

Clinical Implications

Recognition. Paroxysmal AV block is infrequently seen, and the diagnosis can be a challenge because of the following its intermittent character, the frequent absence of abnormalities in AV conduction and QRS configuration outside the episodes of AV block, and its inappropriate and unexpected character, since better conduction would be expected after a prolonged rest.

Organic heart disease. Phase 4 block is usually associated with organic heart disease.

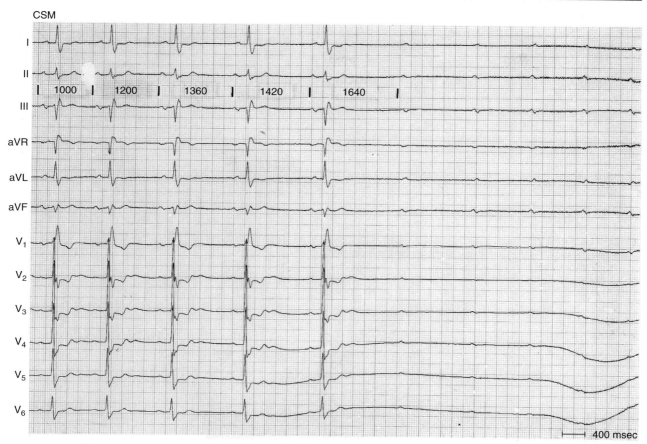

Figure 3-25   Paroxysmal AV block on lengthening of the PP interval by carotid sinus massage *(CSM)*. Note that no change in the PR interval occurs before the block, indicating that the site of block is not within but below the AV node.

Management

Patients with paroxysmal AV block should receive a pacemaker because of the unreliability of the escape mechanism and risk of sudden death.

SUMMARY

The first indication of worsening in AV conduction is a prolonged PR interval with all P waves conducted. Second-degree block has dropped P waves and is divided into type I, type II, and second-degree block with two-to-one conduction. Third-degree AV block is classified according to the QRS width, narrow or broad, a feature that helps determine management. Knowledge of the level of the pathology in the AV conduction system is important in determining prognosis and management. This level can be noninvasively assessed by observing AV conduction on the ECG in response to atropine, carotid sinus massage, and exercise. Immediate pacemaker insertion is usually indicated only in complete (third-degree) AV block with a broad QRS complex and in paroxysmal AV block.

REFERENCES

1. Betge C, Gebhardt-Seehausen U, Mullges W: The human sinus nodal electrogram: techniques and clinical results of intra trial recordings in patients with and without sick sinus syndrome, *Am Heart J* 112:1074-82, 1986.
2. Pisapia A, Le Heuzey JY, Faurre J, et al: Sino atrial dissociation: evidence by intracardiac recordings in man and by microelectrode studies on isolated rabbit atrium, *PACE* 11:23-32, 1988.
3. Narula OS: *Cardiac arrhythmias: electrophysiology, diagnosis and management,* Baltimore, 1979, Lippincott, Williams & Wilkins, pp 85-113.
4. Scherlag BJ, Lau SH, Helfant RH, et al: Catheter technique for recording his bundle activity in man, *Circulation* 39:13-20, 1969.
5. Josephson ME: *Clinical cardiac electrophysiology: techniques and interpretation,* Philadelphia, 2002, Lippincott, Williams & Wilkins, pp 92-109.
6. Wellens HJJ, Gorgels APM, Doevendans PA: *The ECG in acute MI and unstable angina: diagnosis and risk stratification,* Boston, 2003, Kluwer Academic Publishers, p 51.
7. Berger P, Ruocco N, Ryan T, et al: Incidence and prognostic implications of heart block complicating acute inferior MI treated with thrombolytic therapy: results from TIMI II, *J Am Coll Cardiol* 20:533-40, 1992.
8. Kimura K, Kosuge M, Ishikawa T, et al: Comparison of results of early reperfusion in patients with inferior wall acute MI with and without complete atrioventricular block, *Am J Cardiol* 84:731-3, 1999.
9. Braat S, De Zwaan C, Brugada P, et al: Right ventricular involvement with acute MI identifies high risk of developing atrioventricular nodal conduction disturbances, *Am Heart J* 107:1183-7, 1984.
10. Barold SS: American College of Cardiology/American Heart Association guidelines for pacemaker implantation after acute myocardial infarction. What is persistent advanced block at the atrioventricular node? *Am J Cardiol* 80:770-4, 1997.
11. Rosenbaum MB, Elizari MV, Levi RJ, et al: Paroxysmal atrioventricular block related to hypopolarization and spontaneous diastolic depolarization, *Chest* 63:678-84, 1973.
12. Singer DH, Cohen HC: Aberrancy: electrophysiologic aspects and clinical correlation. In Mandel WJ, editor: *Cardiac arrhythmias,* Philadelphia, 1987, Lippincott, Williams & Wilkins.

4

Narrow QRS Tachycardia

EMERGENCY APPROACH

For Regular Narrow QRS Tachycardia
1. Obtain a 12-lead ECG.
2. Assess the hemodynamic situation.

If Hemodynamically Unstable
1. Cardiovert.
2. Obtain a history.
3. Record postconversion ECG.
4. Examine and compare precardioversion and postcardioversion ECGs by a systematic approach to determine the type of SVT.

If Hemodynamically Stable
1. Look for the "frog sign" in the jugular pulse.
2. Perform vagal stimulation. If unsuccessful:
3. Give adenosine or verapamil:
   - Adenosine 6 mg as a rapid intravenous (IV) bolus; if unsuccessful, administer 12 mg IV after 3 minutes.
   - Verapamil 10 mg IV over a 5- to 10-minute period; reduce to 5 mg if the patient is taking a beta-blocker or is hypotensive. If unsuccessful:
4. Give procainamide 10 mg/kg body weight over a 5-minute period. If unsuccessful:
5. Perform electrical cardioversion.
6. Obtain a history.
7. Record a postconversion ECG.
8. Examine and compare the preconversion and postconversion ECGs by a systematic approach to determine the type of SVT.

Narrow QRS tachycardia is a cardiac rhythm with a rate faster than 100 beats/min and a QRS duration of less than 0.12 seconds. The narrow QRS indicates that AV conduction occurs through the AV node. This condition is also called SVT. However, during SVT the QRS may be broad because of preexisting bundle branch block, functional bundle branch block, or AV conduction over an accessory AV pathway (see Chapter 5).

The patient with narrow QRS tachycardia usually seeks medical attention because of palpitation, lightheadedness, shortness of breath, or anxiety. Because of the paroxysmal character of SVT, patients with this condition frequently have years of symptoms before the cause is correctly diagnosed or before they even seek medical attention. ECG documentation of the tachycardia is extremely important so that the mechanism of the SVT can be diagnosed and the patient can receive the correct emergency treatment and possibly a cure by catheter ablation.

This chapter addresses the causes, physical examination, anatomic substrate, mechanism, differential diagnosis, and treatment of narrow QRS tachycardias as well as the effect of carotid sinus massage on SVT.

CAUSES OF NARROW QRS TACHYCARDIA

- Sinus tachycardia
- Atrial tachycardia (nonparoxysmal and paroxysmal)
- Atrial flutter
- Atrial fibrillation
- AV nodal reentry tachycardia (AVNRT)
- Orthodromic circus movement tachycardia (CMT)

THREE MOST COMMON TYPES OF REGULAR SVT

1. AVNRT
2. CMT
3. Atrial tachycardia

Figure 4-1 illustrates the importance of evaluating P-wave position and polarity when making the differential diagnosis in SVT.[1-3] The tachycardias illustrated are usually paroxysmal and occasionally persistent (incessant). Nonparoxysmal atrial tachycardia caused by digitalis intoxication, another cardiac emergency, is discussed in Chapter 6.

SYSTEMATIC APPROACH

To arrive at the correct diagnosis it is important to:
- Carefully search for clues during the physical examination.
- Understand the mechanisms and ECG features of the different types of narrow QRS tachycardia.

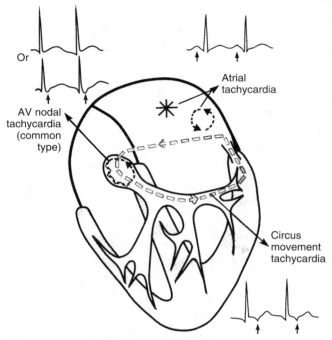

Figure 4-1   Three types of regular SVT, their mechanisms, and the relation between the QRS and P wave during the tachycardia. In atrial tachycardia the P wave precedes the QRS. In AV nodal tachycardia (common type) the P wave is usually buried within the QRS or may distort the end of the QRS *(arrows)*. In circus movement tachycardia by an accessory pathway the P wave follows the QRS *(arrows)*. The site of origin of atrial activation during these three types of SVT determines the width and the polarity (axis) of the P wave.

- Evaluate the ECG during the tachycardia, compared with the sinus rhythm in the same leads, to facilitate the recognition of the P wave during tachycardia.
- Evaluate the ECG during carotid sinus massage.

PHYSICAL EXAMINATION DURING SVT

The clinical findings in SVT are summarized in Table 4-1.

Careful physical examination during tachycardia can help establish the origin of the arrhythmia. Some examples follow.

Pulse, Blood Pressure, and First Heart Sound

In all types of regular SVT, the pulse is regular and the blood pressure and loudness of the first heart sound are constant. In atrial fibrillation and atrial flutter with changing AV conduction and changing intervals between

TABLE 4-1	Clinical Findings and Blood Pressure Behavior in SVT			
Type of SVT	Pulse	Neck Vein Pulsation	Systolic Blood Pressure	Loudness of First Heart Sound
Sinus tachycardia	Regular	Normal	Constant	Constant
Atrial tachycardia	Regular	Normal	Constant	Constant
Atrial flutter	(1) Regular with two-to-one conduction (2) Irregular with variable conduction	Flutter waves	(1) Constant if regular pulse (2) Changing if irregular pulse	(1) Constant if regular pulse (2) Changing if irregular pulse
Atrial fibrillation	Irregular	Irregular	Changing	Changing
AV nodal reentry tachycardia	Regular	Frog sign	Constant	Constant
Circus movement tachycardia	Regular	Frog sign	Constant	Constant

successive QRS complexes, the pulse, blood pressure, and loudness of the first heart sound vary.[4]

Neck Veins

The pulsations in the neck veins often reveal the mechanism of the tachycardia.[4] For example, rapid, regular pulsations (the "frog sign") occur during SVT, flutter waves occur during atrial flutter, and irregular pulsations occur during atrial fibrillation. Sinus tachycardia and atrial tachycardia are the only two SVTs that do not result in abnormal pulsations in the neck veins.

The Frog Sign

In AVNRT or CMT the atria contract against closed AV valves, producing rapid, regular, expansive venous pulsations in the neck that resemble the rhythmic puffing motion of a frog, the result of simultaneous activation of the atria and ventricles. The patient, and perhaps the family, may have noticed the frog sign.

Other Signs and Symptoms

■ Termination of the tachycardia by a vagal maneuver suggests AVNRT or CMT by an accessory pathway but may occasionally occur in atrial tachycardia.
■ Polyuria suggests AVNRT or CMT. When the atria contract against closed AV valves, as they do in AVNRT or CMT, the atria stretch under increased atrial pressure, releasing atrial natriuretic peptide, which acts as a diuretic. This situation also occurs in some cases of paroxysmal atrial fibrillation.
■ Syncope suggests rapid SVT, atrial fibrillation with conduction over an accessory pathway, or concomitant structural cardiac abnormalities.

Different Types of SVT

ATRIAL TACHYCARDIA

During atrial tachycardia the ectopic P wave precedes the QRS complex (Figure 4-2). The configuration of the P wave (axis and width) tells us the site of origin of an atrial tachycardia (Figures 4-3 to 4-5).

The PR interval and the ratio between P waves and QRS complexes depend on the rate of abnormal atrial impulse formation and the AV nodal transmission characteristics.

Paroxysmal atrial tachycardia is the most common type of atrial tachycardia. It is recognized by its sudden onset and offset (Figure 4-6).

Incessant atrial tachycardia is a much rarer type of atrial tachycardia. In this case, the arrhythmia is present for more than 50% of the day. The incessant type is also known as "permanent" atrial tachycardia (Figure 4-7). Incessant atrial tachycardia is a serious arrhythmia because of its persistent nature and the inability to control the rate, which markedly increases during exercise (Figure 4-8). This debilitating arrhythmia will eventually lead to a dilated cardiomyopathy, a so-called *tachycardiomyopathy*.

Because of the pathologic consequences of incessant atrial tachycardia and because a cure is available by catheter ablation, recognition that the arrhythmia is the cause of the cardiomyopathy is important. Destruction of the atrial site of abnormal impulse formation by catheter ablation results in cessation of the arrhythmia and improvement in pump function.

Mechanisms

Paroxysmal atrial tachycardia is caused by either reentry in a small part of the atrium or triggered activity.

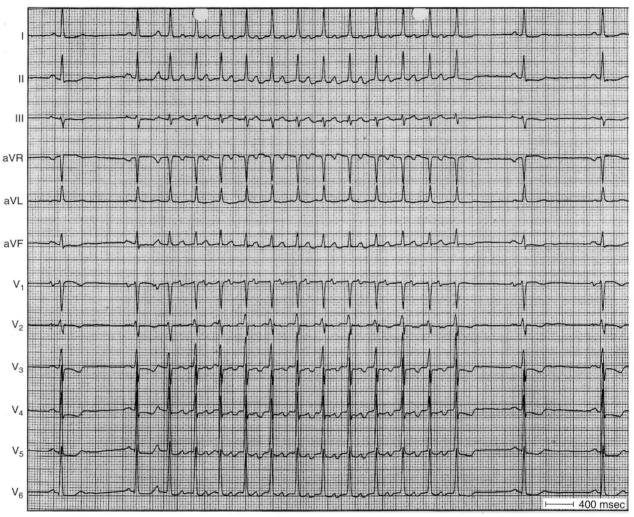

Figure 4-2   Atrial tachycardia. Twelve beats of an atrial tachycardia follow two sinus beats. The P waves preceding the QRS during the tachycardia are different from the sinus P waves.

Incessant atrial tachycardia is caused by abnormal automaticity.

ECG Recognition

Rhythm: Paroxysmal or incessant
Atrial rhythm: Regular
Rate: 120 to 250 beats/min
P waves: Polarity and width depend on the site of origin in atrium
Ventricular rhythm: Regularity and rate depend on AV nodal transmission

ATRIAL FLUTTER

Atrial flutter is a rapid form of atrial tachycardia sustained by a macroreentrant circuit, usually in the right atrium and occasionally in the left atrium.[5] In most cases of right atrial flutter, the slow part of the flutter reentrant circuit is the cavo-tricuspid isthmus, the area between the inferior vena cava's Eustachian valve, tricuspid valve, and coronary sinus. Catheter ablation is performed in this narrow isthmus of slow conduction for the permanent interruption of the reentry circuit and thus the cessation of atrial flutter.

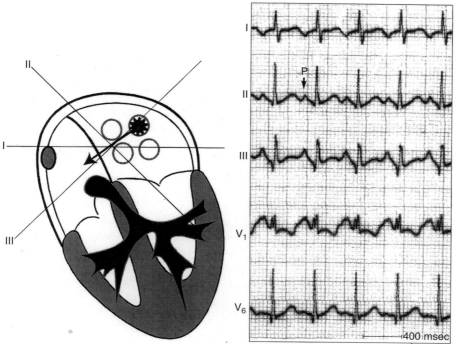

Figure 4-3   Atrial tachycardia. The P waves are negative in lead I and positive in leads II and III, with the highest positivity in III. This indicates *(left panel)* an origin of the tachycardia in the superior part of the left atrium. The P wave has a width of 100 msec, indicating sequential activation of left and right atrium, pointing to an origin close to the lateral wall of the left atrium.

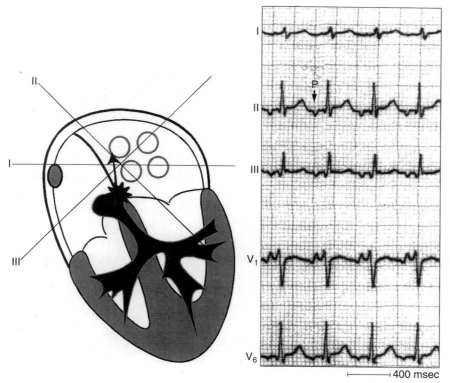

Figure 4-4   Atrial tachycardia. The P waves are negative in leads II and III, indicating an origin of the tachycardia low in the atrium. The P waves are also very narrow (40 msec) because of simultaneous activation of the right and left atria, pointing to an origin close or in the interatrial septum *(left panel).*

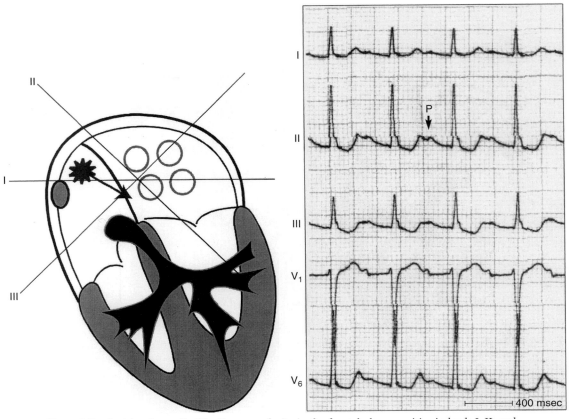

Figure 4-5 Atrial tachycardia. The P-wave polarity in the frontal plane, positive in leads I, II, and III and most positive in II, points to an origin in the high lateral right atrium.

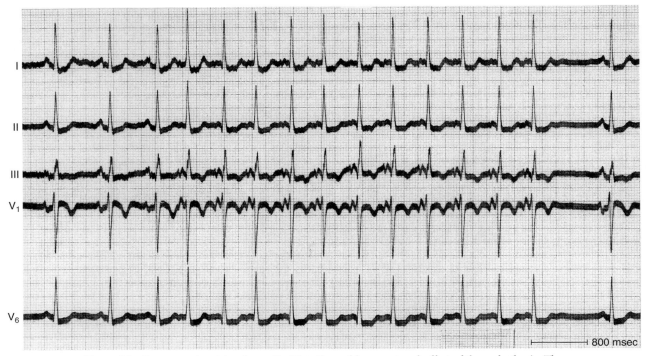

Figure 4-6 Paroxysmal atrial tachycardia. Note the sudden onset and offset of the arrhythmia. The P wave preceding the QRS is clearly different from the sinus P wave.

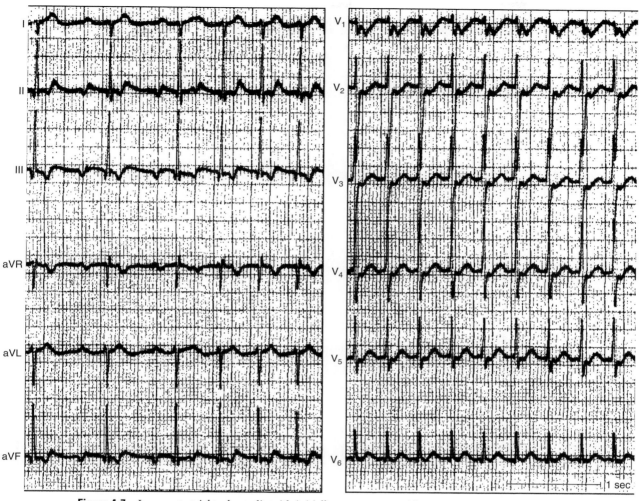

Figure 4-7   Incessant atrial tachycardia with initially two-to-one and later one-to-one AV conduction. The patient had been in tachycardia for 12 years and had a dilated cardiomyopathy.

Counterclockwise Atrial Flutter

During the more common "typical" type of atrial flutter, caudo-cranial activation of the right atrium runs counterclockwise up the intraatrial septum and down the right atrial free wall.

Clockwise Atrial Flutter

During the less common (10%) "reverse typical" type of atrial flutter, the macroreentry circuit rotates in a clockwise direction, that is, down the intraatrial septum and up the right atrial free wall. Figure 4-9 shows examples of the two more common types of atrial flutter.

ECG Recognition

The classic sawtooth pattern of atrial activity is the ECG hallmark of atrial flutter. Its recognition is facilitated by *carotid sinus massage*–induced AV block.

Atrial rhythm: Regular

Rate: 250 to 350 beats/min

Flutter configuration: Depends on the position and direction of the flutter circuit

Ventricular rhythm: Regularity and rate depend on AV transmission characteristics; the possibilities are:

■ Regular (fixed AV conduction ratio)
■ Group beating (Wenckebach conduction)
■ Irregular with no fixed pattern (variable conduction ratio)

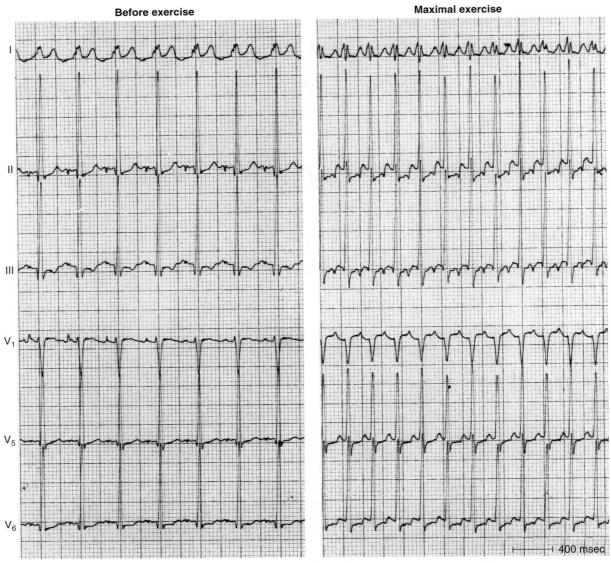

Before exercise   **Maximal exercise**

400 msec

Figure 4-8   Effect of exercise on incessant atrial tachycardia. At rest the heart rate is 150 beats/min, increasing to 220 beats/min during maximal exercise.

ATRIAL FIBRILLATION

The incidence of atrial fibrillation (AF), the most common tachyarrhythmia[6] (Figure 4-10), increases with age. The Framingham study showed the lifetime risk for the development of AF is one in four men and women 40 years and older.[7] AF is a common arrhythmia and a major cause of morbidity and mortality, increasing the risk of death, congestive heart failure, and embolic phenomena, including stroke.[8-10]

Currently, AF is divided into the following four categories:

1. New-onset AF
2. Paroxysmal AF, characterized by spontaneous termination of the arrhythmia
3. Persistent AF, indicating that the arrhythmia does not stop spontaneously but has to be terminated by pharmacologic or electrical conversion
4. Permanent AF

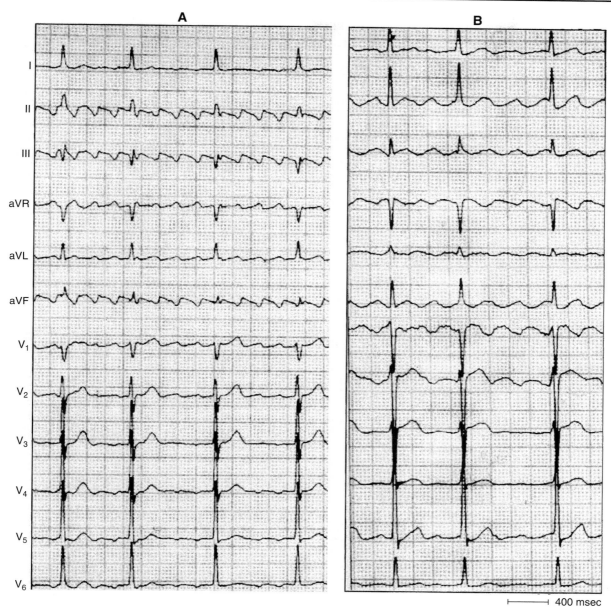

Figure 4-9   Atrial flutter. **A,** Counterclockwise atrial flutter. The flutter waves are negative in leads II, III, and aVF and positive in lead V_1. **B,** Clockwise atrial flutter, showing positive flutter waves in the inferior leads and negative flutter waves in lead V_1.

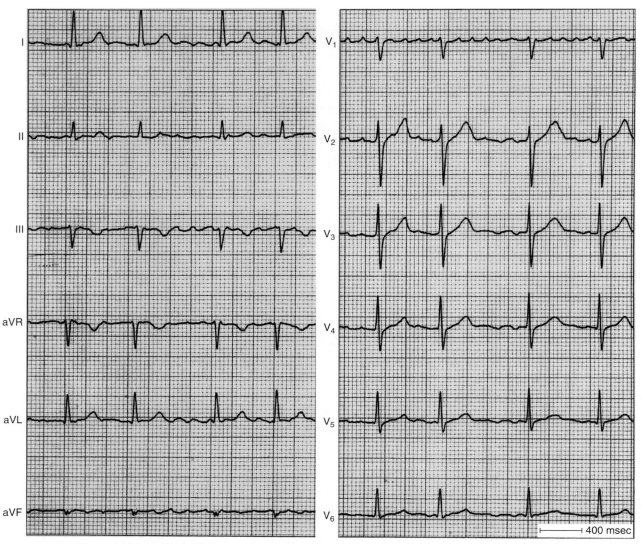

Figure 4-10   Atrial fibrillation. At the atrial level the rhythm is rapid and irregular. At the ventricular level the rhythm is completely irregular.

ECG Recognition

Atrial rhythm: Completely irregular

Atrial rate: 350 to 500 beats/min

Ventricular rhythm: Irregular unless complicated by complete AV block or digitalis toxicity (see Chapter 6); very rapid rates may appear to be regular

Rate: Depends on AV nodal transmission

Mechanisms

Different mechanisms may be responsible for AF, such as focal firing in or close to the pulmonic veins in paroxysmal AF or multiple reentrant wavelets in the atria in permanent AF.[11-13]

AV NODAL REENTRY TACHYCARDIA

AVNRT, the most common form of a regular SVT, is based on a reentry circuit consisting of AV nodal tissue, often also tissue in the low atrium, with usually simultaneous activation of the ventricles and the atria (the common type of AVNRT).

Substrate

In patients with AVNRT, the arrhythmia uses two functionally and anatomically separate atrionodal pathways. They have different refractory periods, one long and one short; different conduction velocities, one slow and one fast; and dissimilar responses to certain drugs.

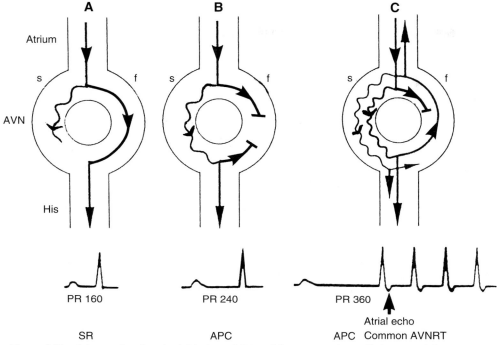

Figure 4-11   Scheme showing the initiation of AV nodal reentry tachycardia by an atrial premature complex *(APC)* during sinus rhythm *(SR)*. **A,** During sinus rhythm, the atrial impulse reaches the bundle of His by the most rapidly conducting (the fast f) pathway. **B,** An APC is conducted to the bundle of His over the slow (s) pathway because of block in the fast (f) pathway. This results in sudden prolongation of the PR interval compared with sinus rhythm. **C,** An even earlier APC with slower conduction in the slow pathway is able to reenter the fast pathway and initiate the common form of AV nodal reentry tachycardia *(AVNRT)*.

Mechanisms

In AVNRT, an impulse circulates through the AV node with activation of the ventricles from the anterograde path of the circuit and activation of the atrium by the retrograde path. The circuit may contain in its proximal part low atrial tissue, but in some patients it is confined entirely to the AV node. Three types of AVNRT are known: the slow-fast (common), fast-slow (uncommon), and slow-slow (uncommon) types.

Slow-fast AVNRT. Figure 4-11 illustrates the mechanism of the common (slow-fast) type of AVNRT. Two atrionodal pathways with different properties are present. The initiating sequence is as follows:

1. A premature atrial beat finds the fast pathway refractory and the slow pathway nonrefractory and is therefore conducted only over the slow pathway to the ventricles.
2. At the distal site of the communication between the two AV nodal pathways, the impulse goes down to the ventricles by the His-Purkinje system and travels back up the fast pathway to reenter the atria.

3. This establishes a circulating wavefront within the AV node and results in simultaneous activation of atria and ventricles and the typical ECG pattern of the common form of AVNRT.

Because of the slow anterograde and fast retrograde conduction within the circuit, atrial activation and ventricular activation are simultaneous and the retrograde P waves are completely or partially hidden within the QRS. This is possible because atrial activation starts low in the atrial septum, resulting in simultaneous activation of both atria, leading to a very narrow (40 to 50 msec) P wave. Such a narrow P wave is easily hidden in the QRS of 80 to 100 msec (Figure 4-12). A partially hidden P wave may lead to a distortion at the end of the QRS (i.e., a pseudo-r′ wave in lead V_1 and a pseudo-s wave in the inferior leads) (Figure 4-13). Rarely, the P wave appears at the beginning of the QRS, resulting in pseudo-q waves in leads II, III, and aVF (Figure 4-14).

A one-to-one relation usually exists between atrial and ventricular events in the slow-fast AVNRT, but occasionally two-to-one block occurs in the journey from the AV node to the ventricle (Figure 4-15). The site of this

APB

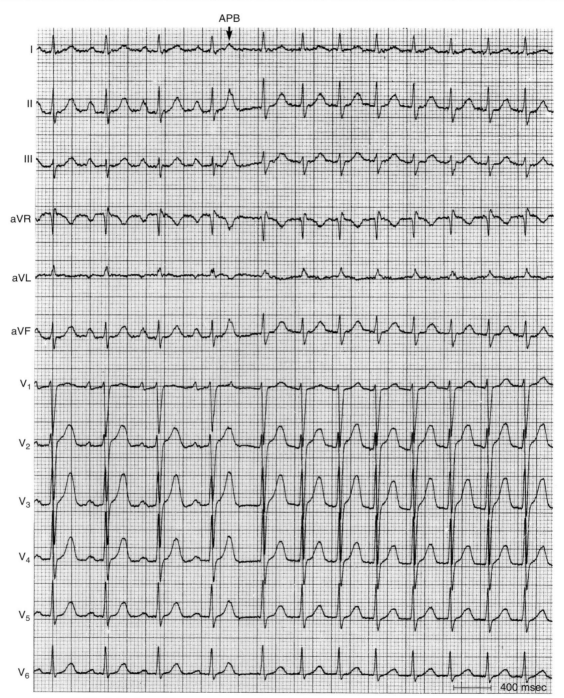

Figure 4-12 Initiation of the common type (slow-fast) of AV nodal reentry tachycardia by an APB distorting the T wave during sinus rhythm. Note the sudden PR prolongation at the time of initiation of the arrhythmia and that during AV nodal reentry tachycardia the P waves are hidden in the QRS complex.

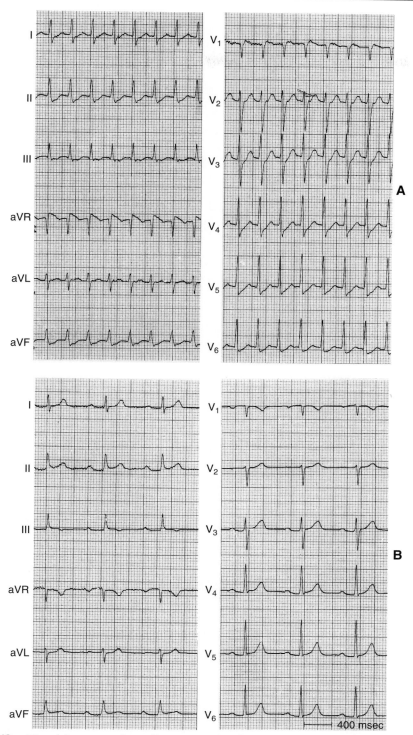

Figure 4-13 AV nodal reentry tachycardia. A comparison between **A** and **B** reveals that during AV nodal reentry tachycardia (**A**) the P wave (negative in leads II, III, and aVF, positive in V$_1$) distorts the end of the QRS, producing a pseudo-S in the inferior leads and a pseudo-incomplete RBBB in lead V$_1$. This same distortion is not found during sinus rhythm (**A**).

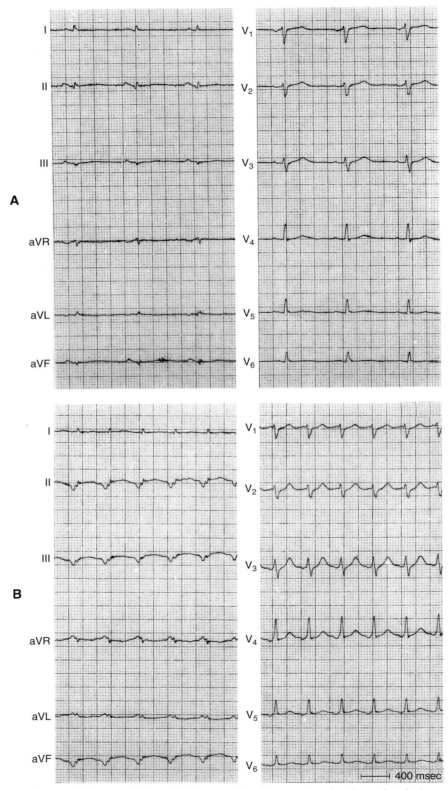

Figure 4-14 AV nodal reentry tachycardia. A comparison between **A** and **B** shows that during AV nodal reentry tachycardia (**B**) the negative P waves in leads II, III, and aVF are located at the beginning of the QRS, producing pseudo-Q waves in the inferior leads. The ventricular complex is very low voltage so that the negative P wave dominates.

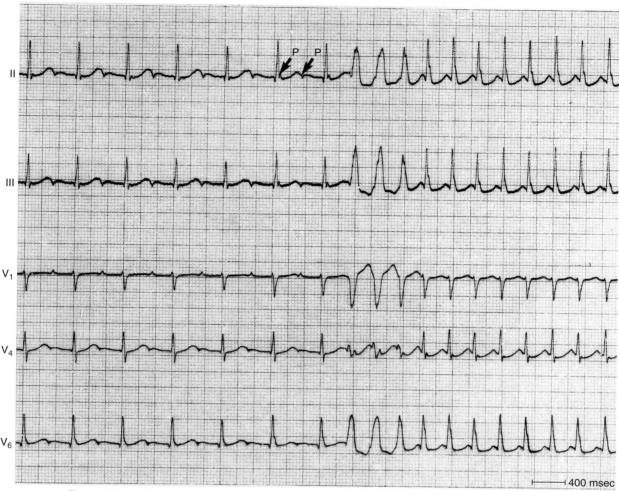

Figure 4-15 AV nodal reentry tachycardia with the left part of the tracing showing two-to-one conduction from the AV node to the ventricle. The P wave not followed by a QRS is exactly between two QRS complexes. In the middle of the tracing is a change to one-to-one conduction. Note the occurrence of phase 3 block in the left bundle branch (aberrant ventricular conduction) when the ventricular rate accelerates because of the change from two-to-one to one-to-one conduction.

two-to-one block is either in the AV node (25%) or is in or below the bundle of His (75%).

Fast-slow AVNRT. Occasionally, an AVNRT can be initiated by a VPB. The sequence is as follows:

1. A ventricular ectopic impulse conducts retro-gradely to the atria by the slow pathway; the fast pathway is still refractory.
2. Once within the atria, the impulse can now return to the ventricles by the now nonrefractory fast pathway.
3. From the ventricles, the impulse once again returns to the atria by the slow pathway and around and around as a reentry circuit is established.

The return of the impulse to the atria over the slow pathway results in a retrograde P wave (negative in leads II, III, and aVF) well beyond the QRS (RP interval greater than PR interval), and because reactivation of the ventricles from the reentry circuit takes place over the fast pathway, the P wave is close to the QRS that follows. This so-called *long RP tachycardia* must be differentiated from a low atrial tachycardia and a CMT by a slowly conducting accessory pathway for ventriculoatrial (VA) conduction (Figure 4-16).

Slow-slow AVNRT. Rarely, both pathways involved in AV nodal reentry are slowly conducting AV nodal fibers. In such a case the P wave occurs well after the

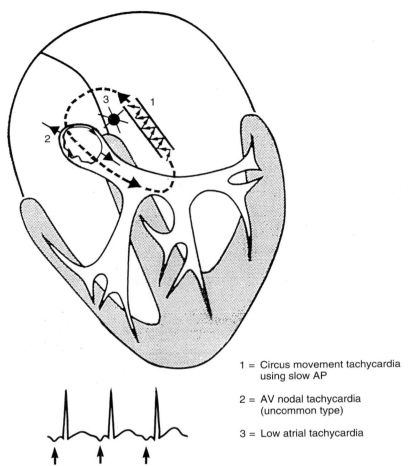

1 = Circus movement tachycardia
    using slow AP

2 = AV nodal tachycardia
    (uncommon type)

3 = Low atrial tachycardia

Figure 4-16 The three types of SVT resulting in an ECG with a negative P wave in front of the QRS complex in the inferior leads. Statistically most likely is a circus movement tachycardia with AV conduction over the AV node and ventriculoatrial conduction over a slowly conducting accessory pathway *(1)*. The other two possibilities are an AV nodal tachycardia of the unusual (fast-slow) type *(2)* or a low atrial tachycardia close to the AV node *(3)*.

QRS, usually in the middle of two QRS complexes (Figure 4-17).

ECG Recognition

Heart rate: 130 to 250 beats/min
Rhythm: Regular, paroxysmal
QRS duration: Less than 0.12 seconds
Retrograde P waves in slow-fast AVNRT: Hidden or partially visible at the end of the QRS (pseudo-r' in V_1 and pseudo-s in inferior leads)
Retrograde P waves in fast-slow AVNRT: Negative in inferior leads with an RP interval longer than the PR interval
Retrograde P waves in slow-slow AVNRT: Negative in inferior leads with an RP interval ≥130 msec

NOTE: Recognition of the retrograde P wave is facilitated by comparing the ECG during tachycardia with the ECG during sinus rhythm (see Figure 4-13 for more information)

Clinical Implications

The tachycardia that results from AV nodal reentry is more common in women and usually not associated with structural heart disease. The episodes are often self-limiting or easily terminated by a vagal maneuver. However, the arrhythmia may recur frequently, cause symptoms, and be refractory to medical therapy. When drug therapy fails to control the arrhythmia, catheter ablation of one of the two AV nodal pathways must be considered.

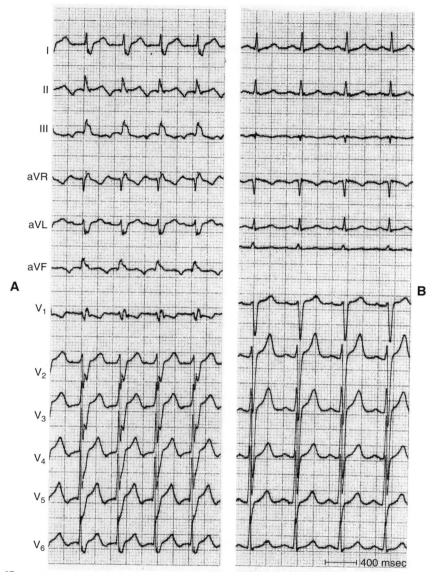

Figure 4-17 **A,** Example of a slow-slow AV nodal reentry tachycardia. Note that the negative P wave (in the inferior leads) is approximately halfway between the QRS complexes. **B,** ECG during sinus rhythm.

Wolff-Parkinson-White Syndrome

Different types of accessory pathways can be present between the atrium, AV node, and ventricle.[14] These pathways lead to earlier activation of the ventricle (preexcitation) after a supraventricular impulse than would have occurred after normal conduction over the AV node. The most common type of preexcitation, Wolff-Parkinson-White (WPW) syndrome, is caused by a direct connection between atrium and ventricle. Such a pathway may be located anywhere atrial and ventricular myocardial tissues are adjacent to each other, such as along the mitral or tricuspid annulus. Left free wall pathways account for approximately 55% of the locations; right free wall, 9%; posteroseptal, 33%; and anteroseptal, 3%.[14]

MECHANISM OF PREEXCITATION

Figure 4-18 illustrates the factors that play a role in the ECG expression of preexcitation in the presence of a direct connection between atrium and ventricle. In the drawing on the left, a short PR, a broad QRS, and a delta wave are present when a major contribution to ventricular activation by AV conduction over the accessory pathway occurs (represented by the black area in the figure).

In the drawing on the right, the contribution to ventricular activation over the accessory pathway is minor (black area in the figure) because the conduction times of the sinus impulse over the AV node and over the accessory pathway to the ventricle are approximately the same.

As shown in Figure 4-19, these differences result in markedly different ECGs. The ECG on the left in Figure 4-19 clearly shows overt preexcitation, which is, however, much more difficult to diagnose in the ECG on the right where the preexcitation is much less apparent.

CONCEALED ACCESSORY PATHWAY

Accessory AV connections frequently do not conduct in both directions (from atrium to ventricle and ventricle to atrium) but may conduct in one direction only, either anterogradely or retrogradely. When conduction over the accessory pathway is possible only in the retrograde direction, the term "concealed" accessory AV pathway is used.

CIRCUS MOVEMENT TACHYCARDIA

Normally, supraventricular impulses are conducted to the ventricles only by way of the AV node, resulting in sufficient delay to allow for maximal atrial contribution to ventricular filling. An accessory AV pathway short circuits this normal delay in AV conduction and often becomes a pathway for a reentry circuit. This is the so-called CMT or AV reciprocating tachycardia.

CMT may result in narrow or broad QRS tachycardia. The narrow QRS (orthodromic) CMT is discussed here. The broad QRS (antidromic) CMT is more extensively discussed under wide QRS tachycardia (Chapter 5).

Pathways of Circus Movement Tachycardia

Orthodromic CMT using a rapidly conducting accessory pathway: AV conduction is over the AV node and VA conduction is over the accessory pathway. The QRS may be narrow or, if aberrant ventricular conduction occurs, a typical bundle branch block pattern will be present.

Orthodromic CMT using a slowly conducting accessory pathway: AV conduction is over the AV node and VA conduction is over a slowly conducting accessory pathway. As with the rapidly conducting accessory pathway, the QRS may be narrow or, if aberrant ventricular conduction occurs, a typical bundle branch block pattern will be present.

Antidromic CMT, type 1: AV conduction is over the accessory pathway and VA conduction is over the bundle of His and the AV node. This sequence produces a broad QRS tachycardia with the morphologic characteristics of a VT.

Antidromic CMT, type 2: AV conduction is over one accessory pathway and VA conduction is over another accessory pathway. This sequence results in a broad QRS tachycardia with the morphologic characteristics of a VT.

ORTHODROMIC CIRCUS MOVEMENT TACHYCARDIA WITH A RAPIDLY CONDUCTING ACCESSORY PATHWAY

Initiation and Perpetuation

Orthodromic CMT with a rapidly conducting accessory pathway is the most common type of CMT and produces a typical ECG pattern. The tachycardia is usually initiated by either an APB or a VPB. Figure 4-20 schematically shows how an orthodromic CMT can be initiated by an APB or VPB.

During orthodromic CMT, activation of the ventricles occurs through the AV node and bundle of His; therefore the QRS is narrow unless bundle branch block is present. Activation of the atria occurs retrogradely by way of the accessory pathway, and thus the polarity of the P wave is determined by the location of the atrial insertion of the accessory pathway. Activation of ventricle and activation of atrium follow sequentially so that the P waves are separated from the QRS complexes. Retrograde conduction to the atria occurs rapidly by way of the accessory pathway, causing the P wave to be closer to the preceding QRS than to the one that follows (RP interval less than PR interval).

ECG Recognition

Rhythm: Regular paroxysmal tachycardia
QRS: Less than 0.12 seconds unless bundle branch block is present

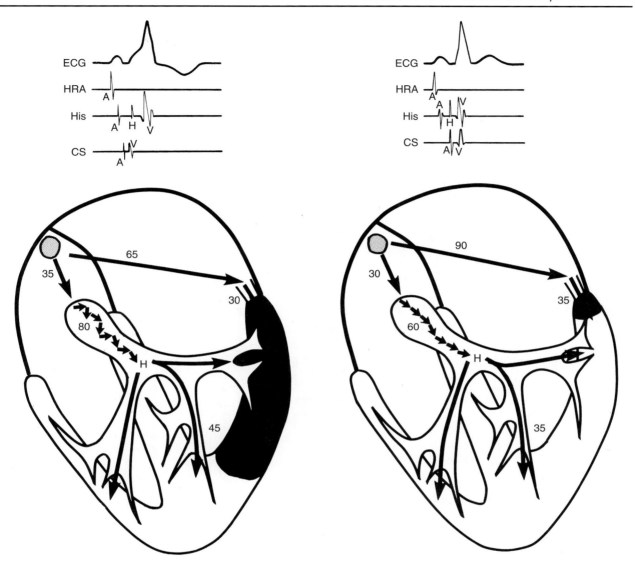

Figure 4-18   Factors determining the degree of ventricular preexcitation in a patient with Wolff-Parkinson-White syndrome during sinus rhythm. The corresponding ECG and intracavitary recordings from the high right atrium *(HRA)*, His bundle region, and coronary sinus *(CS)* are shown at the *top*. *Left*, AV conduction time from the sinus node over the normal AV nodal–His pathway is 160 msec. The time required to travel from the sinus node to the atrial insertion of the accessory pathway is 65 msec, and the left-sided accessory pathway conduction time is 30 msec (total of 95 msec). Because of the shorter conduction time over the accessory pathway, an important part of the ventricle is preexcited, resulting in a short PR interval, a distinct delta wave, and a widened QRS complex. *Right*, A longer conduction time from the sinus node to the atrial insertion of the accessory pathway, a longer conduction time of the accessory pathway itself, and a shorter conduction time over the AV node are shown. Thus the impulse arrives in the ventricles simultaneously by the AV node and the accessory pathway, producing a normal PR interval and a narrow QRS complex.

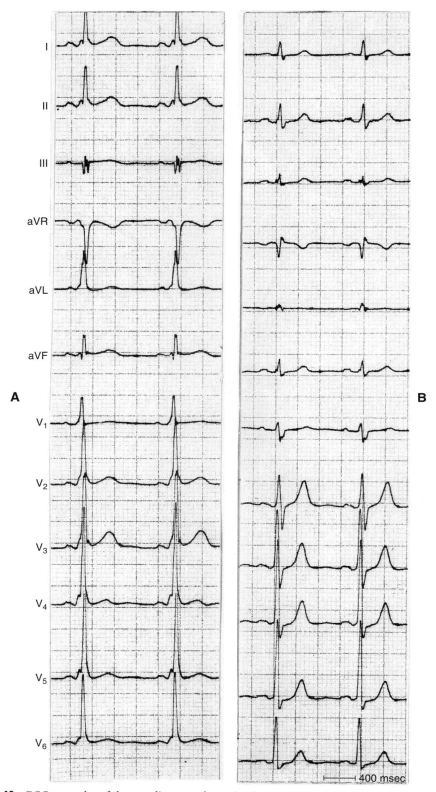

Figure 4-19   ECG examples of the two diagrams shown in Figure 4-18. **A** and **B** correspond to the left and right panels, respectively, of Figure 4-18. Note the prominent delta wave in **A** indicating that a much larger area of the ventricle is preexcited than is shown in **B.**

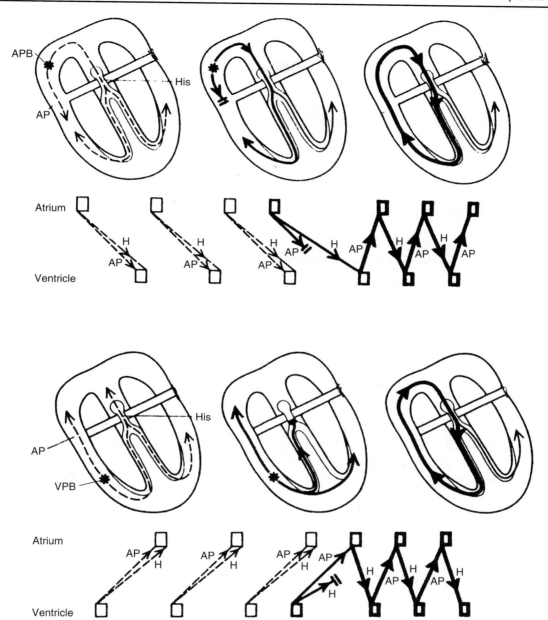

Figure 4-20   The initiation of an orthodromic circus movement tachycardia incorporating an accessory pathway. *Top,* Initiation by an APB. Because the refractory period of the accessory pathway *(AP)* is longer than that of the AV nodal–His axis *(H),* a critically timed APB is blocked in the accessory pathway (fourth event in the scheme). After activation of the ventricle over the AV nodal–His pathway, the impulse is conducted back to the atrium over the accessory pathway in the retrograde direction. The impulse is then conducted again to the ventricles over the AV node and a circus movement tachycardia is initiated. *Bottom,* Initiation of circus movement tachycardia by a VPB. A critically timed VPB finds the bundle branch–His–AV nodal pathway refractory and is conducted retrogradely to the atrium over the accessory pathway. After atrial activation, the impulse returns to the ventricle over the AV nodal–His pathway. Perpetuation of this mechanism results in circus movement tachycardia.

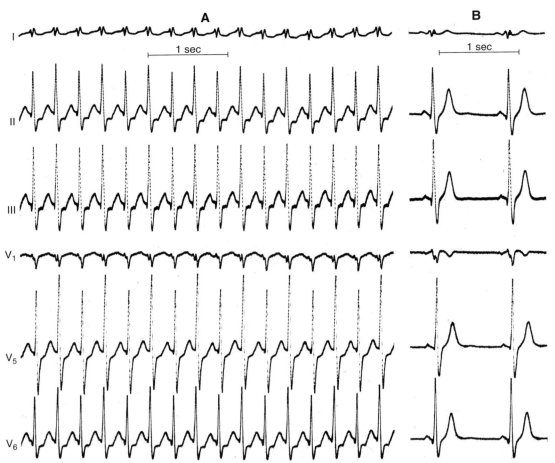

Figure 4-21 **A,** Electrical alternans during a circus movement tachycardia. Several of the leads (II, III, V₅, V₆) show alternation in the height of successive QRS complexes. Note that the amount of electrical alternans may vary considerably from lead to lead; thus careful examination of each lead for the presence of this phenomenon is necessary. **B,** The same patient during sinus rhythm.

P waves: Always separate from the QRS during narrow QRS CMT

Intervals: RP interval less than PR interval

P wave axis: Depends on the location of the accessory pathway. If reentry into the atria is through a left lateral accessory pathway, the P wave is negative in lead I and aVL. If the pathway is posteroseptal, the P waves are negative in leads II, III, and aVF.

QRS alternans: Often present, especially at high tachycardia rates (Figure 4-21), in contrast to AVNRT. QRS alternans only argues in favor of a CMT when present after the tachycardia has lasted for at least 5 seconds.

A 12-lead ECG recording during the tachycardia is important because P waves may be clearly visible in one lead but not in another. The same holds true for the phenomenon of electrical alternans.

Finding the P wave during circus movement tachycardia. In the SVT seen in Figure 4-22, *A,* careful comparison of the ST segment of the tachycardia with that of sinus rhythm (Figure 4-22, *B*) reveals a negative P wave separate from the QRS in leads II, III, and aVF and a positive P wave in leads aVR, aVL, and V₁.

ORTHODROMIC CIRCUS MOVEMENT TACHYCARDIA WITH A SLOWLY CONDUCTING ACCESSORY PATHWAY

Orthodromic CMT with a slowly conducting accessory pathway (also called persistent [incessant] or permanent CMT) is a constantly recurring tachycardia sustained by

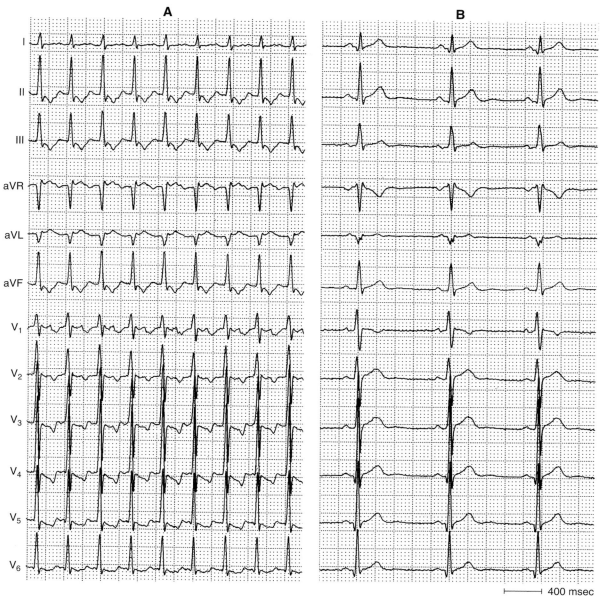

Figure 4-22 A circus movement tachycardia by a concealed accessory pathway. **A,** The diagnosis is made on the basis of the position of the P waves in relation to the QRS during the tachycardia and the absence of preexcitation during sinus rhythm (**B**). When compared with sinus rhythm (**B**), negative P waves are clearly visible in leads II, III, and aVF, following and separate from the QRS complex. The P waves during the tachycardia are positive in leads aVR and aVL, indicating a posteroseptal atrial insertion of the accessory pathway.

⊢――――――⊣ 400 msec

using a reentry circuit by the AV node in the anterograde direction and a slowly conducting accessory pathway in the retrograde direction. It is important to recognize this relatively rare condition because it frequently does not respond to drugs and may, because of its persistent nature, lead to a dilated cardiomyopathy with congestive heart failure. The arrhythmia can be cured by catheter ablation of the accessory pathway.

Anatomic Substrate

The accessory pathway conducts the impulse only from ventricle to atrium (concealed accessory pathway) and is

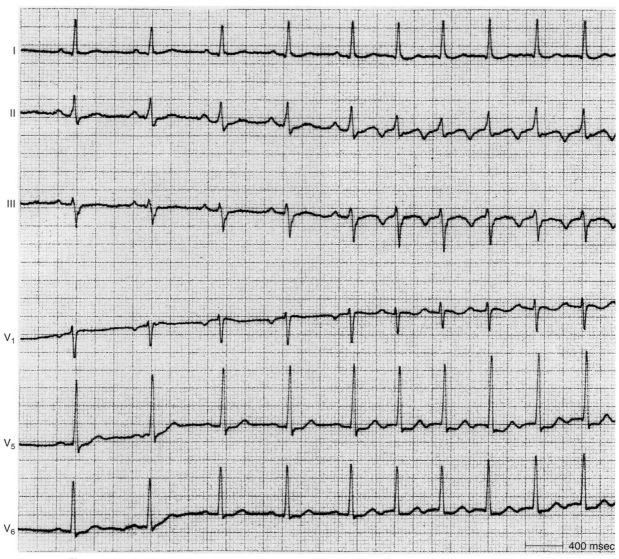

Figure 4-23   Initiation of an incessant circus movement tachycardia using a slowly conducting concealed accessory pathway. An increase in sinus rate is sufficient to initiate the tachycardia. During tachycardia the P waves are negative in leads II, III, V_5, and V_6, and the RP interval is longer than the PR interval.

usually located posteroseptally, with its atrial insertion close to the ostium of the coronary sinus, producing a typical ECG pattern.

Mechanism

Orthodromic CMT with a slowly conducting accessory pathway is persistent; that is, the patient has tachycardia most of the day.

Impulse conduction over the slowly conducting accessory pathway can be accelerated by atropine, isoprenaline,

and exercise. Carotid sinus massage can terminate the circulating impulse both in the AV node and in the accessory pathway. These properties, which do not apply to rapidly conducting accessory pathways, suggest that the slowly conducting accessory pathway behaves like AV nodal tissue.

An APB is not necessary to begin this tachycardia; it can start spontaneously after a sinus beat (Figure 4-23). The impulse passes in an anterograde direction down the AV node to activate the ventricles and then returns

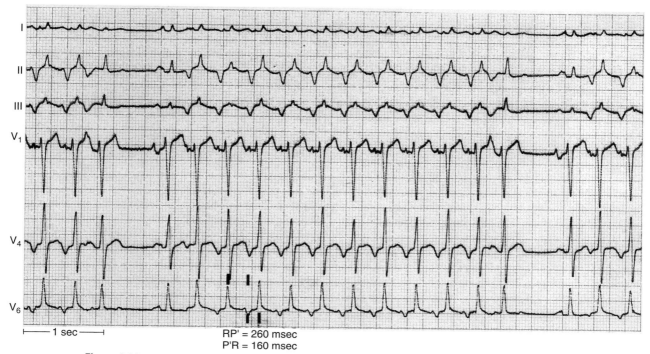

RP' = 260 msec
P'R = 160 msec

Figure 4-24   Incessant circus movement tachycardia by a slowly conducting concealed accessory pathway for retrograde conduction. The diagnosis is made because the patient is in tachycardia most of the time with an RP interval greater than the PR interval. The tachycardia is temporarily terminated by an APB, which is conducted to the ventricle. This QRS is followed by a pause because of retrograde block in the accessory pathway. After one sinus beat the circus movement tachycardia starts again.

to the atria by way of the slowly conducting accessory pathway.

ECG Recognition

Rhythm: Regular and persistent
Rate: 110 to 220 beats/min, increasing with exercise
QRS width: Less than 0.12 seconds unless bundle branch block is present
P waves:

- Always separate from the QRS
- Negative in leads II, III, aVF, and V_3 to V_6 (posteroseptal insertion)

PR interval: RP interval greater than PR interval

The tachycardias shown in Figures 4-23 and 4-24 are examples of CMT using a slowly conducting concealed accessory pathway in the retrograde direction. The diagnosis is made because of the (1) incessant nature of the tachycardia, (2) polarity of the P waves during the tachycardia, and (3) the long RP interval.

The negative P waves in the inferior leads indicate that activation of the atria is initiated low in the atrium close to the mouth of the coronary sinus. Because retro-

grade conduction over the accessory pathway is slow, the P wave is closer to the QRS that follows than to the preceding one (RP interval > PR interval). Table 4-2 summarizes the ECG features of narrow QRS tachycardia.

Systematic Approach to the Patient with a Narrow QRS Tachycardia

A systematic approach permits correct identification of the site of origin or pathway of the narrow QRS tachycardia in 85% of patients.[15] Such a four-step approach during tachycardia is summarized in Table 4-3 and involves an evaluation of the following:

1. Spontaneous AV block versus that induced by carotid sinus massage
2. Presence of QRS alternans
3. P-wave location
4. P-wave polarity

IS AV BLOCK PRESENT?

AV block rules out CMT. When AV block is present, the atrial rate helps make the differential diagnosis between

TABLE 4-2	Summary of the ECG Features of Narrow QRS Tachycardia		
ECG Signs	AV Nodal Reentry Tachycardia	Circus Movement Tachycardia (Incorporating Accessory Pathway)	Atrial Tachycardia
AV block (spontaneous or by carotid sinus massage)	Usually not but two to one is possible	Rules out circus movement tachycardia	If present, atrial rate 250 = atrial flutter; atrial rate <250 = atrial tachycardia
Electrical alternans	Rare	Common (especially at high rates)	Rare
P-wave location	Hidden in the QRS or distorting the distal (common) or proximal (uncommon) portion of the QRS	Present between the R waves; common form (fast accessory pathway); RP less than PR; uncommon form (slow accessory pathway) RP greater than PR	Present between R waves; PR duration varies with site of origin and AV nodal conduction time
P polarity	Always negative in leads II, III, and aVF	Varies according to location of the accessory pathway	Varies with the location of the atrial focus, but in digitalis toxicity, often almost identical to sinus P wave
P width	Narrow	Varies according to a trial insertion site of the accessory pathway	Varies with the location of the atrial focus
Aberrancy	Rare	Common	Rare

TABLE 4-3	Steps in the Diagnosis of a Regular Narrow QRS Tachycardia	
Question	Answer	Diagnosis
If second-degree AV block (spontaneous or after carotid sinus massage), what is the atrial rate?	250/min or more <250/min	Atrial flutter Atrial tachycardia AVNRT with two-to-one block (rare)
Is QRS alternation present?	No Yes	Inconclusive CMT
Where is the P wave located?	PR greater than RP P in R PR less than RP	CMT with fast AP AVNRT Atrial tachycardia or CMT with slow AP
What is the frontal P-wave axis?	Superior	Low atrial tachycardia or CMT with slow or fast (septal) AP
	Other	Atrial tachycardia or CMT with fast AP (right or left)
What is the horizontal P-wave axis?	Right to left Left to right	Right atrial tachycardia or CMT with a right-sided AP Left atrial tachycardia or CMT with a left-sided AP

AP, Accessory pathway; *AVNRT*, AV nodal reentry tachycardia; *CMT*, circus movement tachycardia.

atrial flutter and atrial tachycardia; rates greater than 250 beats/min suggest atrial flutter, and rates less than that suggest atrial tachycardia. AV nodal reentry with two-to-one block below the AV node is rare but possible (Figure 4-25).

IS QRS ALTERNANS PRESENT?

QRS alternans during narrow QRS tachycardia has been demonstrated to have a high degree of specificity for orthodromic CMT and is therefore helpful in differenti- ating this type of tachycardia from other types of tachy-cardia.[16]

QRS alternans, which is particularly found at high heart rates (greater than 180 beats/min), occurs in approximately 30% of CMTs and is rare in AV nodal reentry. However, the finding of QRS alternans can only be used as a clue to the diagnosis of CMT if the alternans is still present after the first 5 seconds of the tachycardia. This is because changes in height and configuration of the QRS are common in the first seconds after the start of any type of SVT.

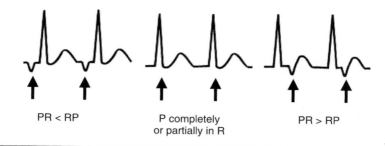

	PR < RP	P completely or partially in R	PR > RP
Atrial Tachy	Common	Uncommon	Uncommon
AVNRT	Uncommon	Common	Uncommon
CMT with fast Acc P	–	–	+
CMT with slow Acc P	+	–	–

Figure 4-25   The relation between the QRS and the P wave in different types of a regular SVT. As shown, in atrial tachycardia the P wave precedes the QRS complex. In AV nodal reentry tachycardia *(AVNRT)* the P wave is usually completely or partially hidden in the QRS. In the circus movement tachycardia *(CMT)* by a fast accessory pathway *(Acc P)* for retrograde conduction the RP interval is less than the PR interval. The reverse is true in CMT using a slowly conducting accessory pathway.

WHERE IS THE P WAVE RELATIVE TO THE QRS?

See Figure 4-25 for the relation of the P wave to the QRS.

P wave within the QRS. If the P wave is within or distorting the beginning or end of the QRS, the arrhythmia can be diagnosed as AVNRT.

P wave separate from the QRS and RP interval less than the PR interval. If the P wave is separate from the QRS and the RP interval is less than the PR interval, the mechanism is CMT (using a fast accessory pathway).

P wave separate from QRS and RP interval greater than the PR interval. If the P wave is separate from the QRS and the RP interval is greater than the PR interval, the mechanism may be one of three possibilities:

1. CMT by a slowly conducting accessory pathway
2. The uncommon form of AVNRT
3. Atrial tachycardia

Figure 4-26 illustrates two cases of SVT. In *A,* AV nodal reentry is present; note that the P wave is distorting the end of the QRS during the tachycardia, looking like an r′ wave in lead V_1 and an S wave in leads II, III, and aVF. Figure 4-26, *B,* shows orthodromic CMT. The P waves are clearly separate from the QRS with an RP interval less than the PR interval.

WHAT IS THE POLARITY (AXIS) OF THE P WAVE?

Inferior (frontal plane). A frontal plane P axis that is inferior (positive P waves in leads II, III, and aVF) rules out both AVNRT and CMT and indicates atrial tachycardia. (See Chapter 6 for atrial tachycardia caused by digitalis toxicity.)

Superior (frontal plane). A frontal plane P-wave axis that points superiorly (negative P waves in leads II, III, aVF) could be the result of either AVNRT or CMT using a posteroseptal accessory pathway.

Right to left (horizontal plane). In the horizontal plane, a right-to-left P-wave axis (positive P wave in leads I and aVL) rules out AV nodal reentry. Such an axis can be found in either right atrial tachycardia or CMT using a right-sided accessory pathway.

Left to right (horizontal plane). A left-to-right axis (negative P wave in leads I and aVL) could be CMT using a left-sided accessory pathway or left atrial tachycardia.

ABERRANT VENTRICULAR CONDUCTION, A HELPFUL CLUE

The appearance of aberrant ventricular conduction (functional bundle branch block) during SVT is helpful

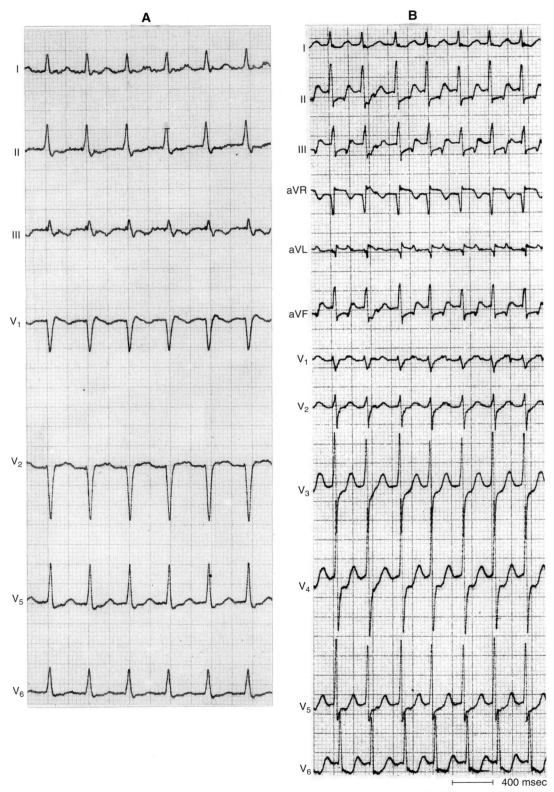

Figure 4-26   AV nodal reentry tachycardia (**A**) and circus movement tachycardia (**B**) are shown for comparison. Note that during AV nodal reentry tachycardia the P wave is distorting the end of the QRS (pseudo-S in leads II and III and pseudo-r′ in lead V$_1$). In circus movement tachycardia the P waves are clearly separate from the QRS and can easily be seen in leads II, III, aVL, and aVF. Their polarity indicates a posteroseptal atrial insertion of the accessory pathway.

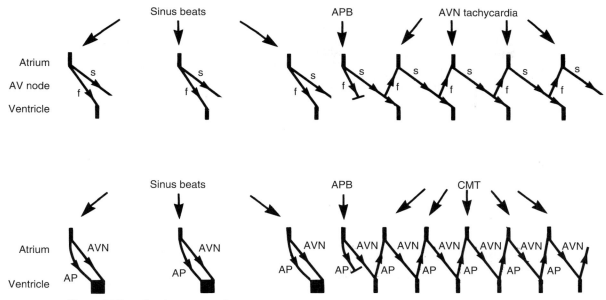

Figure 4-27   Why aberrant conduction is more common in circus movement tachycardia *(CMT)* than in AV nodal reentry tachycardia. *Top,* A ladder diagram of initiation of the common type of AV nodal reentry tachycardia by an APB. After the APB the change from conduction over the fast to the slow AV nodal pathway results in a relatively long coupling interval at the ventricular level between the conducted ABP and the preceding QRS, making phase 3 block in the bundle branch unlikely. *Bottom,* Initiation of a circus movement tachycardia by an APB. Initiation occurs because the APB is blocked in the accessory pathway in the anterograde direction. Conduction over the AV node results in a relatively short coupling interval of the conducted APB to the preceding QRS complex, favoring the occurrence of phase 3 block in the bundle branch. Persistence of aberrant conduction during tachycardia is frequently based on retrograde invasion into the bundle branch (see Appendix D).

in the differential diagnosis between AV nodal reentry tachycardia and CMT.

The presence of aberrant ventricular conduction in SVT. The presence of aberrant ventricular conduction (functional bundle branch block) in itself favors a diagnosis of CMT because aberrancy is more common during that mechanism than during AVNRT. This is because of the difference in the duration of the PR interval of the APB and its ventricular response in the two mechanisms. The onset of AVNRT is preceded by a long PR interval, allowing the ventricles more time to repolarize so that functional bundle branch block is unlikely to occur. The onset of CMT, on the other hand, is preceded by a shorter PR interval, making it more likely that there will be block in one of the bundle branches that has not had time to repolarize (Figure 4-27).

The heart rate during the aberrancy. When episodes of aberrant and nonaberrant ventricular conduction occur

in the same patient during SVT, a comparison of the two heart rates is important. If these rates differ, the location of the accessory pathway is known.

When the functional bundle branch block is on the same side as the accessory pathway, the rate will be slower during aberrancy than without aberrancy. This is because of the longer intraventricular distance the impulse must travel to complete the circuit, as demonstrated in Figure 4-28.

Such a finding is diagnostic of CMT and identifies the accessory pathway as inserting in the free wall of either the RV or LV.[17] For example, a slowing of the rate during CMT because of RBBB (Figure 4-29) indicates a right free wall accessory pathway; a slowing because of LBBB (Figure 4-30) indicates a left free wall accessory pathway. Of course, if bundle branch block is on one side and the accessory pathway on the other, no slowing will be evident during bundle branch block.

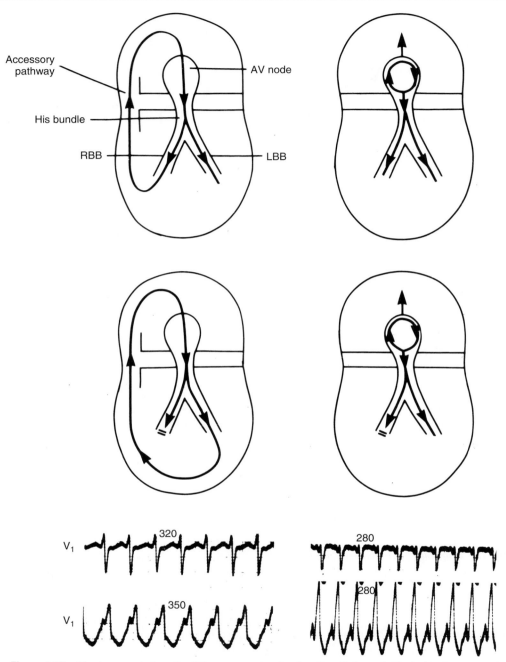

Figure 4-28   The increase in length of the reentry circuit when bundle branch block develops during circus movement tachycardia using an accessory pathway on the same side as the bundle branch block. **A,** A right-sided accessory pathway is present. **B,** The tachycardia circuit is confined to the dual pathways in the AV node. When RBBB develops in the patient with a right-sided accessory pathway, the circuit becomes longer and the tachycardia rate slows (compare lead V_1 before and after RBBB on the left). In contrast **(B),** nothing happens with the tachycardia rate when bundle branch block develops during AV nodal reentry tachycardia because the bundle branch is not incorporated in the tachycardia circuit (measurements are in milliseconds).

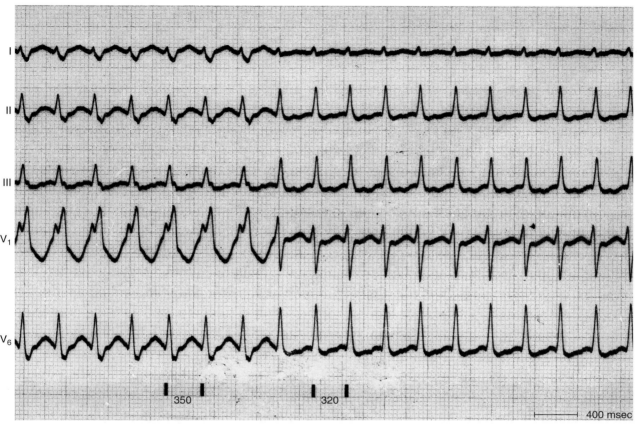

Figure 4-29 Circus movement tachycardia with RBBB aberration. The rate is slower during the aberration than during the narrow QRS tachycardia, indicating the presence of a right-sided accessory pathway (measurements are in milliseconds). QRS alternans is also noted in lead V_1 during narrow QRS tachycardia.

Systematic Approach to Treatment of Regular SVT

1. Record a 12-lead ECG.
2. Physical examination: if the ECG does not allow proper diagnosis of the site of origin of the regular narrow QRS tachycardia because P waves cannot be identified, evaluate the jugular pulse; the frog sign indicates either AVNRT or CMT. Flutter waves in the jugular pulse indicate atrial flutter.
3. Apply a vagal maneuver. If unsuccessful:
4. Inject 6 mg of adenosine over a 1- to 2-second period. If SVT is not terminated in 3 minutes, inject 12 mg of adenosine as a rapid IV bolus. Adenosine has a half-life of less than 1.5 seconds, so the adverse reactions

(facial flushing, dyspnea) last only a short time. If adenosine is not available:

5. Inject 10 mg of verapamil IV over a 5- to 10-minute period. In case of previous use of a beta-blocking drug or hypotension, reduce the dose of verapamil to 5 mg (inject over a 5- to 10-minute period).
6. When the tachycardia is not terminated, inject procainamide IV (10 mg/kg body weight) over a 5- to 10-minute period.
7. Cardiovert if the tachycardia persists and the patient is deteriorating hemodynamically.
8. Once the tachycardia has been terminated, record the 12-lead ECG in sinus rhythm so that P waves during the tachycardia can more easily be located; this is best done by comparing the QRS and ST-T segments during tachycardia with those of the sinus rhythm.

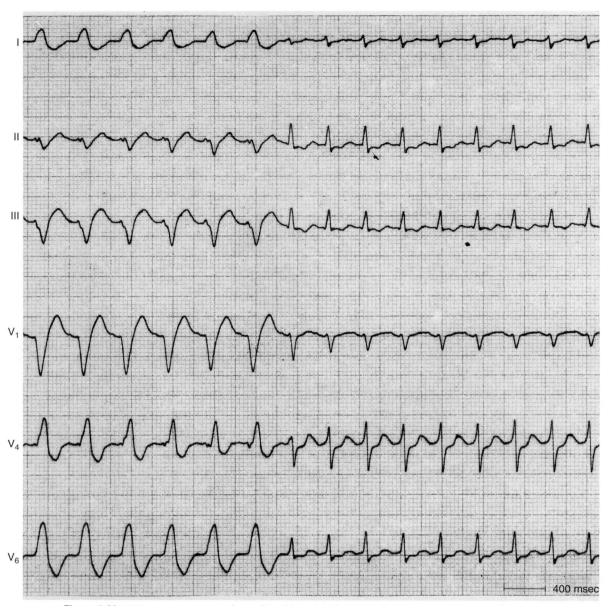

Figure 4-30 Circus movement tachycardia with and without LBBB aberration. The rate of the tachycardia is slower during LBBB, indicating the presence of a left-sided accessory pathway.

VAGAL STIMULATION

The vagal nerve is part of the parasympathetic nervous system, the mediator of which is acetylcholine. Both the sinus and AV nodes are richly supplied with autonomic nerves and are especially sensitive to acetylcholine. Vagal maneuvers cause the parasympathetic nerves to release acetylcholine, which blocks or delays conduction in the AV node.

When a vagal maneuver causes complete AV nodal block, it terminates CMT or AVNRT. If the tachycardia mechanism does not involve the AV node (atrial tachycardia, atrial flutter, or AF), the vagal maneuver exposes the type of arrhythmia when AV block is created.

TYPES OF VAGAL MANEUVERS

Vagal maneuvers include the following:
- Carotid sinus massage
- Gagging (by placing the finger in the throat)
- Valsalva maneuver (blowing against a closed glottis; squatting)
- Trendelenburg position
- The dive reflex (facial immersion in cold water)
- Coughing

Eyeball pressure is **not** an acceptable vagal maneuver; it is unpleasant for the patient, rarely effective, and may cause retinal detachment.

CAROTID SINUS MASSAGE

The carotid sinus is located at the bifurcation of the carotid artery just below the angle of the jaw (Figure 4-31). In the hands of the informed health professional, carotid sinus stimulation is an excellent diagnostic and therapeutic vagotonic maneuver. Its purpose is to create an elevation of blood pressure in the carotid sinus so that acetylcholine is released, causing a slowing or block of AV conduction, which will terminate AVNRT and CMT and expose the atrial activity of atrial flutter and AF.

HOW TO PERFORM CAROTID SINUS MASSAGE
Palpate and Auscultate the Carotid Arteries

1. Before beginning carotid sinus massage, try to exclude stenosis of one of the carotid arteries by palpation and listen for carotid bruits.
2. If possible, take a history that will reveal any transient ischemic attacks. Such a finding is a contraindication for carotid sinus massage.
3. Monitor the effect of carotid sinus massage on the ECG. If an ECG is not available:
4. Listen to the heart with the stethoscope as you massage the carotid sinus.

Precautions

- Pressure applied for longer than 5 seconds may be dangerous.
- Beware of performing this maneuver in patients older than 65 years because long sinus pauses may result (pauses of 3 to 7 seconds may occur).

Correct Positioning of the Patient

1. Place the patient in a horizontal position with the neck extended by placing either a small pillow or an arm under the patient's shoulders.
2. Turn the patient's head away from the side to be massaged.

Correct Technique

1. Locate the bifurcation of the carotid artery just below the angle of the jaw. Figure 4-31 shows an approach from behind the patient.
2. Massage one side at a time.
3. Begin with only slight pressure in the event of a hypersensitive patient. Thereafter, apply firm pressure with a massaging action for no more than 5 seconds. Firm pressure is achieved by pressing the carotid sinus against the lateral processes of the vertebrae. Such a maneuver will cause pain, and the patient should be warned of this and told that it will last for only a few seconds.

EFFECT OF CAROTID SINUS MASSAGE ON SVT

- Either temporary slowing of the ventricular rate from AV block (Figure 4-32) *or*
- No effect in atrial flutter, AF, and the incessant form of atrial tachycardia
- Occasional conversion of atrial flutter to AF
- Gradual and temporary slowing of the heart rate during sinus tachycardia (Figure 4-33)

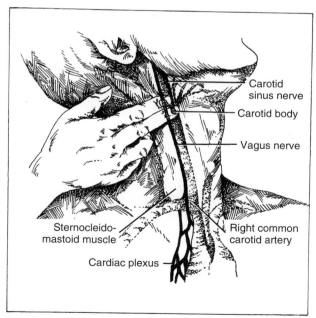

Figure 4-31 Location of the carotid body and position of the fingers for carotid sinus massage. (Reprinted from Conover M: *Understanding electrocardiography,* ed 8, St Louis, 2003, Mosby.)

CSM

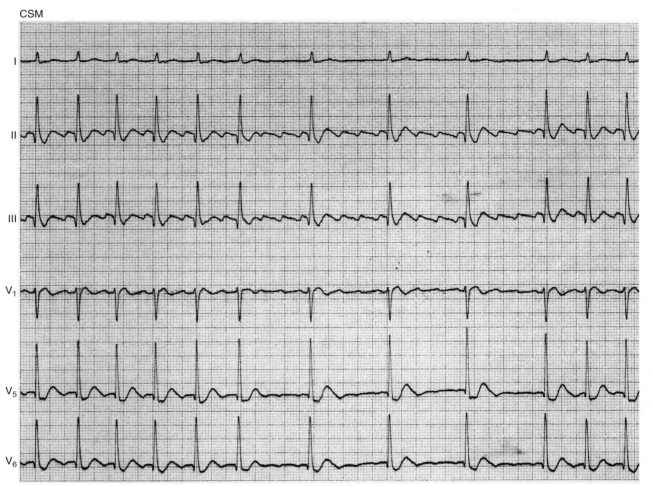

Figure 4-32 Carotid sinus massage *(CSM)* slows conduction through the AV node, revealing an underlying atrial flutter.

■ Abrupt cessation of AVNRT and CMT (Figure 4-34) or no effect. Carotid sinus massage terminates these tachycardias because of block in the AV node. The effect of carotid sinus massage on SVT is summarized in Table 4-4.

Emergency Management of Atrial Fibrillation

The emergency management of AF is determined by several factors, such as the duration of AF and the

hemodynamic consequences and presence and type of heart disease.[18]

ATRIAL FIBRILLATION PRESENT LESS THAN 48 HOURS

If AF has been present for less than 48 hours and no significant heart disease is present, pharmacologic cardioversion of AF to sinus rhythm should be attempted. Drugs can be given intravenously, such as:

■ Flecainide (1.5 to 3.0 mg/kg over a 10- to 20-minute period)

CSM

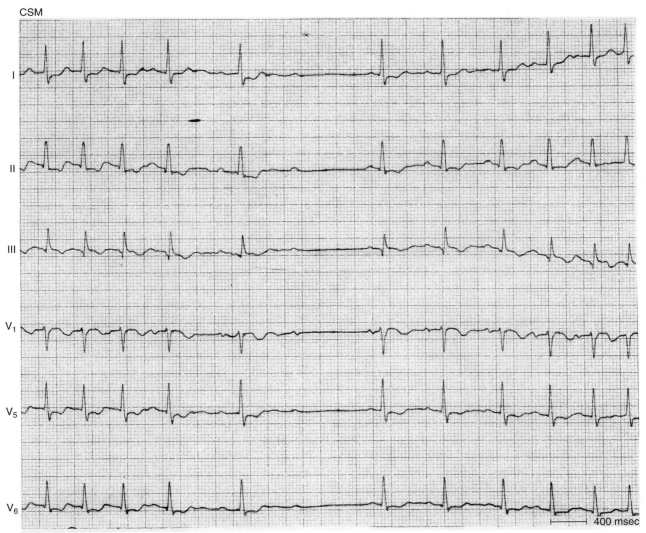

Figure 4-33 Carotid sinus massage *(CSM)* causes gradual slowing of the rate of the sinus node and one blocked P wave during sinus tachycardia.

- Propafenone (1.5 to 2.0 mg/kg over a 10- to 20-minute period)
- Procainamide (5 to 10 mg/kg over a 10- to 20-minute period)
- Ibutilide (1 mg over a 10-minute period, repeat 1 mg when necessary)
- Amiodarone (5 to 7 mg/kg over a 30- to 60-minute period)

Several of these drugs, as well as others such as quinidine and dofetilide, can also be administered orally.[18]

RECENT ONSET ATRIAL FIBRILLATION: HEMODYNAMICALLY UNSTABLE

If AF is of recent onset and hemodynamically poorly tolerated (angina, MI, shock, or pulmonary edema), immediate cardioversion should be performed without prior anticoagulation.

ATRIAL FIBRILLATION PRESENT MORE THAN 48 HOURS: HEMODYNAMICALLY STABLE

If AF has been present for more than 48 hours or is of unknown duration, a decision must be made whether to

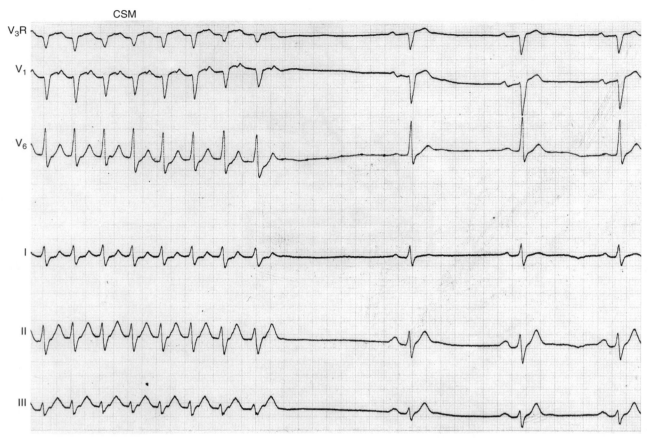

Figure 4-34 Carotid sinus massage *(CSM)* causes block in the AV node, thereby interrupting a circus movement tachycardia by a concealed accessory pathway for VA conduction.

TABLE 4-4	Effect of Carotid Sinus Massage on SVT
Type of SVT	**Effect of CSM**
Sinus tachycardia	Gradual and temporary slowing in heart rate
Atrial tachycardia	
Paroxysmal	Cessation of tachycardia or no effect
Incessant	Temporary slowing of ventricular rate (AV block) or no effect
Atrial flutter	Temporary slowing of ventricular rate (AV block), conversion into atrial fibrillation, or no effect
Atrial fibrillation	Temporary slowing of ventricular rate (AV block) or no effect
AV nodal reentry tachycardia	Cessation of tachycardia or no effect
Circus movement tachycardia	Cessation of tachycardia or no effect

accept the arrhythmia, control the ventricular rate, and give anticoagulant therapy or to perform a cardioversion attempt in the future. In the latter case, cardioversion is performed at least 3 weeks later after adequate anticoagulation has been achieved.

In both situations, the initial pharmacologic approach is to control the ventricular rate by drugs such as beta-blockers, calcium antagonists, digoxin, and amiodarone, alone or in combination, together with anticoagulant therapy.

Aspirin can be given only to patients with lone AF, that is, AF with no risk factors (such as heart failure, history of thromboembolism, hypertension, or diabetes). In all other patients with AF, oral anticoagulation should be prescribed, maintaining the international normalized ratio at 2.0 to 3.0 for at least 3 weeks.

ATRIAL FIBRILLATION PRESENT MORE THAN 48 HOURS: HEMODYNAMICALLY UNSTABLE

When AF has been present for more than 48 hours and is hemodynamically poorly tolerated, a transesophageal echocardiogram should be performed.

When No Left Atrial Thrombus Is Found by Transesophageal Echocardiogram

- Anticoagulation with an IV bolus injection of unfractionated heparin should be given.
- The patient is then cardioverted.
- Cardioversion is followed by continuation of unfractionated heparin by infusion in a dose adjusted to prolong the activated partial thromboplastin time at one and one half to two times the reference control value.
- This should be followed by oral anticoagulation, maintaining the international normalized ratio at 2.0 to 3.0 for at least 3 weeks.

When a Left Atrial Thrombus Is Found by Transesophageal Echocardiogram

- The patient should receive heparin followed by oral anticoagulation.
- The ventricular rate should be controlled pharmacologically.
- Cardioversion is performed when transesophageal echocardiogram shows resolution of the thrombus.

SUMMARY

Narrow QRS tachycardia is faster than 100 beats/min with a QRS duration of less than 0.12 seconds. It may be caused by sinus or atrial tachycardia, atrial flutter or AF, AV nodal tachycardia, or orthodromic CMT. The two most common causes of a regular SVT are AV nodal reentry and orthodromic circus movement using an accessory pathway in the retrograde direction and the AV node in the anterograde direction.

A systematic approach to the differential diagnosis during SVT involves queries as to regularity of the rhythm, the presence or induction (by vagal maneuvers) of AV block, QRS alternans, observations regarding the position and polarity of the P wave, and the response to vagal maneuvers.

A systematic approach to the treatment of SVT requires a 12-lead ECG, physical examination, and a vagal maneuver. When vagal maneuvers are unsuccessful, pharmacologic therapy is used and electrical cardioversion performed when necessary.

REFERENCES

1. Orejarena LA, Vidaillet H Jr, De Stefan F, et al: Paroxysmal supraventricular tachycardia in the general population, *J Am Coll Cardiol* 31:150-7, 1998.
2. Kalbfleisch SJ, el-Atassi R, Calkins H, et al: Differentiation of paroxysmal narrow QRS complex tachycardias using the 12-lead electrocardiogram, *J Am Coll Cardiol* 32:85-9, 1999.
3. Blomstrom-Lundqvist C, Scheinman MM, Aliot EM, et al: ACC/AHA/ESC guidelines for the management of patients with supraventricular arrhythmias—executive summary. A report of the American College of Cardiology/American Heart Association task force on practice guidelines and the European Society of Cardiology committee for practice guidelines (writing committee to develop guidelines for the management of patients with supraventricular arrhythmias) developed in collaboration with NASPE-Heart Rhythm Society, *J Am Coll Cardiol* 42:1493-531, 2003.
4. Harvey WP, Ronan JA: Bedside diagnosis of arrhythmias, *Prog Cardiovasc Dis* 8:419-31, 1966.
5. Puech P, Latour M, Grolleau R: Le flutter et ses limites. *Arch Mal Coeur* 63:116-25, 1970.
6. Wolf PA, Abbott RD, Kannel WB: Atrial fibrillation: a major contributor to stroke in the elderly: the Framingham study, *Arch Intern Med* 147:1561-4, 1987.
7. Lloyd-Jones DM, Wang TJ, Leip EP, et al: Lifetime risk for development of atrial fibrillation. The Framingham study, *Circulation* 110:142-6, 2004.
8. Benjamin EJ, Wolf PA, D'Agostino RB, et al: Impact of atrial fibrillation on the risk of death: the Framingham Heart Study, *Circulation* 98:946-52, 1998.
9. Stewart S, Hart CL, Hole DJ, et al: A population based study of the long term risks associated with atrial fibrillation: 20 year follow-up of the Renfrew/Paisley Study, *Am J Med* 113:359-64, 2002.
10. Wolf PA, Abbott RD, Kannel WB: Atrial fibrillation as an independent risk factor for stroke: the Framingham Study, *Stroke* 22:983-1, 991.
11. Allessie MA, Lammers WJEP, Bonke FIM, et al: Experimental evaluation of Moe's multiple wavelet hypothesis of atrial fibrillation. In Zipes DP, Jalife J, editors: *Cardiac arrhythmias*, New York, 1985, Grune & Stratton, pp 265-76.
12. Falk RH, Podrid PJ: *Atrial fibrillation: mechanism and management*, New York, 1991, Raven.
13. Haissaguerre M, Jais P, Shah DC, et al: Spontaneous initiation of atrial fibrillation by ectopic beats originating in the pulmonary veins, *N Engl J Med* 139:659-64, 1998.
14. Wellens HJJ, Brugada P, Penn OC: The management of preexcitation syndromes, *JAMA* 257:2325-33, 1997.
15. Bar FW, Brugada P, Dassen WRM, et al: Differential diagnosis of tachycardia with narrow QRS complex (shorter than 0.12 sec.), *Am J Cardiol* 54:555-60, 1984.
16. Green M, Heddle B, Dassen W, et al: Value of QRS alternation in determining the site of origin of narrow QRS supraventricular tachycardia, *Circulation* 68:368-73, 1983.
17. Coumel PH, Attuel P: Reciprocating tachycardia in overt and latent pre-excitation: influence of functional bundle branch block on the rate of tachycardia, *Eur J Cardiol* 1:423-9, 1974.
18. Fuster V, Ryden LE, Asinger RW, et al: ACC/AHA/ESC: guidelines for the management of patients with atrial fibrillation, *Eur Heart J* 22:1852-923, 2001.

5

Wide QRS Tachycardia

EMERGENCY APPROACH

1. Do not panic when confronted with the broad QRS tachycardia.
2. Obtain a 12-lead ECG.

If Hemodynamically Unstable

1. Cardiovert.
2. Obtain a history.
3. Examine the precardioversion and postcardioversion ECGs to determine the cause of the arrhythmia.

If Hemodynamically Stable

1. Examine the patient for clinical signs of AV dissociation.
2. Systematically evaluate the 12-lead ECG.
3. Obtain a history.

If VT

1. Give procainamide 10 mg/kg body weight intravenously (IV) over a 5-minute period unless the tachycardia is ischemia related; then give lidocaine. If unsuccessful:
2. Cardiovert.
3. Examine the ECG during the VT and during sinus rhythm to determine the cause of the tachycardia.

If SVT with Aberration

1. Perform vagal stimulation. If unsuccessful:
2. Give adenosine 6 mg by rapid IV bolus; if unsuccessful, follow with a 12-mg IV bolus 3 minutes later. If unavailable:
3. Give verapamil 10 mg IV over a 5- to 10-minute period; reduce to 5 mg if the patient is taking a beta-blocker or is hypotensive. If unsuccessful:
4. Give procainamide 10 mg/kg body weight IV over a 5-minute period; if unsuccessful:
5. Cardiovert.
6. Examine SVT and postconversion ECGs to determine mechanism.

If in Doubt
1. Do not give verapamil.
2. Give IV procainamide.
If Wide QRS and Irregular
1. Do not give digitalis or verapamil.
2. Give IV procainamide unless torsades de pointes is present (see Chapter 7).

Because a drug given for the treatment of SVT may be deleterious to a patient with VT,[1,2] the differential diagnosis in broad QRS tachycardia is critical. Errors are made because emergency care professionals wrongly consider VT unlikely if the patient is hemodynamically stable,[3] and they are often unaware of the ECG findings that quickly and accurately distinguish VT in more than 90% of cases. This chapter describes both the physical examination and ECG findings that help differentiate aberrant ventricular conduction (bundle branch block) from ventricular ectopy.[4-6] Treatment is also discussed. For mechanisms of aberrant ventricular conduction, see Appendix D.

To arrive at the correct diagnosis the ECG features of VT and SVT with aberration must be understood and clues carefully searched for during the physical examination.

CAUSES

The different types of wide QRS tachycardia are illustrated in Figure 5-1 and include the following:

- *SVT* with preexisting or functional bundle branch block, including sinus tachycardia, atrial tachycardia, atrial flutter, atrial fibrillation, and AV nodal reentry tachycardia.
- *Orthodromic circus movement tachycardia (CMT)* by the AV node in the anterograde direction and an accessory pathway in the retrograde direction with preexisting or functional bundle branch block.
- *SVT, including atrial fibrillation,* with conduction over an accessory pathway.
- *Antidromic CMT tachycardia* by an accessory pathway in the anterograde direction (including a Mahaim fiber) and the AV node or another accessory pathway in the retrograde direction.
- *VT.*

NOTE: 80% of wide QRS tachycardias presenting in the emergency department are VT.

PHYSICAL EVALUATION FOR AV DISSOCIATION

AV dissociation is present in approximately 60% of VTs. The other 40% show some form of retrograde conduction to the atria. Thus the finding of AV dissociation is an important diagnostic clue. Physical evaluation for AV dissociation can be found on the ECG and be diagnosed during the physical examination of the patient.[7] The three physical signs of AV dissociation are the following:

1. Irregular cannon A waves in the jugular pulse
2. Varying intensity of the first heart sound
3. Beat-to-beat changes in systolic blood pressure

Any one of these three indicates AV dissociation. In the absence of such clues, VT is still not ruled out; the possibility of coexistent atrial fibrillation or ventriculoatrial (VA) conduction remains, in which case none of the signs of AV dissociation will be present. Theoretically, an AV junctional tachycardia with bundle branch block and retrograde block can have AV dissociation; however, in view of the rarity of such a rhythm, AV dissociation remains a valuable diagnostic clue for VT.

The Jugular Pulse

In VT with independent beating of atria and ventricles, the atria occasionally beat against closed AV valves because of simultaneous ventricular contraction. This causes a backflow of blood into the jugular vein, producing cannon A waves. Inspection of the jugular vein reveals the characteristic occasional expansive pulsation.

Varying Intensity of the First Heart Sound

The first heart sound marks the onset of ventricular systole and is caused by the closing of the mitral and tricuspid valves. It is usually loudest at the apex but may be louder at the fourth left intercostal space.

During AV dissociation a beat-to-beat change in the loudness of the first heart sound is present because of the varying position of the AV valves at the time of ventricular contraction. Thus the first heart sound varies in intensity during VT with AV dissociation and complete

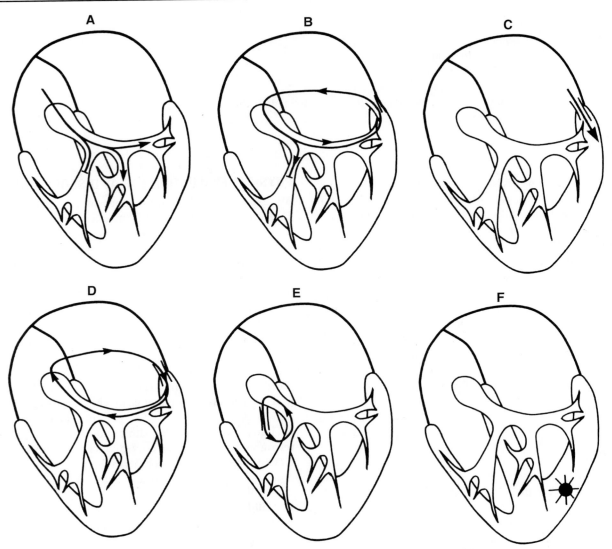

Figure 5-1 The different types of tachycardia with a wide QRS complex. **A,** SVT (sinus tachycardia, atrial tachycardia, atrial flutter, atrial fibrillation, AV nodal reentry tachycardia), with preexisting or tachycardia-related bundle branch block. **B,** CMT with AV conduction over the AV node and ventriculoatrial conduction over an accessory pathway in the presence of preexisting or tachycardia-related bundle branch block. **C,** SVT (sinus tachycardia, atrial tachycardia, atrial flutter, atrial fibrillation) with AV conduction over an accessory AV pathway. **D,** Circus movement tachycardia with AV conduction over an accessory AV pathway and ventriculoatrial conduction over the AV node or a second accessory AV pathway (not shown). **E,** Tachycardia with anterograde conduction over a nodoventricular (Mahaim) fiber and retrograde conduction over the bundle of His or an SVT with AV conduction over a nodoventricular fiber (not shown). **F,** VT.

heart block as well as during AV Wenckebach and atrial fibrillation.

Changes in Systolic Blood Pressure

During AV dissociation, ventricular filling from the atria varies depending on the time lapse between atrial and ventricular contraction. These differences in ventricular filling lead to a beat-to-beat change in systolic stroke volume into the aorta, which in turn causes beat-to-beat changes in systolic blood pressure (Figure 5-2). This sign of AV dissociation can easily be picked up at the bedside by the blood pressure recorder. Thus a typical finding in

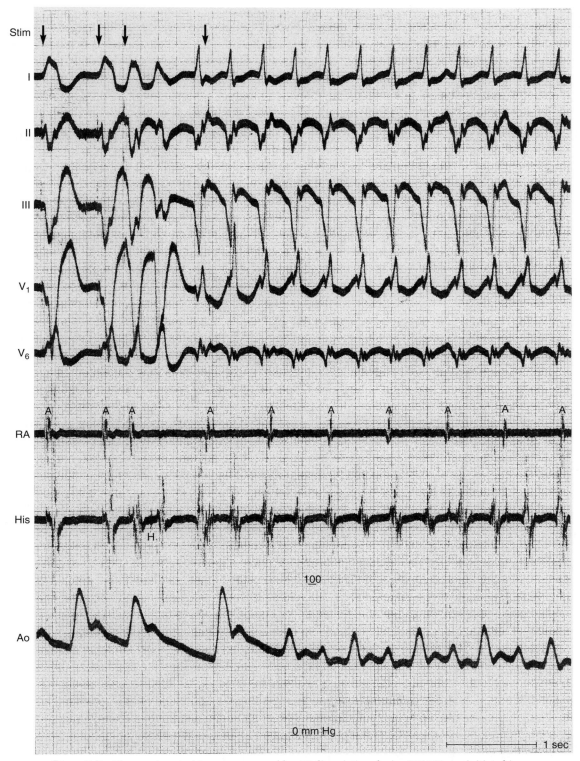

Figure 5-2 Changes in arterial pressure caused by AV dissociation during VT. VT was initiated in the catheterization laboratory by delivering two premature ventricular beats during ventricular pacing. In the aortic pressure tracing *(Ao)* the systolic pressure changes relative to the timing of atrial contraction in relation to ventricular contraction. *RA* is a recording from inside the right atrium. The His bundle lead records the electrical activity of the heart at the site of the bundle of His.

VT with AV dissociation is a regular rhythm, whereas the systolic blood pressure differs from beat to beat.

ECG Findings of Value in Differentiating Causes of a Wide QRS Tachycardia

AV DISSOCIATION

Independent atrial and ventricular activity (AV dissociation) during a wide QRS tachycardia is a hallmark of VT,

as shown in Figure 5-3, where independent P waves can be seen. However, during VT some form of VA conduction may be present, especially when the VT rate is relatively slow (Figures 5-4 and 5-5). Also, another arrhythmia may be present at the atrial level, such as atrial fibrillation.

When AV dissociation is present during VT, the atrial rate is usually slower than the ventricular rate, except when atrial tachycardia, atrial flutter, or atrial fibrillation

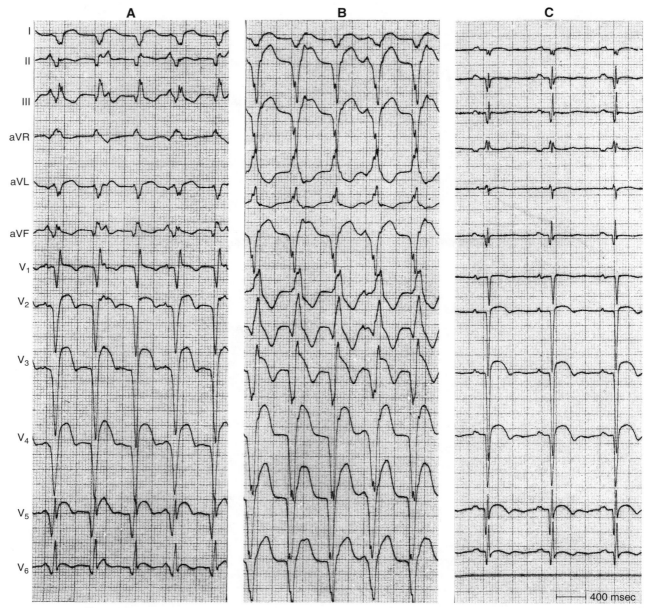

Figure 5-3   Two types of VT in a patient with an old anteroseptal MI (**C**). Both VTs (**A** and **B**) have an RBBB shape and clearly show AV dissociation. Independent sinus P waves are nicely seen in the inferior leads and in lead V₁.

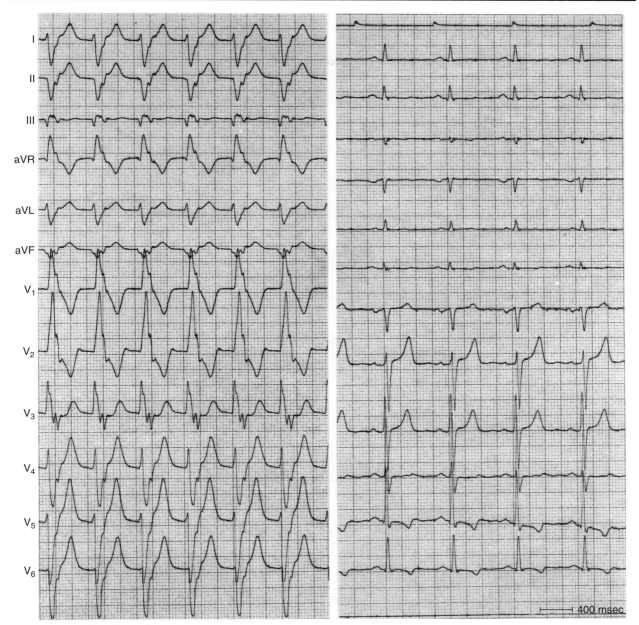

Figure 5-4 VT manifesting four diagnostic clues. There is one-to-one VA conduction (negative P waves in the inferior leads immediately after the QRS). The QRS shows a monophasic R in lead V_1 and an rS complex in V_6. The frontal plane QRS axis is northwest.

is present. During VT, part or all of the ventricle may occasionally be activated by a supraventricular impulse (e.g., a sinus beat), which is conducted through the AV conduction system when the ventricle is excitable. This typically occurs when the VT rate is relatively slow. This phenomenon results in "capture" beats (complete activation over the AV conduction system, as show in Figure 1-45, p. 45) or "fusion" beats (activation of the ventricle by both ectopic impulse formation and activation over the AV conduction system) (Figure 5-6).

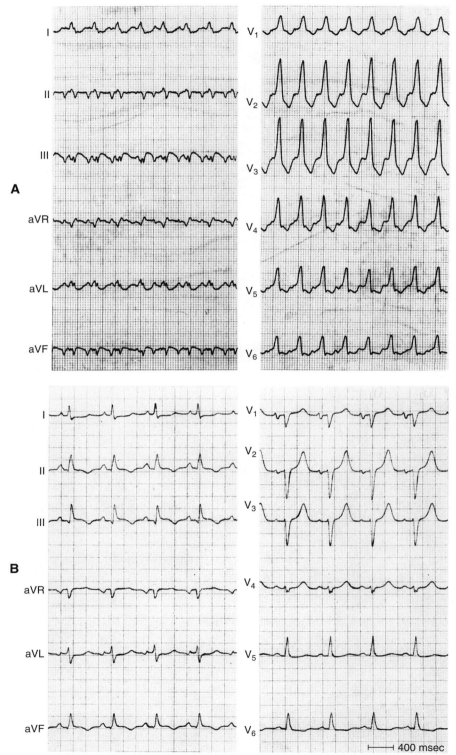

Figure 5-5 VT with retrograde Wenckebach type conduction to the atrium (**A**). Note the positive concordant pattern in the precordial leads. The patient had an old inferior MI (**B**).

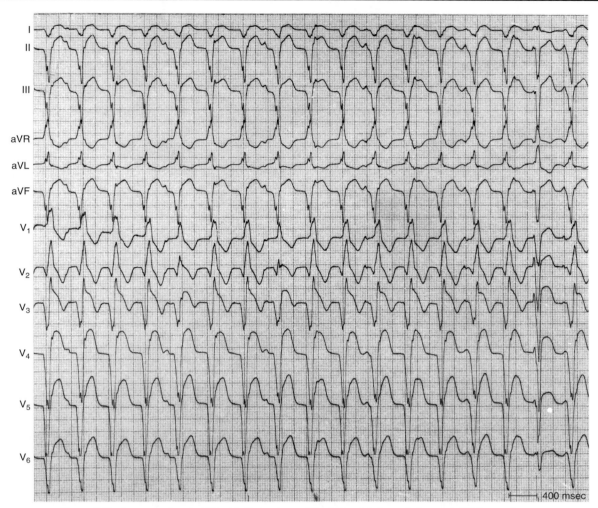

Figure 5-6 An example of a VT with fusion beats. The fifth, eighth, and sixteenth QRS complexes (best seen in leads V_1 and V_2) are narrower when compared with the other QRS complexes because of different degrees of fusion between a ventricular ectopic complex and a conducted supraventricular beat.

CONFIGURATIONAL CHARACTERISTICS OF THE QRS COMPLEX

The following configurational characteristics of the QRS complex help in the differential diagnosis of wide QRS tachycardia:

- RBBB shapes versus LBBB shapes (the rules for the two patterns are not interchangeable)
- Concordant precordial patterns
- Q waves
- QRS onset to S nadir duration

RBBB-Shaped QRS Complex

Leads V_1 and V_6 are the important ECG leads in distinguishing VT from SVT with RBBB.

SVT with RBBB

- Leads V_1 and V_6 usually have a triphasic pattern.[4,8]
- Lead V_1 has an rSR′ pattern, with the initial r reflecting normal septal activation, the S wave reflecting LV activation, and the R′ wave reflecting delayed activation of the RV.
- Lead V_6 shows a narrow q wave resulting from normal septal activation, an R wave representing LV activation, and an S wave reflecting delayed RV activation. In lead V_6 the RS ratio is typically greater than one (Figure 5-7).

VT with an RBBB shape

- Lead V_1 shows a monophasic or biphasic QRS complex (R, qR, QR, or RS).

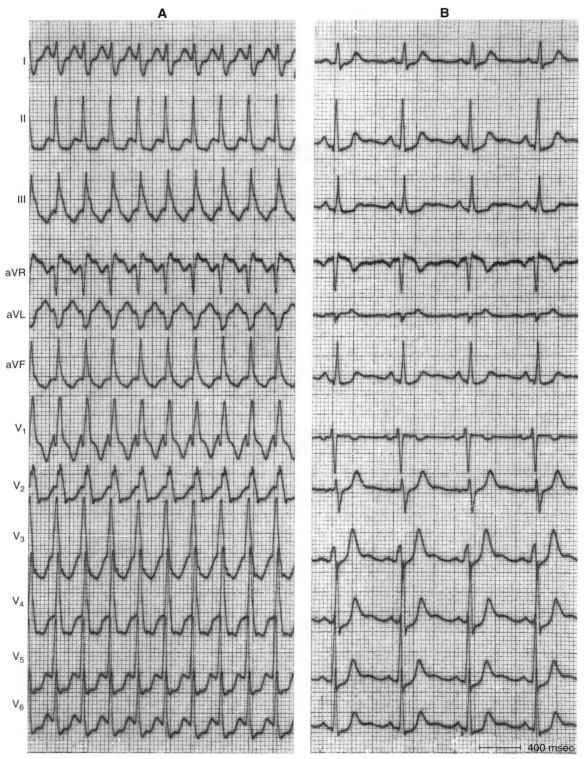

Figure 5-7 **A,** SVT with RBBB. Note the typical QRS features in leads V$_1$ (rSR′) and V$_6$ (qRs). **B,** Sinus rhythm in the same patient.

- In lead V_6, the presence of a deep S wave with an R:S ratio of less than one supports the diagnosis of VT.[4] This situation is typical when left axis deviation is present. In cases of right axis deviation, the R:S ratio in lead V_6 is usually greater than one (Figure 5-8).

Limitations. Approximately 10% of VTs with an RBBB shape have a triphasic (rSR′) complex in lead V_1, such as the one seen in SVT with RBBB. However,

the differential diagnosis can still be made because other ECG characteristics, as well as physical findings already discussed, usually lead to the correct diagnosis.

LBBB-Shaped QRS Complex

Leads V_1, V_2, and V_6 are the important ECG leads in distinguishing VT from SVT with LBBB.[5]

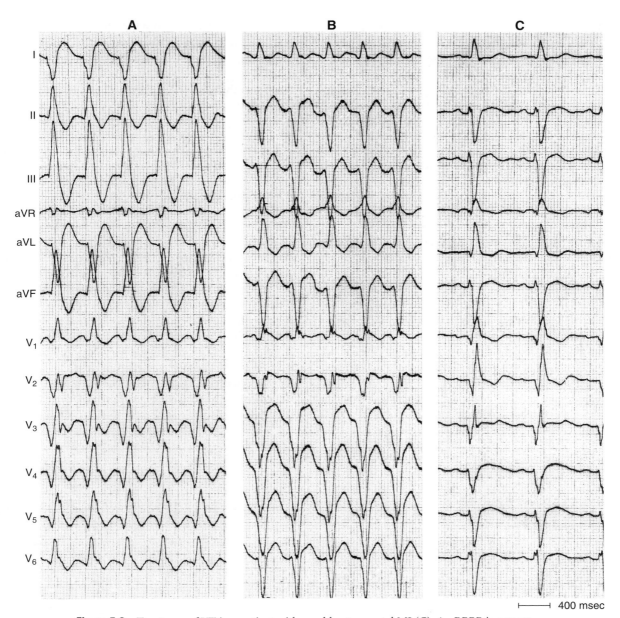

Figure 5-8 Two types of VT in a patient with an old anteroseptal MI (**C**). An RBBB is present (**A** and **B**), with a QR pattern in lead V_1. QRS negativity or positivity in lead V_6 is determined by the frontal plane axis. In **A**, a QR complex is seen in lead V_6 during left axis deviation. In **B**, a QS complex is seen in lead V_6 during left axis deviation.

SVT with an LBBB shape

- If an r wave is present in either lead V_1 or V_2, it is narrow (less than 0.03 seconds) (Figure 5-9, *A*).
- The downstroke of the S wave is fast, without slurring or notching.
- The distance from the beginning of the QRS to the nadir of the S wave is 0.06 seconds or less.

VT with an LBBB shape

- Lead V_1 or V_2 has an R wave longer than 0.04 seconds in duration *and*
- The downstroke of the S wave in lead V_1 or V_2 is slurred and delayed, the distance from the beginning of the QRS to the nadir of the S wave being more than 0.06 seconds (Figures 5-10 and 5-11)
- A Q wave in lead V_6 is diagnostic of VT[5]

Both leads V_1 and V_2 should be evaluated in this type of broad QRS tachycardia because initial forces may be isoelectric in lead V_1, leading to misclassification. When lead V_1 has supraventricular morphologic features (narrow r and clean downstroke), examination of leads V_2 and V_6 is especially important before making a diagnosis of SVT.

Limitations

The following limitations are associated with the criteria for the differential diagnosis in LBBB-shaped broad QRS tachycardia:

- LBBB in SVT having the same morphologic features as VT (broad r, slurred downstroke in leads V_1 or V_2). This situation may be found in patients with preexisting LBBB and severe fibrotic disease of the LV. In such a situation, a comparison of the sinus rhythm tracing with that of the tachycardia provides the correct diagnosis.
- Antidromic CMT with anterograde conduction over an accessory pathway inserting in the RV. Such

a mechanism produces a tachycardia morphologically identical to the LBBB-shaped VT.

- The use of antiarrhythmic drugs that cause slow intraventricular conduction, such as class IA drugs (procainamide, quinidine, as well as disopyramide) or class IC drugs (flecainide and propafenone). These drugs may broaden the R wave and produce a delayed S nadir in lead V_1 and/or lead V_2.

Concordant Pattern in the Precordial Leads

Leads V_1 to V_6 may all show positive or negative QRS complexes, referred to as positive and negative concordance.

- Negative precordial concordance is diagnostic of VT (Figure 5-12, *A*).
- Positive precordial concordance occurs in VT originating in the posterobasal area of the LV (Figure 5-12, *B*), but positive precordial concordance may also be seen in SVT with AV conduction over an accessory pathway inserting into the posterobasal LV (Figure 5-13).

Presence of Q Waves During Tachycardia

As a rule, QR complexes during a wide QRS tachycardia are highly suggestive of VT (Figures 5-8 and 5-14) unless, of course, identical QR complexes are present in the same leads during sinus rhythm.[9] In patients with VT after MI, approximately 40% have a QR complex in one or more ECG leads. These QR complexes are usually in the same leads that the Q waves are located in during sinus rhythm. QR complexes during VT therefore typically occur in patients with a localized ventricular scar, such as those with a previous MI or localized infiltrative or inflammatory myocardial disease.

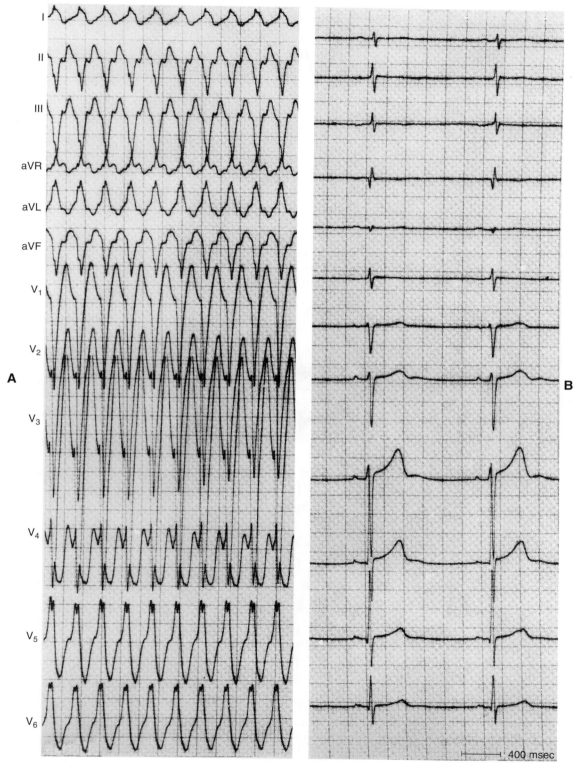

Figure 5-9 SVT with LBBB aberration (**A**). Note the typical QRS features in leads V_1 and V_2 (rapid, clean downstroke, early S nadir, and the absence of a Q in lead V_6). **B,** The same patient during sinus rhythm.

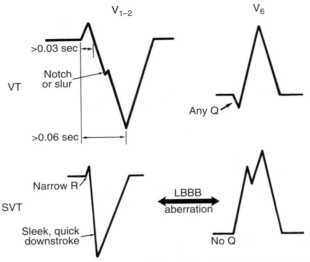

Figure 5-10 Typical configuration of the QRS during VT and SVT in leads V_1, V_2, and V_6 when lead V_1 is predominantly negative. In leads V_1 and V_2, a narrow r and a clean, rapid downstroke support the diagnosis of SVT; a broad r, slurred downstroke, or delayed S nadir support the diagnosis of VT. In lead V_6 a Q wave supports a diagnosis of VT.

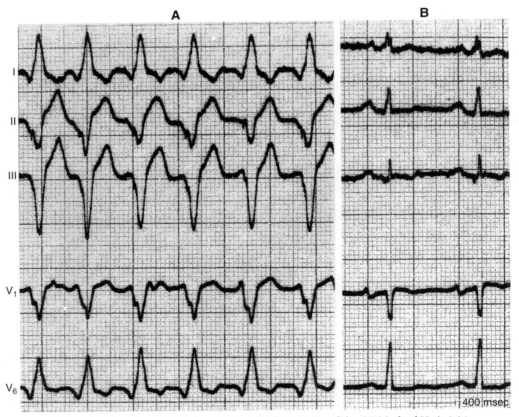

Figure 5-11 VT (**A**) with an LBBB shape. Note initial positivity of the QRS in lead V_1 (>0.04 seconds), slurring of the S wave in lead V_1, and a distance from the beginning of the QRS to the nadir of the S wave in lead V_1 of 140 msec. Lead V_6 shows a qR complex. **B,** ECG during sinus rhythm.

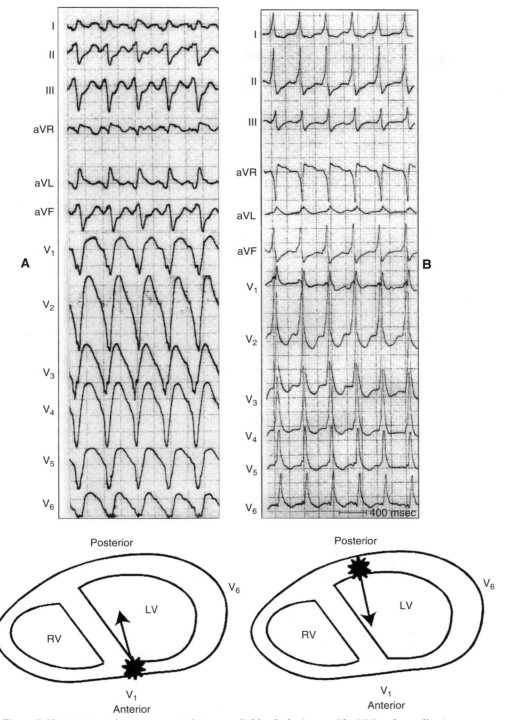

Figure 5-12 A concordant pattern in the precordial leads during a wide QRS tachycardia. **A,** Negative precordial concordance in a patient with an old apical MI. **B,** Positive precordial concordance in a patient with an old posterior wall MI. The drawings below the ECGs indicate the site of origin of VT in the horizontal plane.

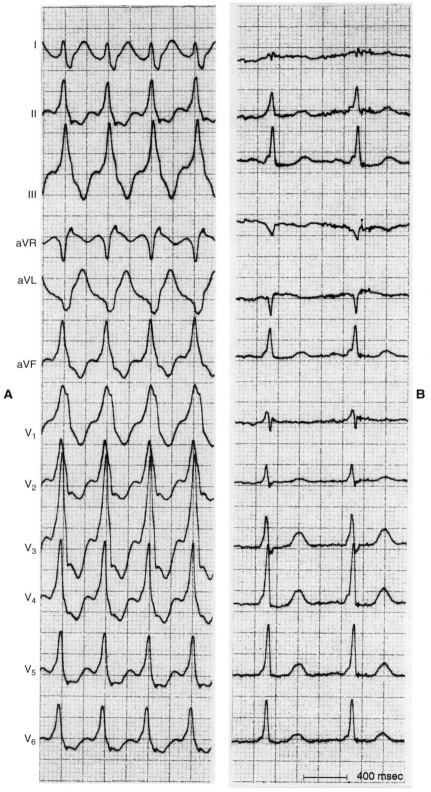

Figure 5-13 **A,** Antidromic circus movement tachycardia with AV conduction over a left posterior accessory pathway. Note the positive precordial concordance. **B,** The same patient during sinus rhythm.

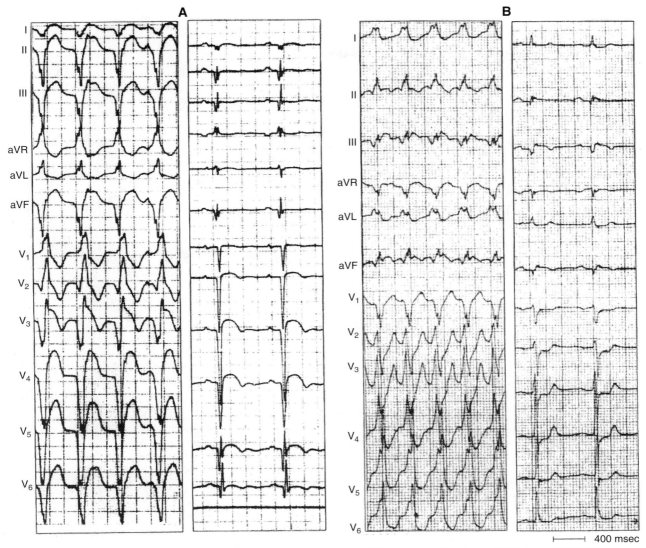

Figure 5-14 Q waves during tachycardia. **A,** QR complexes in the precordial leads V_2 and V_3 in an RBBB-shaped VT. *Right,* Pattern of an anteroseptal MI during sinus rhythm. **B,** QR complexes in the inferior leads in an LBBB-shaped VT. Note the QR complexes of the tachycardia are in the same leads as the Q waves during sinus rhythm.

Interval from Onset of QRS to Nadir of the S Wave in Precordial Leads

As already indicated, in LBBB-shaped QRS tachycardia the interval from the onset of the QRS to the nadir of the S wave in precordial leads is increased in VT. Brugada et al[10] postulated that an RS interval of >100 msec in one or more precordial leads is highly suggestive of VT.

The clinician must be careful, however, because such a duration sometimes may occur during the following situations:

■ SVT with AV conduction over an accessory pathway

■ SVT during the administration of drugs that slow intraventricular conduction (Figure 5-15)
■ SVT with preexisting bundle branch block, especially LBBB

OTHER DIAGNOSTIC CLUES
Width of the QRS Complex

Two facts are of value in distinguishing SVT from VT:

1. Block or delay in conduction through the right bundle branch during a supraventricular rhythm results in an RBBB configuration and a QRS complex with a width of 120 msec.

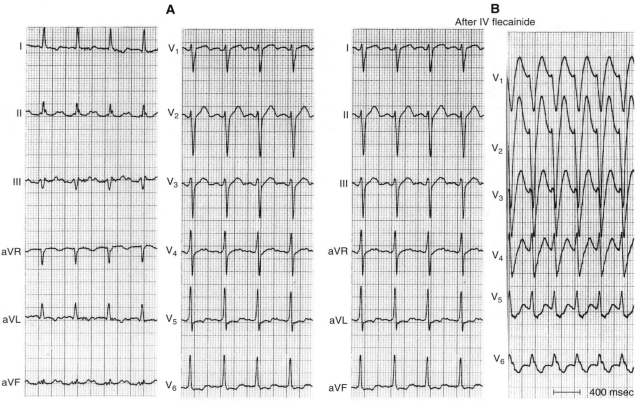

Figure 5-15 A pseudo-VT pattern after the administration of flecainide during an SVT. **A,** Left atrial tachycardia with two-to-one AV conduction. **B,** ECG recorded after IV flecainide was given. This resulted in slowing of impulse formation of the atrial tachycardia with one-to-one AV conduction. The rate-related intraventricular slowing in conduction velocity by flecainide resulted in marked widening of the QRS and the development of ECG features suggesting a ventricular origin of the tachycardia.

2. When conduction in the left bundle branch is blocked, width of the QRS complex may become as long as 140 msec.

Thus *the wider the QRS complex, the more likely that the tachycardia is ventricular in origin.* This situation is typically the case when ectopic ventricular impulse formation occurs in the free wall of the RV or LV and activation of the two ventricles occurs sequentially rather than simultaneously.

However, the following situations may result in an SVT with a QRS width of more than 140 msec in RBBB and more than 160 msec in LBBB:

- SVT in the presence of bundle branch block with additional intramyocardial conduction delay
- SVT with AV conduction over an accessory pathway
- Marked QRS widening during SVT from antiarrhythmic drugs that prolong intraventricular conduction

VT may also have a QRS width of less than 140 msec, such as VTs that originate in or close to the intraventricular septum of the LV (Figure 5-16).

QRS Axis in the Frontal Plane

When impulse formation originates in the ventricle, the frontal plane QRS axis is frequently abnormal, depending on the site of origin of the VT. A frontal plane axis to the left of −30 degrees during tachycardia has been shown to be suggestive of a VT.[4] This observation still holds true in VT with an RBBB configuration but remains questionable in VT with an LBBB shape.[5]

The cause of VT with an LBBB shape is usually one of the following:

1. An anterior or inferoposterior scar from a previous MI in or close to the interventricular septum
2. An idiopathic VT arising from the outflow tract of the RV

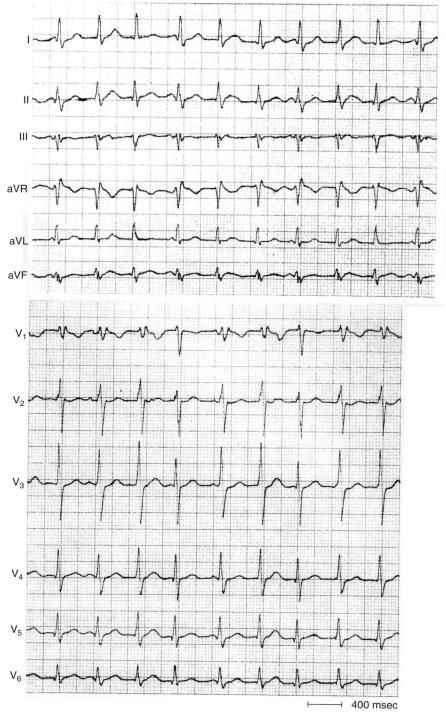

Figure 5-16   A relatively narrow VT (QRS of 120 msec) because of an origin on the left side of the interventricular septum. Note AV dissociation with capture beats (QRS complexes 3 and 9 in the limb leads and 4 and 7 in the precordial leads). Capture beats are identified because of the shorter preceding cycle, and the P wave that is conducted can be seen distorting the previous T wave.

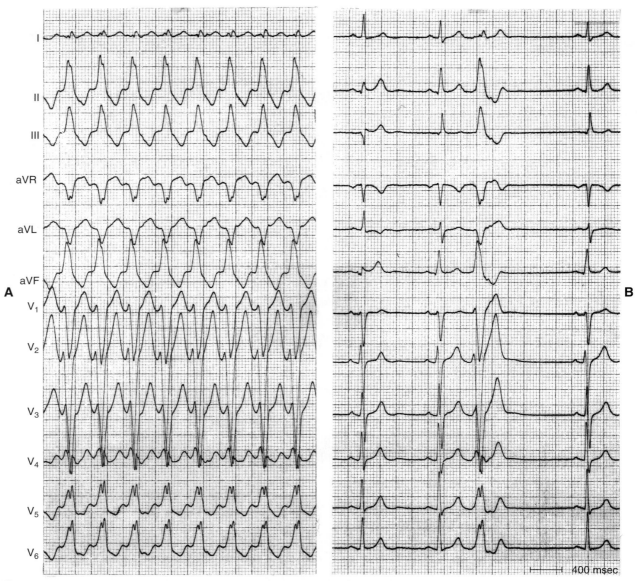

Figure 5-17 **A,** Idiopathic VT originating in the outflow tract of the RV. The QRS has an LBBB shape with a vertical frontal plane axis. Note the initial positivity in leads V_1 and V_2 (80 msec) and a long interval (110 msec) between the beginning of the QRS and the nadir of the S in the same leads. **B,** Same patient during sinus rhythm. Note the presence of a VPB with the same QRS configuration as the QRS during tachycardia.

3. A VT in arrhythmogenic RV dysplasia

In the first and third causes the exit point of the VT, and therefore the QRS axis, may vary. In idiopathic VT from the RV outflow tract the frontal plane axis is typically vertical or to the right (Figure 5-17). In general, in a patient with a wide LBBB-shaped tachycardia, marked left axis deviation (i.e., to the left of −60 degrees) or marked right axis deviation (i.e., to the right of +90 degrees) suggests a VT (Figure 5-18).

Narrow Beats During a Wide QRS Tachycardia

Three mechanisms for a smaller beat during VT are:

1. Conducted sinus beats leading to capture or fusion
2. Echo beats

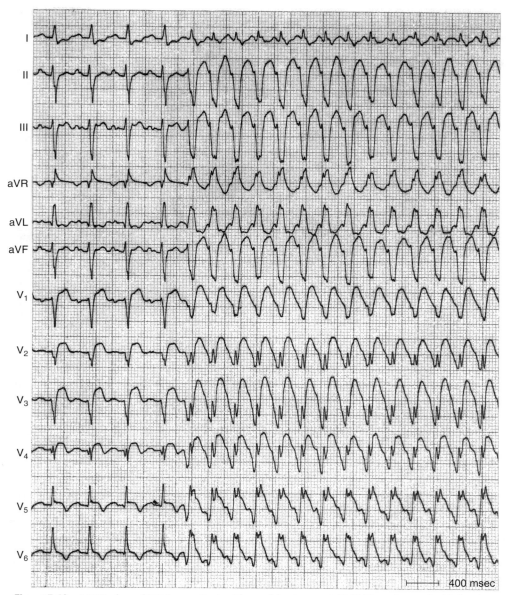

Figure 5-18 LBBB-shaped VT in a patient with an old anteroseptal MI. Note the marked left axis deviation and the Q waves in leads aVL and V_4 to V_6.

3. Another ventricular focus firing simultaneously, or nearly so, in the other ventricle

Echo Beats

During VT, the impulse can enter the bundle branch system and be conducted retrogradely through the AV node to produce an echo beat that, on return to the ventricles, produces a narrow QRS complex. In Figure 5-19, the three ventricular beats at the beginning of the tracing show retrograde conduction to the atria with progressive lengthening of the RP or VA interval. This is followed by reentry down the AV node and return to the ventricle.

Two Ventricular Ectopic Foci

A narrower beat during VT may be produced, not only by the fusion of supraventricular and ventricular beats within the ventricular chamber, as already discussed, but also when fusion occurs between the impulse responsible for VT and a ventricular ectopic impulse arising in the other ventricle.

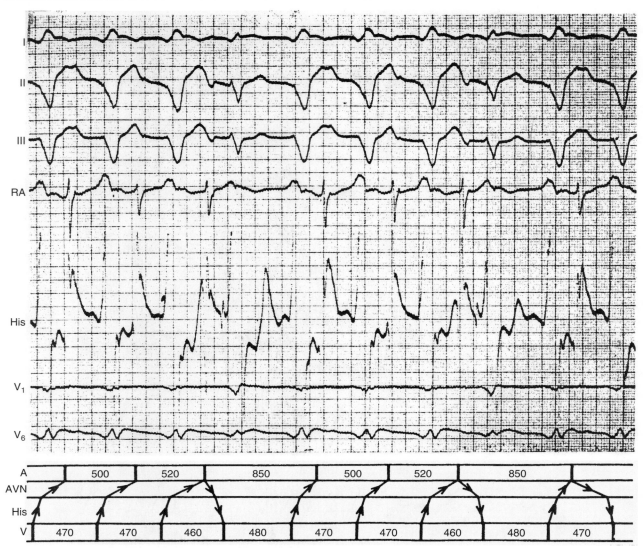

Figure 5-19 VT with retrograde conduction to the atria (A) followed by a ventricular echo beat. Note the progressive lengthening of the RP interval after the first three VT complexes, best seen in leads II and III. This is followed by a retrograde P wave and a ventricular echo. That is, the retrograde P wave is conducted back down the AV node (AVN) to the ventricles (V), producing a narrow QRS. The same sequence is repeated thereafter. To facilitate recognition of these phenomena, both right atrial (RA), and His bundle recordings are shown.

Narrow Beats During Wide QRS SVT

A narrower beat occurring during a wide QRS tachycardia is not always an indication of VT; in addition to the conditions already mentioned, it may occur during SVT with bundle branch block and VPBs arising in the ventricle having the bundle branch block. It may also occur during atrial fibrillation in the patient with an accessory pathway when AV conduction of an occasional impulse over the AV node/bundle of His axis is present.

Difference Between the Bundle Branch Block Shape in Tachycardia and Sinus Rhythm

Figure 5-20 shows a bundle branch pattern during the wide QRS tachycardia (A) that is different from that seen during sinus rhythm (B). During the tachycardia the QRS shape is that of RBBB (positive complex in lead V_1), whereas during sinus rhythm LBBB is present. Such a finding indicates that the wide QRS tachycardia must be VT because an SVT would have shown (in this particular example) an LBBB pattern.

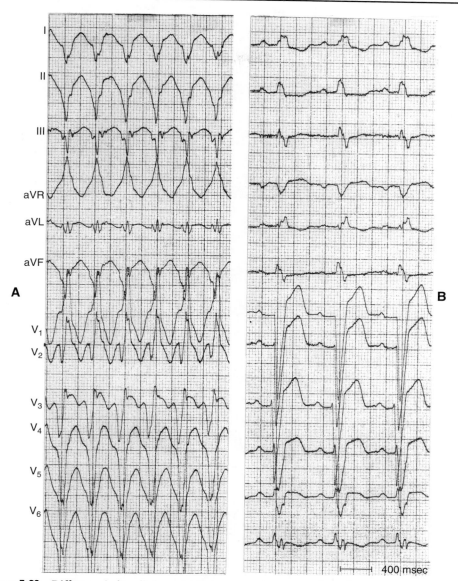

Figure 5-20 Difference in bundle branch block patterns between tachycardia and during sinus rhythm. **A,** VT with an RBBB shape. However, during sinus rhythm (**B**) an LBBB is present. That finding rules out the possibility that the tachycardia in **A** is SVT with RBBB.

QRS Width During Tachycardia Less Than During Sinus Rhythm

Figure 5-21, *A,* shows a patient with a very wide QRS during sinus rhythm, whereas the QRS during tachycardia (Figure 5-21, *B*) is not as wide. Therefore the tachycardia must be VT. During sinus rhythm sequential (first right then left) ventricular activation takes place, resulting in a broad QRS. VT has its origin closer to the interventricular septum, resulting in more simultaneous

activation of both ventricles and a narrower QRS complex.

THREE SIGNS AND SYMPTOMS THAT CANNOT BE USED IN THE DIFFERENTIAL DIAGNOSIS OF BROAD QRS TACHYCARDIA

Hemodynamic Status and Age

In the differential diagnosis of broad QRS tachycardia, hemodynamic status and age should not be used as crite-

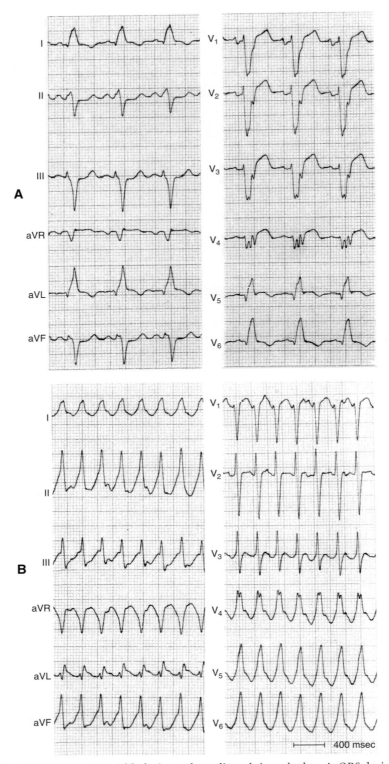

Figure 5-21 Difference in QRS width during tachycardia and sinus rhythm. **A,** QRS during sinus rhythm. The QRS width measures 200 msec because of a marked delay in LV activation in a patient with an old anteroseptal MI and LBBB. **B,** In the same patient, tachycardia with a QRS width of 170 msec. This indicates more symmetrical ventricular activation during tachycardia than during sinus rhythm, which can only be explained by impulse formation closer to the interventricular septum, indicating that this tachycardia is VT. Note the independent P waves (AV dissociation).

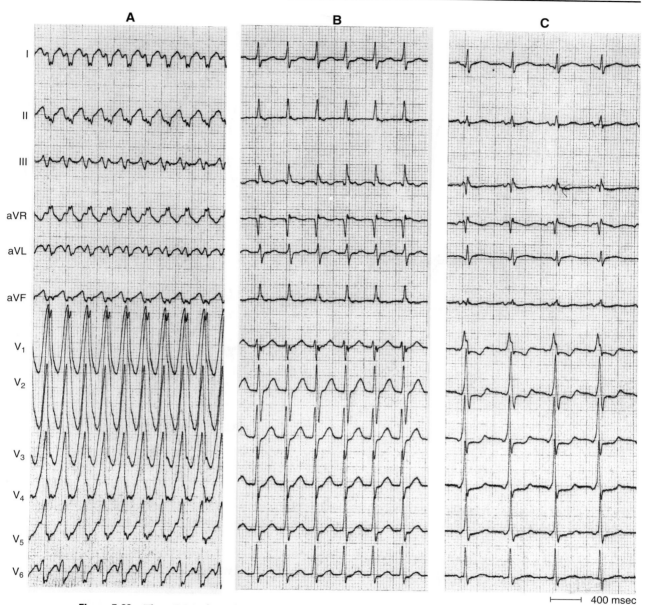

Figure 5-22   Three ECGs from the same patient. **A,** Atrial flutter with one-to-one AV conduction over a left free wall accessory pathway. **B,** An orthodromic circus movement tachycardia with AV conduction over the AV node and ventriculoatrial conduction over the left-sided accessory pathway. **C,** ECG during sinus rhythm showing ventricular preexcitation over a left-sided accessory pathway.

ria because VT can occur at all ages, and some patients are hemodynamically stable in spite of VT and hemodynamically compromised during SVT. More emphasis should be placed on ECG findings in broad QRS tachycardia.

Ventricular Rate During the Tachycardia

Heart rate is not helpful in distinguishing between SVT and VT. Although SVT tends to be faster than VT, too much overlap occurs to make this a useful criterion.

Regularity

Regular rhythm. A regular broad QRS tachycardia may be any of the following: VT, SVT with bundle branch block, or SVT with AV conduction over an accessory pathway.

Irregular rhythm. An irregular rhythm during a wide QRS tachycardia suggests bundle branch block during atrial fibrillation or atrial fibrillation with AV conduction over an accessory AV pathway. Occasionally, how-

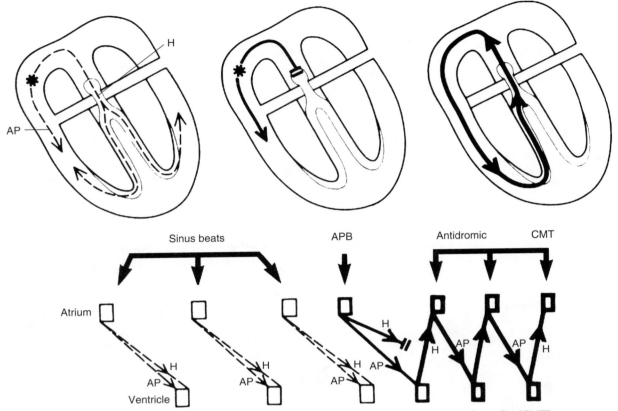

Figure 5-23 Scheme showing the initiation of an antidromic circus movement tachycardia *(CMT)* by an APB. At a critical premature beat interval the AV node–His *(H)* pathway becomes refractory, with AV conduction going exclusively over the accessory AV pathway *(AP)*. This is followed by retrograde conduction to the atrium over the His AV node pathway and antidromic CMT.

ever, VT, especially when drug-induced, may be quite irregular (as in polymorphic VT or torsades de pointes).

Wide QRS Tachycardias in Patients with an Accessory AV Pathway

In patients having an accessory AV pathway in addition to the normal AV connection through the AV node/His bundle–bundle branch system, tachycardias may occur with AV conduction over the accessory pathway (Wolff-Parkinson-White syndrome). These tachycardias have a wide QRS complex because the accessory AV pathway inserts into ventricular tissue, and ventricular activation, as in VT, starts outside the normal AV conduction system. The rhythm may be regular or irregular.

REGULAR TACHYCARDIAS

Regular wide QRS tachycardias in patients with an accessory AV pathway include antidromic CMT tachycardia and SVTs such as atrial tachycardia, atrial flutter

(Figure 5-22), and AV nodal reentrant tachycardia with AV conduction over the accessory pathway.

Antidromic Circus Movement Tachycardia

Antidromic CMT is based on a reentry circuit by an accessory pathway in the anterograde AV direction and the bundle branch–His–AV node pathway or a secondary accessory pathway in the retrograde direction. Figure 5-23 illustrates the initiation of an antidromic tachycardia by an APB. This tachycardia, because ventricular activation starts outside the normal AV conduction system, is indistinguishable from VT. Figure 5-13 is another example of an antidromic CMT in a patient with Wolff-Parkinson-White syndrome.

Emergency Response

1. Record a 12-lead ECG.
2. If hemodynamically unstable, cardiovert.
3. If hemodynamically stable, give IV procainamide 10 mg/kg over a 5-minute period.
4. If a sinus rhythm is not restored, cardiovert.

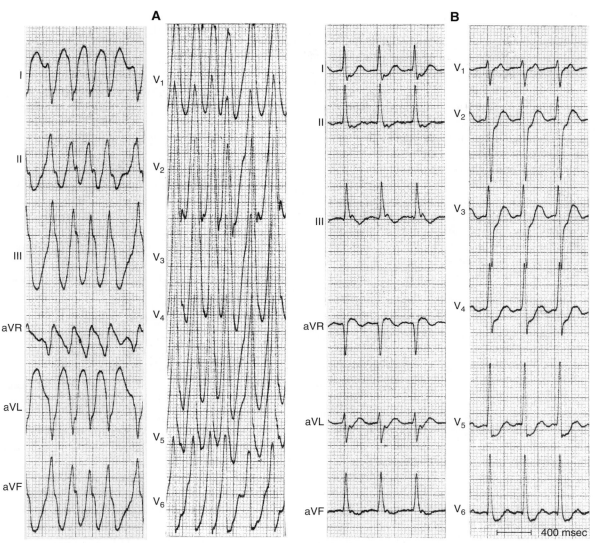

Figure 5-24 **A,** Atrial fibrillation in a patient with a left-sided accessory pathway. Note the very rapid ventricular rate because of a short anterograde refractory period of the accessory pathway. **B,** The same patient during orthodromic circus movement tachycardia using the left-sided accessory pathway for ventriculoatrial conduction.

IRREGULAR WIDE QRS TACHYCARDIA: ATRIAL FIBRILLATION WITH CONDUCTION OVER AN ACCESSORY PATHWAY

When atrial fibrillation occurs in a patient with Wolff-Parkinson-White syndrome, the resulting arrhythmia is fast, broad, and irregular.

The *ventricular rate* is fast and dependent on the refractory period of the accessory pathway; the shorter the refractory period, the faster the rate. Patients with atrial fibrillation and a short anterograde refractory period of the accessory pathway are at risk of

dying suddenly because atrial fibrillation with a very high ventricular rate may deteriorate into ventricular fibrillation.

The *broad QRS complexes* resemble those of VT in morphology, as shown in Figure 5-24, because the accessory AV pathway inserts into the ventricle, causing ventricular activation to begin as if from an ectopic focus at the location of ventricular insertion.

The *irregularity* of the ventricular rhythm is the result of many of the chaotic atrial fibrillatory impulses being conducted to the ventricles over the accessory pathway.

Emergency Response

A broad QRS tachycardia that is irregular with a ventricular rate of more than 200 beats/min and QRS morphologically identical to that of VT should immediately arouse the suspicion of atrial fibrillation with conduction over an accessory pathway.[4]

Emergency response to this arrhythmia is as follows:
1. Record a 12-lead ECG.
2. If hemodynamically unstable, cardiovert.
3. If hemodynamically stable, give IV procainamide 10 mg/kg over a 5-minute period.
4. If the ventricular rate does not slow with procainamide, cardiovert.
5. If the ventricular rate slows and sinus rhythm is restored, the patient should either be treated with drugs to prolong the refractory period of the accessory pathway and prevent the occurrence of premature beats that initiate atrial fibrillation, or, preferentially, referred for catheter ablation of the accessory pathway.

DANGER: Do not use digitalis or a calcium channel blocker in Wolff-Parkinson-White syndrome and atrial fibrillation. Such treatment may lead to a further increase in the ventricular rate. Digitalis may shorten the refractory period of the accessory pathway, and a calcium channel blocking agent such as verapamil may depress pump function, and subsequent sympathetic stimulation may lead to a further increase in ventricular rate.

Emergency Treatment of the Wide QRS Tachycardia

WHEN IN DOUBT

When a patient has a broad QRS tachycardia, diagnostic errors can be avoided by using a calm and systematic approach.

- If the patient is in poor hemodynamic condition, cardiovert; otherwise, follow the diagnostic steps that will differentiate a supraventricular from a ventricular origin of the tachycardia.
- When in doubt about the origin of the tachycardia, do not use verapamil; use IV procainamide instead.

One study observed a 44% incidence (11 of 25 patients) of severe hemodynamic deterioration when IV verapamil 5 to 10 mg was administered during VT, necessitating immediate cardioversion.[1,2] Hypotension with resulting ischemia may render the arrhythmia impossible to cardiovert.

Procainamide has advantages in both VT and SVT. It prolongs the refractory period of the ventricles and that of an accessory AV pathway and the retrograde fast AV nodal pathway. Procainamide may therefore terminate VT, CMT by an accessory pathway, and the common form of AV nodal reentry.

WHEN VT IS THE DIAGNOSIS

1. Give IV procainamide 10 mg/kg body weight over a 5-minute period; this prolongs the ventricular refractory period, slows conduction in the ventricle, and frequently terminates the arrhythmia.
2. Use lidocaine only if acute myocardial ischemia (as in acute MI) is considered the cause of the VT.[11]
3. If antiarrhythmic drug therapy is unsuccessful, cardiovert.

WHEN SVT IS THE DIAGNOSIS

1. Use vagal stimulation to prolong the refractory period of the AV node. A good vagal maneuver in prehospital emergencies is to ask the patient to cough; other vagal maneuvers include carotid sinus massage, gagging, Valsalva maneuver, Trendelenburg position, squatting, and facial immersion in cold water. If unsuccessful:
2. Give adenosine 6 mg IV over a 1- to 2-second period; if unsuccessful, give 12 mg IV 3 minutes later. If adenosine is not available:
3. Give verapamil 10 mg IV over a 5- to 10-minute period to block conduction in the AV node; reduce to 5 mg if the patient is taking a beta-blocking agent or is hypotensive. If unsuccessful:
4. Give IV procainamide 10 mg/kg body weight over a 5-minute period. This may lead to block of the retrograde AV nodal pathway if the mechanism is AV nodal reentry tachycardia; it may lead to retrograde block of the accessory pathway if the mechanism is CMT. Procainamide also prolongs the anterograde refractory period of an accessory AV pathway, thereby reducing the ventricular rate when the mechanism of the broad QRS tachycardia is atrial fibrillation with conduction over an accessory pathway. If unsuccessful:
5. Cardiovert.

SUPERIORITY OF PROCAINAMIDE OVER LIDOCAINE IN VT OUTSIDE AN EPISODE OF ACUTE CARDIAC ISCHEMIA

In a randomized study of sustained VT occurring outside an episode of acute ischemia, procainamide was found to be superior to lidocaine in terminating VT. In that study, patients were randomly given either lidocaine 1.5 mg/kg IV in 3 minutes or procainamide 10 mg/kg IV in 5 minutes. When one drug failed to convert the VT, the other drug was given 20 minutes later. Procainamide was far superior, both when given as initial treatment and after failure of lidocaine.[11]

SYSTEMATIC APPROACH TO WIDE QRS TACHYCARDIA

A calm demeanor and a well-established, orderly, and correct protocol are important. Hemodynamic status is not a clue to the mechanism of the arrhythmia. Hemodynamic instability means only that the patient must be immediately cardioverted, not that VT is present.

When the Patient Is Hemodynamically Unstable

1. Cardiovert
2. Stabilize
3. Evaluate systematically
4. Diagnose

Once the hemodynamically unstable patient has been cardioverted and stabilized, the preconversion 12-lead ECG should be evaluated for QRS configuration and signs of AV dissociation, QRS width, QRS axis, precordial concordance, and fusion beats to determine the mechanism of the tachycardia. Remember that every broad QRS tachycardia that is hemodynamically unstable is not necessarily VT. If it is SVT with aberration, important decisions must be made about the underlying mechanism (see Chapter 4).

When the Patient Is Hemodynamically Stable

1. Evaluate systematically
2. Diagnose
3. Treat

FOLLOW-UP CARE

When Cardioversion Was the First Therapeutic Response

1. Obtain a postcardioversion 12-lead ECG.
2. Carefully evaluate the preconversion and postconversion tracings to determine the site of origin and (if possible) the pathway of the tachycardia.
3. Examine the tracing during sinus rhythm for:
   - **MI,** which makes VT the most likely diagnosis
   - **Delta waves,** which, during sinus rhythm (preexcitation), suggest that the mechanism of a wide QRS during SVT is either CMT with bundle branch block or AV conduction over an accessory pathway.
   - **Bundle branch block.** In cases of preexisting bundle branch block, carefully compare the QRS during sinus rhythm with that during the tachycardia to diagnose VT or SVT with aberrant ventricular conduction. In SVT with preexisting bundle branch block, the QRS complex is identical to that of the sinus rhythm (Figure 5-25).
4. Take a careful history to establish the absence or presence of heart disease. Ask about how the arrhythmia was tolerated and events that may have triggered the episode, which may be prevented in the future. The answers to such questions are important because they help determine the significance and prognosis of the attacks of tachycardia as well as the most appropriate therapy. Thus the patient who has had a sustained episode of a tachycardia should be asked:
   - Have you had heart disease?
   - Have you had tachycardia before? If so,
   - At what age was the onset? (If the tachycardia was experienced initially at a young age, it is more likely to be SVT than VT.)
   - How often does the tachycardia occur and how long does it last?
   - Is there anything in particular that seems to trigger the onset of the tachycardia?
   - Did you have angina or dyspnea before or during the tachycardia?
   - Did you feel faint or pass out during the tachycardia?

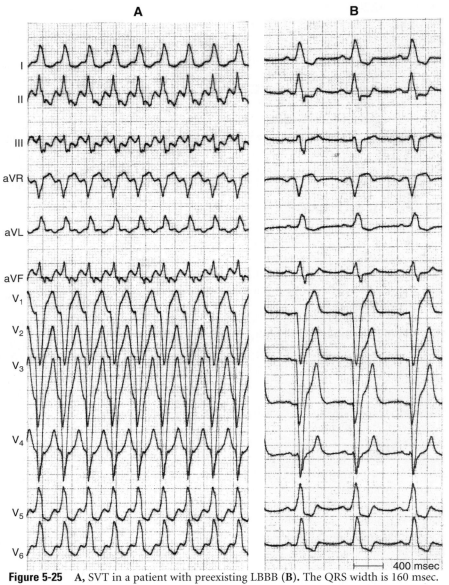

Figure 5-25 **A,** SVT in a patient with preexisting LBBB (**B**). The QRS width is 160 msec.

TABLE 5-1	Limitations of ECG Signs Suggestive of a Ventricular Origin of a Wide QRS Tachycardia
Signs	**Limitations**
AV dissociation during tachycardia	1. VA conduction during VT 2. Coexisting atrial fibrillation 3. AV junctional rhythm with bundle branch block
QRS width: >0.14 seconds in RBBB shape >0.16 seconds in LBBB shape	1. Preexisting bundle branch block, especially LBBB 2. SVT with AV conduction over an accessory pathway 3. Use of drugs slowing intraventricular conduction
Left axis deviation (<−30 degrees) in RBBB-shaped QRS	1. SVT with left anterior hemiblock 2. SVT during class IC drug administration
qR pattern in lead V_1 in RBBB-shaped QRS	SVT after anteroseptal MI
R/S <1 in lead V_6 in RBBB-shaped QRS	Frequently not present in RBBB-shaped QRS with right axis
R nadir S more than 100 msec in one or more precordial leads	1. SVT with drugs (especially class IC) slowing intraventricular conduction 2. SVT with AV conduction over an accessory pathway 3. Preexisting bundle branch block, especially LBBB
Concordant pattern in the precordial leads	Positive concordance may occur during SVT with AV conduction over a left posterior accessory pathway
Presence of q (Q) R complexes during tachycardia in leads other than aVR	Only in VT with localized scar (MI, sarcoidosis, amyloidosis)

When VT Was the Diagnosis

When VT is diagnosed, establish the cause of heart disease by the appropriate noninvasive and invasive tests and select long-term therapy accordingly.

When SVT Was the Diagnosis

When SVT is diagnosed, carefully study the preconversion tracings to determine the mechanism of the tachycardia. If an accessory pathway is involved, refer the patient to a cardiologist experienced in the study and management of tachycardias in Wolff-Parkinson-White syndrome (see Chapter 4).

SUMMARY

The systematic approach outlined in this chapter is essential when analyzing ECGs of patients with a wide QRS tachycardia. Table 5-1 reviews the different signs that should be checked and also indicates the possible limitations of the different signs. Correctly diagnosing the tachycardia is imperative because incorrectly diagnosing a SVT may lead to selecting inappropriate antiarrhythmic drugs and to deleterious results. Familiarity with the criteria described in this chapter should prevent such a misdiagnosis.

REFERENCES

1. Stewart RB, Bardy GH, Greene HL: Wide complex tachycardia: misdiagnosis and outcome after emergent therapy, *Ann Intern Med* 104:766-71, 1986.
2. Buxton AE, Marchlinski FE, Doherty JU, et al: Hazards of intravenous verapamil for sustained ventricular tachycardia, *Am J Cardiol* 59:1107-10, 1987.
3. Dancy M, Camm AJ, Ward D: Misdiagnosis of chronic recurrent ventricular tachycardia, *Lancet* 2:320-3, 1985.
4. Wellens HJJ, Bar FWHM, Lie KI: The value of the electrocardiogram in the differential diagnosis of a tachycardia with a widened QRS complex, *Am J Med* 64:27-36, 1978.
5. Kindwall E, Brown J, Josephson ME: Electrocardiographic criteria for ventricular tachycardia in wide complex left bundle branch block morphology tachycardia, *Am J Cardiol* 61:1279-83, 1988.
6. Wellens HJJ: Electrophysiology: ventricular tachycardia. Diagnosis of broad QRS complex tachycardia, *Heart* 86:579-85, 2001.
7. Harvey WP, Ronan JA: Bedside diagnosis of arrhythmias, *Prog Cardiovasc Dis* 8:419-31, 1966.
8. Marriott HJL: Differential diagnosis of supraventricular and ventricular tachycardia, *Geriatrics* 25:91-7, 1970.
9. Coumel P, Leclercq JF, Attuel P, et al: The QRS morphology in post-myocardial infarction ventricular tachycardia. A study in 100 tracings compared with 70 cases of idiopathic ventricular tachycardia, *Eur Heart J* 5:792-9, 1984.
10. Brugada P, Bruguda J, Mont L, et al. A new approach to the differential diagnosis of a regular tachycardia with a wide QRS complex, *Circulation* 83:1649-56, 1991.
11. Gorgels AP, van den Dool A, Hofs A, et al: Procainamide is superior to lidocaine in terminating sustained ventricular tachycardia, *Circulation* 80(suppl II):2590, 1989.

C H A P T E R

6

Digitalis-Induced Emergencies

EMERGENCY APPROACH

Systematic Diagnostic Approach

1. Obtain periodic 12-lead ECGs for all patients taking digitalis.
2. Question the patient regarding noncardiac symptoms of digitalis toxicity and concomitant medication that may interact with digitalis.
3. Know the ECG signs of digitalis arrhythmias.
4. Look specifically for bradycardia, tachycardia, inappropriate regularity (such as in atrial fibrillation or flutter), or group beating.

Emergency Management

1. Stop digitalis administration.
2. Prescribe bed rest (no sympathetic stimulation).
3. Initiate continuous ECG monitoring.
4. If hemodynamically unstable, phenytoin is indicated unless digitalis antibodies are available.
5. Ventricular pacing is indicated in the following situations:
   - Symptomatic bradycardia
   - During treatment with phenytoin because suppression of the tachycardia may be followed by asystole
6. Evaluate kidney function and correct potassium and magnesium deficits.

Avoid

   - Sympathetic stimulation (stress, anxiety, exercise, sympathomimetic drugs)
   - Carotid sinus massage
   - Fast or sudden cessation of ventricular pacing

Digitalis has a class I grading with an A classification because of evidence outlined in the American College of Cardiology and American Heart Association guidelines for chronic heart failure treatment.[1] Digitalis use is likely to increase in patients with atrial fibrillation after the outcome of studies comparing the effects of repeated attempts to obtain sinus rhythm versus accepting atrial fibrillation with adequate ventricular rate control.[2,3]

However, it is important to remember that digitalis has a narrow therapeutic window, with women requiring a lower dosage than men.[4] The mortality rate of unrecognized digitalis intoxication is high[5-7] and often unacknowledged because the patient is considered to have died from a "bad heart."

Because the complaints of patients with digitalis intoxication can be nonspecific and serum drug levels do not correlate well with toxicity, it is essential that health professionals caring for patients taking digitalis be familiar with the ECG findings suggestive of digitalis intoxication and know what to do in that situation.

ACTIONS

Digitalis, most commonly in the form of digoxin, is frequently used in heart failure and atrial fibrillation. As recently reviewed by Rahimtoola,[8] this inexpensive drug, which is more than 200 years old, has multiple actions such as the following:

- Positive inotropy
- Slowing of the ventricular rate during atrial fibrillation
- Vasodilatory effects
- Increase in baroreceptor sensitivity
- Reduction of plasma neurohormones
- Increase in vagal tone
- Diuresis

MECHANISM OF DIGITALIS TOXICITY

The arrhythmias of digitalis toxicity are the result of (1) a block in conduction, which may be located in the SA or AV nodal regions, or (2) rapid impulse formation in the atrium, AV junction, and ventricular Purkinje system.

Digitalis inhibits the enzyme sodium-potassium adenosine triphosphatase[9] and thus interferes with the sodium pump, causing sodium to accumulate within the cell, which in turn alters the sodium-calcium exchange. This results in a buildup of calcium within the cell, which explains the positive inotropic effect of the drug.[9] In an effort to rid the cell of excess calcium, after full repolarization (end of phase 3 of the action potential), a transient electrogenic sodium-calcium exchange occurs that briefly reduces the membrane potential (makes it less negative). It is this sodium/calcium exchange that mediates the delayed afterdepolarization, which may result in a propagated action potential called "triggered activity."[10] The result of this activity is the perpetuation of the typical tachycardias seen clinically in digitalis toxicity, such as atrial tachycardia, junctional tachycardia, and fascicular VT.

Figure 6-1 illustrates delayed afterdepolarization. The action potential in Figure 6-1, A, is followed by hyperpolarization of the membrane (marked negativity) and then a delayed afterdepolarization, which in this case does not reach threshold potential. In Figure 6-1, B, the delayed afterdepolarization reaches threshold potential and results in triggered activity. As the cycle length of the basic rhythm increases, so does that of the triggered rhythm.[10,11]

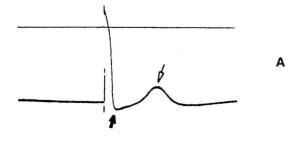

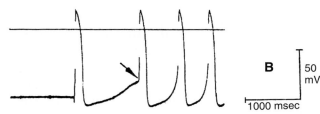

Figure 6-1 Delayed afterdepolarization and triggered activity. The *top line* is the reference 0 potential. **A,** A driven action potential is followed by hyperpolarization *(solid arrow)* and then delayed afterdepolarization *(open arrow).* **B,** A driven action potential is followed by a delayed afterdepolarization that reaches threshold potential. Nondriven action potentials *(arrow)* arise from the peak of each subsequent delayed afterdepolarization.

CONDITIONS THAT MAY PROMOTE DIGITALIS TOXIC ARRHYTHMIAS

Conditions that are capable themselves of producing triggered activity and therefore may promote arrhythmic expressions of digitalis intoxication include the following[12]:

- Increased sympathetic stimulation, which induces intracellular calcium overload
- Hypokalemia
- Hypercalcemia
- Hypomagnesemia
- Diuretics
- Ischemia and reperfusion
- Increased wall tension
- Heart failure

SUPPRESSANTS OF TRIGGERED ACTIVITY

- Beta-blockers
- Calcium antagonists
- Phenytoin
- Lidocaine
- Caffeine

ST-T SEGMENT CHANGES DURING DIGITALIS USE

- There is a concave depression of the ST-T segment in many ECG leads, especially leads II, III, AVF, and V_4 to V_6.
- There may be ST segment elevation in leads aVR and V_1.
- The QT interval is shortened.
- The height of the T wave is diminished.
- Usually U waves are present.

This effect of digitalis on the ST-T segment may last for 2 weeks after the drug is discontinued.

TYPICAL FEATURES OF DIGITALIS ARRHYTHMIAS

As indicated, digitalis excess can lead to conduction abnormalities in the SA and AV nodal region and enhanced impulse formation in the atria (usually close to the sinus node), the AV junction, and the ventricle (usually in the bundle branch–Purkinje system).

In healthy hearts digitalis intoxication (as in a suicide attempt or accidental ingestion) results in conduction abnormalities only, whereas in the sick heart both conduction abnormalities and enhanced impulse formation occur.[13] To recognize digitalis intoxication, clinicians should be alert for the following four ECG features:

1. The appearance of bradycardia when the heart rate was previously normal or fast (causes: SA or AV block)
2. The occurrence of tachycardia when the rate was previously normal (causes: atrial tachycardia, AV junctional tachycardia, and VT)
3. Unexpected rhythm regularity in a patient known to have an irregular rhythm (cause: complete AV block with a regular AV junctional rhythm in the patient with atrial fibrillation or atrial flutter)
4. The appearance of an irregular rhythm that regularly repeats itself, also called group beating (causes: ventricular bigeminy, SA or AV Wenckebach conduction, or combinations of these)

SLOW RHYTHMS
Sinus Bradycardia and SA Block

Digitalis suppresses phase 4 depolarization and causes conduction problems in the SA region. Thus sinus bradycardia, sinus arrest, and SA Wenckebach conduction may result from digitalis toxicity. SA Wenckebach conduction is diagnosed when group beating of the P waves is present with progressive shortening of the PP interval before the blocked beat. The ECG features of SA Wenckebach conduction and complete SA block are illustrated in Figures 6-2 and 6-3, respectively.

AV Nodal Block

Digitalis lengthens the refractory period of AV nodal tissue, which may lead to a prolonged PR interval, AV nodal Wenckebach conduction, or complete AV nodal block. An example of complete AV nodal block during atrial fibrillation is given in Figure 6-4.

In digitalis intoxication conduction disturbances in the SA and AV nodal regions are often combined, resulting in very challenging and complicated tracings (Figure 6-5).

RAPID RHYTHMS
Atrial Tachycardia with Block Caused by Digitalis Toxicity

- Atrial rate is 130 to 250 beats/min.
- Two-to-one AV block or AV Wenckebach conduction are usually present.
- P axis is usually directed inferiorly (P wave positive in leads II, III, and aVF).
- Ventriculophasic PP alternation is often present.

When digitalis is discontinued, AV conduction may improve before the atrial tachycardia abates, resulting in transient one-to-one AV conduction prior to conversion to sinus rhythm. Because the focus is usually high in the

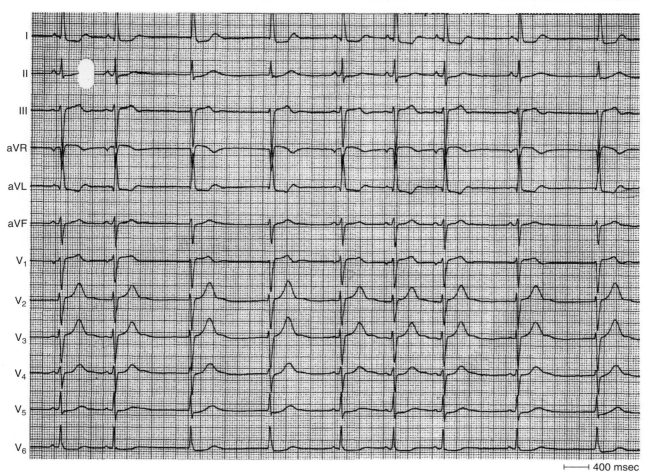

├────┤ 400 msec

Figure 6-2   This 12-lead ECG shows the presence of SA Wenckebach conduction in the beginning and middle of the tracing.

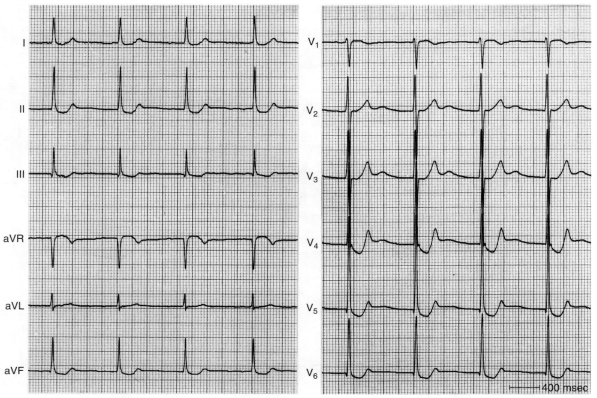

Figure 6-3   Complete SA block in digitalis intoxication. No sinus P waves are present.

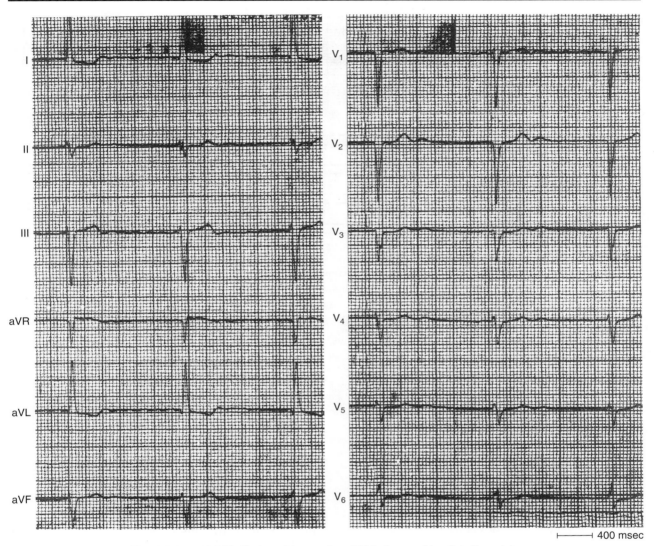

├────┤ 400 msec

Figure 6-4 Atrial fibrillation with complete AV block caused by digitalis toxicity.

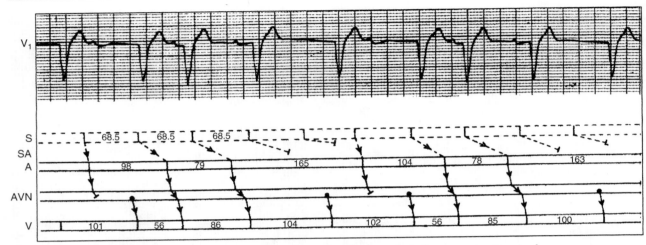

Figure 6-5 Complex arrhythmia presenting as a "regular irregularity" or group beating. As shown in the ladder diagram, SA Wenckebach conduction is present at the atrial level with second-degree AV nodal block and enhanced impulse formation in the AV junction.

right atrium close to the sinus node, the P waves closely resemble sinus P waves, causing the rhythm to mimic that of sinus tachycardia (Figure 6-6).

Ventriculophasic PP Intervals

Ventriculophasic behavior of PP intervals often occurs in atrial tachycardia caused by digitalis toxicity. That is, the PP interval embracing the R wave is shorter than the PP interval without an R wave. The fact that the P wave following the QRS is somewhat premature may cause a misdiagnosis of bigeminal nonconducted premature atrial complexes.

The mechanism of ventriculophasic alternation in PP intervals is the same as that seen when ventriculophasic alternation of PP intervals occurs in complete heart block. That is, peak vagal activity occurs just after the aortic pressure wave reaches the baroreceptors of

the carotid body. This causes the next atrial cycle (without a QRS complex) to lengthen.[14]

Figure 6-6, *A*, shows an atrial tachycardia with two-to-one AV block in a patient taking digitalis. The distance between the P waves on either side of the QRS is shorter than that between the P waves without the QRS (ventriculophasic PP alternation). Another feature of digitalis toxicity in these patients is the polarity of the P waves. They are similar to sinus P waves, (positive in leads II, III, and aVF), suggesting an origin close to the sinus node area.

AV Junctional Tachycardia Caused by Digitalis Toxicity

■ Ventricular rate is 70 to 140 beats/min.
■ Rhythm is nonparoxysmal.
■ The rate increases with exercise.

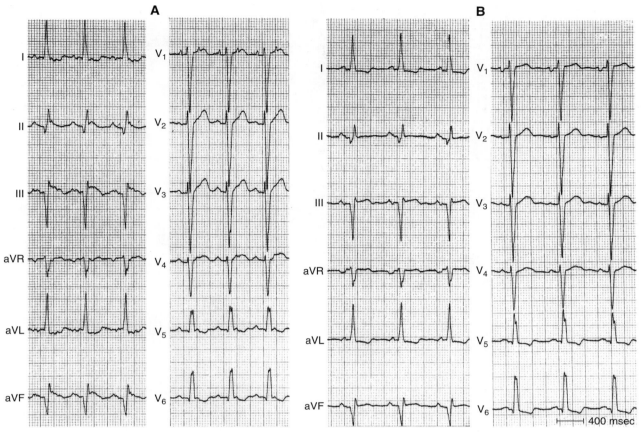

Figure 6-6   **A,** Atrial tachycardia with two-to-one AV block caused by digitalis toxicity. **B,** Same patient during sinus rhythm. In **A,** note the typical features of digitalis-induced atrial tachycardia: superior/inferior atrial activation, indicating an origin high in the right atrium, and ventriculophasic alternation of the PP interval during two-to-one AV block (i.e., the PP interval embracing the QRS is shorter than the PP without a QRS).

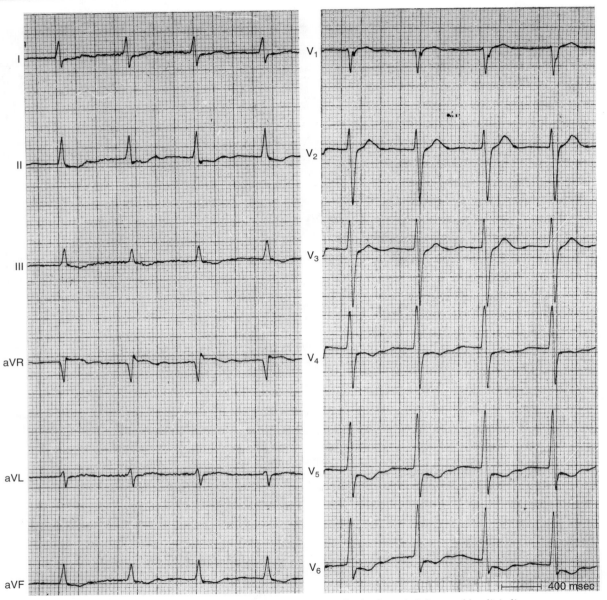

Figure 6-7   Atrial fibrillation with AV junctional tachycardia (95 beats/min) caused by digitalis toxicity. Note the absolute regularity of the rhythm.

- Carotid sinus massage has no effect or nodoventricular block may occur.
- AV dissociation is usually present.

Because of its gradual onset, this tachycardia is called *nonparoxysmal.*[15] Its rate, which is related to the severity of digitalis intoxication, rarely exceeds 140 beats/min and becomes apparent when the AV junctional discharge rate is faster than that of the sinus rhythm, usually at approximately 70 beats/min.

AV dissociation is common, and the term *accelerated AV junctional rhythm* is generally applied (Figure 6-7). When the rate exceeds 100 beats/min, it is called an *AV junctional tachycardia.* The arrhythmia is based on triggered activity in the AV junction. As shown in Figure 6-8, during AV junctional tachycardia anterograde Wenckebach conduction is often present. Note that in Figure 6-8, *B,* because of the discontinuation of digitalis, the rate of the junctional tachycardia slows, allowing one-to-one conduction to the ventricles and causing an increase in the heart rate.

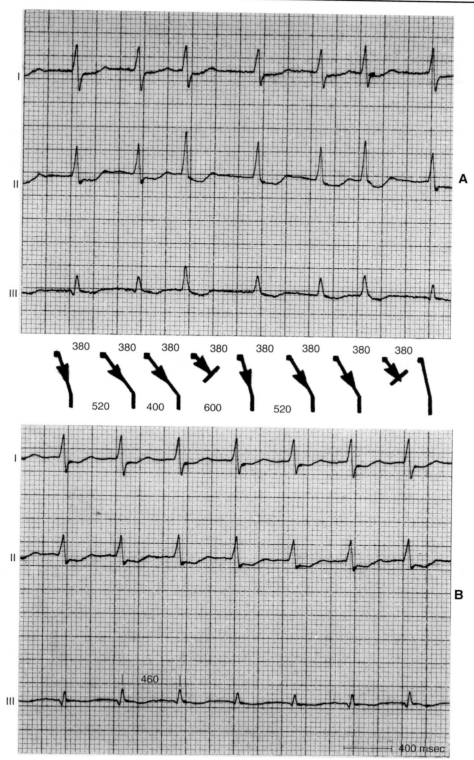

Figure 6-8 Atrial fibrillation and AV junctional tachycardia with Wenckebach conduction to the ventricles. **A,** Four-to-three Wenckebach conduction between the AV junction and the ventricles is present. **B,** One day later, AV junctional tachycardia is recorded at a slower rate, allowing one-to-one conduction from the AV junction to the ventricles.

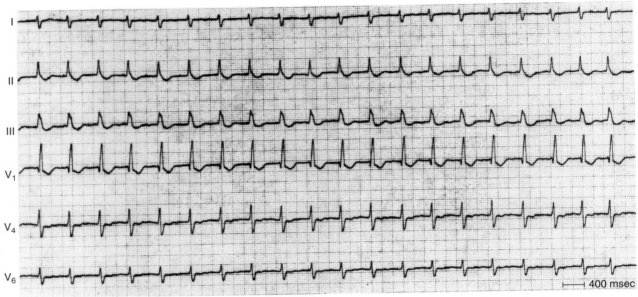

Figure 6-9 Fascicular VT caused by digitalis toxicity. Note the typical features of this arrhythmia: a QRS less than 0.14 seconds and an RBBB pattern. The right-axis deviation indicates an origin of the arrhythmia in the left anterior fascicle.

Fascicular VT Caused by Digitalis Toxicity

■ Ventricular rate is 90 to 160 beats/min.

■ QRS duration is 0.12 to 0.14 seconds.

■ The QRS usually has an RBBB shape.

■ Right- or left-axis deviation of the QRS is usually present.

In digitalis toxicity the site of impulse formation in the ventricle is located in bundle branch–Purkinje tissue, usually in the anterior or posterior fascicle of the left bundle branch; thus the term *fascicular VT* is applied. This results in a relatively narrow QRS complex (0.12 to 0.14 seconds), an RBBB-shaped QRS with either marked left-axis deviation (an origin in the posterior fascicle), or marked right-axis deviation (an origin in the anterior fascicle).

During tachycardia, changes may occur in QRS configuration from one beat to the next because of competition between Purkinje fibers for the pacing role. As with the other digitalis-toxic arrhythmias, its emergence is promoted by the shortening of the cycle length of preceding beats and by catecholamines. Short cycle lengths and increased sympathetic tone cause an otherwise "dormant" delayed afterdepolarization to reach threshold potential and produce triggered activity.

Figure 6-9 is an example of atrial fibrillation with a fascicular VT caused by digitalis toxicity. Note the relatively narrow QRS, the RBBB pattern in lead V_1, and the right-axis deviation. Figure 6-10 shows a double tachycardia, that is, atrial tachycardia and fascicular VT.

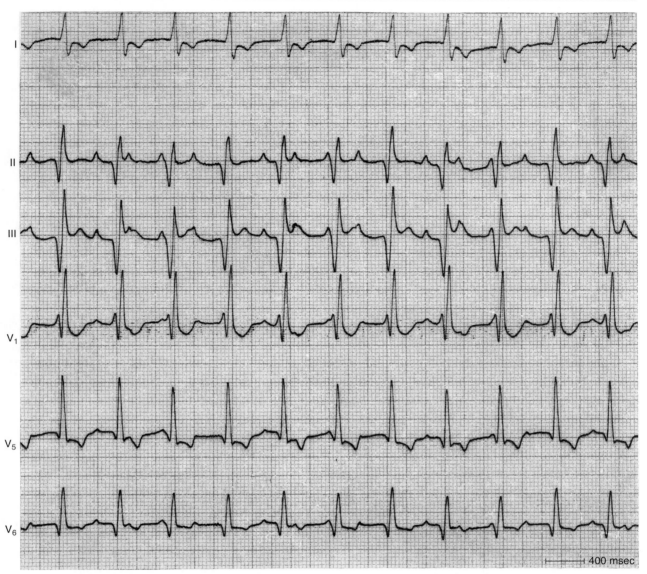

Figure 6-10   Double tachycardia: fascicular VT (110 beats/min) and atrial tachycardia (180 beats/min) caused by digitalis toxicity. Note the typical ECG signs of fascicular VT (RBBB pattern with a relatively narrow QRS) and the typical sign of digitalis-toxic atrial tachycardia (P-wave morphologic features similar to that of sinus P waves).

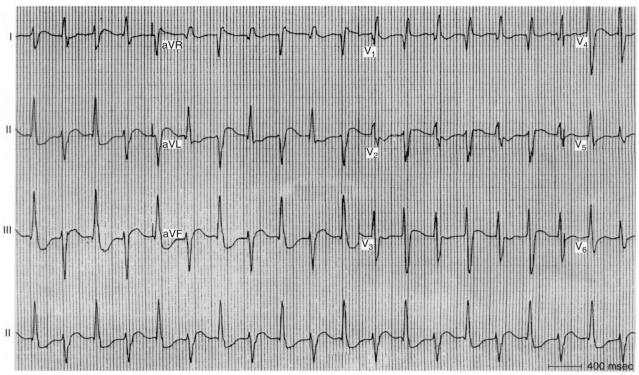

Figure 6-11 Bidirectional VT caused by digitalis toxicity. Note the typical features: RBBB pattern, relatively narrow QRS (0.12 seconds), and alternating left- and right-axis deviation, indicating alternating impulse formation in the left posterior and anterior fascicle.

ECG Features of Bifascicular VT

- Ventricular rate is 90 to 160 beats/min.
- QRS has an RBBB shape.
- QRS duration is 0.12 to 0.14 seconds.
- QRS axis alternates from right to left.

Bifascicular VT has long been recognized clinically as one of the signs of severe digitalis toxicity. The focus is alternating between the anterior and posterior fascicles of the left bundle branch, causing the frontal plane axis to alternate from left to right and giving the tachycardia a "bidirectional" look. As shown in Figure 6-11, the alternating frontal plane axis causes the height and shape of the ventricular complex in lead V_1 to alternate as well.

VENTRICULAR BIGEMINY

Figure 6-12 shows multimorphic ventricular bigeminy caused by digitalis toxicity. However, ventricular bigeminy is usually caused by coronary artery disease, in which case the bigeminal QRS complexes would be monomorphic.[16]

When ventricular bigeminy occurs during digitalis intoxication, because the Purkinje fibers compete for the pacing role, a typical finding is the changing QRS configuration of the bigeminal VPBs while the coupling interval stays fixed (Figure 6-12). Such a finding should immediately raise suspicion for digitalis intoxication.

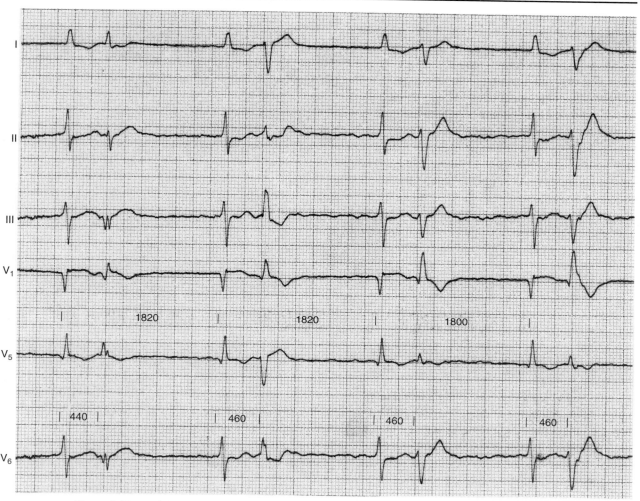

Figure 6-12 Multimorphic ventricular bigeminy caused by digitalis toxicity. The patient has atrial fibrillation with high-degree AV block. Despite small or no changes in coupling interval, the VPBs differ in QRS configuration because of different sites of origin in the Purkinje system of the LV.

ATRIAL FIBRILLATION WITH DIGITALIS TOXICITY

The ECG signs of digitalis toxicity in patients with atrial fibrillation include either regularization or group beating of the ventricular rhythm.

Possible Causes When the Rhythm Is Regular

- Complete AV block with a junctional escape rhythm (narrow QRS with a ventricular rate of fewer then 70 beats/min) (see Figure 6-4).
- Complete AV block with junctional tachycardia (narrow QRS with a ventricular rate of 70 to 140 beats/min) (see Figure 6-7).
- Complete AV block with (fascicular) VT (QRS, 0.12 to 0.14 seconds; RBBB shape; right- or left-axis

deviation; ventricular rate, 90 to 140 beats/min) (see Figure 6-9).

Possible Mechanism for Group Beating

Delay in conduction from a junctional focus (narrow QRS) to the ventricles may occur in a Wenckebach conduction mode. In this situation group beating, one of the hallmarks of Wenckebach conduction, occurs (see Figure 6-8). It is very important to be aware of this mechanism and to rule it out when evaluating a patient with atrial fibrillation, because at first glance the rhythm appears appropriately irregular, when although irregular, it actually has a uniform pattern of repetitive groups. Typically, when digitalis toxicity decreases and the AV junctional

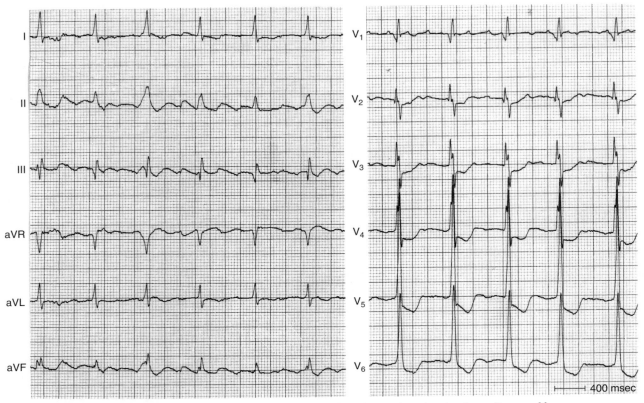

Figure 6-13 Atrial flutter with AV dissociation because of an AV junctional tachycardia caused by digitalis toxicity. No fixed relation between the flutter waves and the QRS complex is present (the ECG sign of AV dissociation during atrial flutter).

discharge rate slows, one-to-one conduction to the ventricle typically occurs (see Figure 6-8).

ATRIAL FLUTTER

The emergence of a junctional tachycardia caused by digitalis toxicity in atrial flutter is more difficult to diagnose than in atrial fibrillation, and toxicity may continue for days without being recognized on the ECG. Toxicity typically may occur in the critical care unit after cardiac or pulmonary surgery.

In uncomplicated atrial flutter conduction between the atria and the ventricles is usually in a two-to-one or Wenckebach mode. When the conduction ratio is constant (e.g., two to one or four to one) the time interval between the flutter wave and the R wave should be the same every time. In digitalis intoxication, however, no conduction between atria and ventricles exists, and the atrial flutter rhythm has no relation to the escape or accelerated AV junctional rhythm. Both rhythms are regular but unrelated (Figure 6-13).

ECG Signs of Digitalis Toxicity in Atrial Flutter

- Atrial flutter with complete AV block and a junctional escape rhythm (narrow QRS with a ventricular rate of fewer than 60 beats/min)
- Atrial flutter with a junctional tachycardia and AV dissociation (narrow QRS with a ventricular rate of 70 to 140 beats/min)
- Atrial flutter with fascicular VT (QRS of 0.12 to 0.14 seconds with an RBBB shape and a ventricular rate of 90 to 160 beats/min; right- or left-axis deviation)

SYMPTOMS OF DIGITALIS INTOXICATION

- Gastrointestinal (nausea, vomiting, diarrhea, abdominal pain, anorexia)
- Visual (ptosis; changes in color vision, especially red and green; reduced vision because of diminished accommodation; binocular central scotoma)
- Neuropsychiatric (hallucinations, nightmares, restlessness, insomnia, pseudodementia, and depression)
- Muscular (fatigue, weakness)

Many factors determine whether a given blood level of digitalis is actually toxic. Thus serum concentrations should not be used as the sole basis for evaluating toxicity. The ECG and symptoms are valuable to the clinician in making these decisions.

The patient and family should be questioned specifically regarding any medication the patient is taking, noticeable changes in bowel habits, any changes in reading ability, and changes in behavior, such as lack of energy, depression, and pseudodementia. Usually, neither the patient nor the family members volunteer these symptoms, and they must be prompted with questions regarding a change in the clearness of the colors on television, clearness of the print when reading the newspaper, forgetfulness, and loss of interest in surroundings.

MORTALITY RATE IN UNDIAGNOSED DIGITALIS TOXICITY

The mortality rate of unrecognized digitalis arrhythmias has been shown to be very high.[6-8] In one study, when atrial tachycardia with block went unrecognized and digitalis was continued, 100% (7 of 7 patients) died.[8] When the drug was stopped, a 6% mortality rate was present (1 of 16 patients). When junctional tachycardia was not recognized as a digitalis arrhythmia, 81% died (25 of 31 patients); when the diagnosis was made and the drug was stopped, the mortality rate was 16% (7 of 43 patients).

FACTORS AFFECTING DOSAGE REQUIREMENTS IN PATIENTS TAKING DIGITALIS
Drug Interaction

Among other factors, the arrhythmias of digitalis toxicity may result from the interaction of digitalis with other drugs that the patient is taking. These factors are summarized in Table 6-1, which shows some frequently prescribed cardioactive drugs that need a somewhat longer discussion. Heininger-Rothbucher et al[17] found in a review of emergency department records that simply because of the higher number of concurrent medications being taken by the elderly, potential adverse drug interactions were more common.

Quinidine. When quinidine is added to digoxin therapy, the dose of digoxin should be decreased by approximately 50%. In this clinical setting, the serum digoxin concentration increases because of a reduction in both the volume of distribution of digoxin and its renal and nonrenal clearance.[18]

Amiodarone. Depending on the dose, amiodarone increases plasma digoxin concentration partly because of

a decrease in renal and nonrenal clearance of digoxin and an increase in digoxin half-life.[18]

Verapamil. Both renal and nonrenal clearance of digoxin decrease when digoxin and verapamil are combined. This effect develops gradually during the first few days and reaches a steady state within 7 days.[19]

Diltiazem. A 22% increase in steady-state plasma digoxin concentration occurs when diltiazem 180 mg/day is added to digoxin.

Drugs That Do Not Appear to Affect Digoxin Concentration

- Beta-blocking agents (these agents may, however, potentiate the bradycardiac effects of digitalis)
- Angiotensin-converting enzyme inhibitors
- Angiotensin II receptor blockers
- Aldosterone antagonists
- Procainamide
- Disopyramide
- Mexiletine
- Flecainide
- Nifedipine

TREATMENT OF DIGITALIS ARRHYTHMIAS

Treatment of digitalis-toxic arrhythmias depends on the clinical condition rather than the serum drug level.

Management varies from temporary withdrawal of the medication to administration of digoxin-specific Fab fragments for life-threatening cardiovascular arrhythmias,[20] or when digitalis antibodies are not available, other ectopic impulse formation–suppressing drugs such as phenytoin or lidocaine. The treatment process is as follows:

1. Discontinue digitalis.
2. Prescribe bed rest (no sympathetic stimulation).
3. Perform continuous ECG monitoring.
4. Correct electrolyte abnormalities.
5. Actively treat a rapid ventricular rhythm depending on the site of origin of the arrhythmia and its hemodynamic consequences.
6. If the arrhythmia is ventricular in origin, especially when a bidirectional tachycardia is present, administer digitalis antibodies or phenytoin.
7. Insert a ventricular pacing lead if phenytoin is used because the drug may not only suppress the arrhythmia, thereby exposing high-degree block, but also prevent escape rhythms from occurring because digitalis depresses phase 4 depolarization in His-Purkinje cells.
8. Ventricular pacing is indicated when digitalis-induced bradycardia by SA block or AV block leads to hemodynamic deterioration.

TABLE 6-1	Factors Influencing Dosage Requirements in Patients Receiving Digitalis	
Factor	**Higher Dosage Needed**	**Lower Dosage Needed**
Intestinal resorption	Malabsorption Antacids Oral antibiotics Cholestyramine Colestipol	Anticholinergic drugs
Body clearance (renal and nonrenal)	Hyperthyroidism	Renal disease Old age Hypothyroidism Quinidine Amiodarone Spironolactone Verapamil Diltiazem
Volume of distribution	Hyperthyroidism	Small physical size Women Old age Renal disease Hypothyroidism Chronic pulmonary disease Quinidine Spironolactone
Binding to cardiac muscle	Hyperkalemia Reserpine	Hypokalemia Hypomagnesemia
Unexplained sensitivity or tolerance	Young age Hypocalcemia	Congestive heart failure Myocardial ischemia Chronic pulmonary disease Hypercalcemia

9. Determine the kidney function to estimate how long the intoxicating effect of digitalis will last (Box 6-1).

Digitalis Antibodies

Digoxin-immune antibody fragments (Fab) for treatment of digitalis intoxication were introduced in 1976. Administration of Fab according to the manufacturer's dosage recommendation immediately reverses the tachyarrhythmia of digitalis toxicity and reestablishes a normal level of serum potassium within minutes.

BOX 6-1

Estimation of the Creatinine Clearance by the Crockroft and Gault Formula[21]

Creatinine clearance = [(140 − Age in yr) + Weight in kg)] + [72 × Serum creatinine in mg/L]
Multiply the creatine clearance by 0.85 for women.

Prompt treatment with digoxin-specific Fab fragment may be life saving.[20]

DANGERS OF PACING AND CAROTID SINUS MASSAGE

- Rapid pacing in a patient with an arrhythmia based on delayed afterdepolarizations may cause acceleration of the arrhythmia.
- Sudden cessation of pacing may cause asystole because of failure of escape beats from the depressed phase 4 depolarization in His-Purkinje cells.
- In patients with digitalis intoxication, carotid sinus massage has been reported to result in worsening of the arrhythmias and induction of ventricular fibrillation.

A SYSTEMATIC EVALUATION OF PATIENTS TAKING DIGITALIS

The arrhythmias in the setting of digitalis toxicity may be complex because more than one focus of abnormal impulse formation may be present (e.g., atrial tachycardia in combination with junctional or fascicular VT).

A combination of blocks, such as AV nodal block and SA nodal block, may also be present. Thus the interpretation of the ECG should be approached systematically after the history is taken. Box 6-2 and the following points provide a guide for evaluating the ECG of patients who are taking digitalis:

1. Talk to your patient, inquiring about the dose of digitalis, additional medication, and symptoms such as visual and gastrointestinal disturbances.
2. Talk to the patient's family, inquiring about the patient's symptoms and personality changes.
3. Before looking at the ECG, review what abnormalities can be encountered as arrhythmic expressions of digitalis toxicity.
4. Evaluate the ECG systematically (see Box 6-2), starting at the atrial level (SA nodal conduction? Atrial tachycardia?) and then down through the AV node (AV block? Junctional tachycardia?), into the His-Purkinje system (Fascicular VT? Bidirectional VT? Ventricular bigeminy?). Such an approach helps identify the different ectopic rhythms and conduction abnormalities that may occur during digitalis intoxication.
5. When the patient with atrial fibrillation is taking digitalis, although the rate slows, the rhythm should remain totally irregular. Regularization indicates either a junctional or ventricular rhythm. A junctional rhythm can be rapid (70 to 140 beats/min) or slow, as in complete AV block. A fascicular ventricular rhythm can be 90 to 160 beats/min.
6. Group beating in atrial fibrillation with a narrow QRS suggests junctional tachycardia with Wenckebach conduction to the ventricle.
7. If atrial flutter is present, the flutter/R-wave relation should be constant or vary in a repetitive fashion as it would with Wenckebach conduction; this is not the case when digitalis toxicity causes complete AV block and accelerated AV junctional impulse formation. The ECG then shows varying flutter/R-wave relations with a regular ventricular rhythm.

BOX 6-2

Systematic Evaluation of the ECG for Digitalis Toxicity

P-Wave Regularity, Rate, and Axis
- If slow, regular, or irregular, suspect SA block.
- If atrial rate >120 beats/min, evaluate the P-wave axis to recognize atrial tachycardia.
- In case of two-to-one AV conduction during atrial tachycardia, look for P-P ventriculophasic alternation.

AV Conduction
- Signs of AV conduction disturbances (prolonged PR, Wenckebach conduction, complete AV block)?

AV Junctional Rhythm
- Is AV conduction present?
- If not, what is the rate of the AV junctional focus?
- Is the tachycardia paroxysmal or nonparoxysmal?
- If nonparoxysmal and the rate is 70-130 beats/min, suspect digitalis toxic AV junctional tachycardia.

Atrial Fibrillation
- Is the ventricular rhythm intermittently or continuously regular, slow, normal, or rapid?
- Suspect digitalis toxicity when the ventricular rhythm is slow and regular; this suggests AV block. When the ventricular rate is normal or high, suspect accelerated AV junctional rhythm.

Atrial Flutter
- Suspect digitalis toxicity when both the flutter and the ventricular rhythm are regular but without a fixed interval between the flutter wave and the QRS complex.

Fascicular VT
- Are the widened QRS complexes conducted from the atrium?
- If not, what is the rate?
- If 90-150 beats/min, suspect fascicular VT, especially when the QRS shows an RBBB-like shape, has a width of 0.12-0.14 seconds, and a frontal plane axis suggesting an origin in one of the fascicles of the left bundle branch.

Ventricular Bigeminal Rhythm
- Suspect digitalis toxicity when during a ventricular bigeminal rhythm the QRS is relatively narrow (0.12-0.14 seconds) and shows changes in configuration while the coupling interval stays fixed.

SUMMARY

The mortality rate associated with digitalis toxicity often goes unrecognized because the poisoning process is slow and the patient is being treated for heart problems, which are ultimately blamed for the patient's symptoms and death. Toxicity is diagnosed by subjective and ECG symptoms because digitalis blood level is unreliable as a sole indicator. Digitalis causes SA and AV conduction problems. The foci for abnormal impulse formation can be located in the atrium, AV junction, and the fascicles of the bundle branches.

These arrhythmias have the following typical diagnostic features:

- In atrial tachycardia the P waves are usually positive in leads II, III, and aVF; the rate is between 130 and 250 beats/min; and two-to-one AV block is present, often with ventriculophasic behavior of the PP intervals.
- In junctional tachycardia retrograde block (AV dissociation) is usually present; the rate is between 70 and 140 beats/min and depends on the degree of digitalis toxicity with a gradual (nonparoxysmal) onset and offset.
- In fascicular VT the rate is between 90 and 160 beats/min and the QRS shows RBBB configuration measuring between 0.12 and 0.14 seconds.

Emergency management consists of discontinuation of digitalis, bed rest, and correction of electrolyte abnormalities. The use of digitalis antibodies, phenytoin, and ventricular pacing depends on the site of origin and hemodynamic consequences of the arrhythmia.

REFERENCES

1. Hunt SA, Baker DW, Clin MH, et al: ACC/AHA guidelines for the evaluation and management of chronic heart failure in the adult: executive summary, *J Am Coll Cardiol* 38:2101-13, 2001.
2. Wyse DG, Waldo AL, DiMarco JP, et al: A comparison of rate control and rhythm control in patients with atrial fibrillation, *N Engl J Med* 347:1825-33, 2002.
3. Van Gelder IC, Hagens VE, Bosker HA, et al: A comparison of rate control and rhythm control in patients with recurrent persistent atrial fibrillation, *N Engl J Med* 347:1834-40, 2002.
4. Adams KF J., Georghiade M, Uretsky BF, et al: Clinical benefits of low serum digoxin concentration in heart failure, *J Am Coll Cardiol* 39:946-53, 2002.
5. Williamson KM, Trasher KA, Fulton KB, et al: Digoxin toxicity: an evaluation in current clinical practice, *Arch Int Med* 158:2444-9, 1998.
6. Gandhi AJ, Vlasses PH, Morton DJ, et al: Economic impact of digoxin toxicity, *Pharmacoeconomics* 12(2 pt 1):175-81, 1997.
7. Dreyfus LS, McKnight EH, Katz M, et al: Digitalis intolerance, *Geriatrics* 18:494-502, 1963.
8. Rahimtoola SH: Digitalis therapy for patients in clinical heart failure, *Circulation* 109:2942-6, 2004.
9. Katz AM: Effects of digitalis on cell biochemistry: sodium pump inhibition, *J Am Cardiol* 5:16A, 1985.
10. Rosen MR: The relationship of delayed after depolarizations to arrhythmias in the intact heart, *PACE* 6:1151-62, 1983.
11. Gadsby DC, Wit AL: Normal and abnormal electrical activity in cardiac cells. In Mandel WJ, editor: *Cardiac Arrhythmias*, Philadelphia, 1987, Lippincott, pp 53-80.
12. Gorgels APM, Vos MA, Brugada P, et al: The clinical relevance of abnormal automaticity and triggered activity. In Brugada P, Wellens HJJ, editors: *Cardiac Arrhythmias: Where to Go from Here?* Mount Kisco, 1987, Futura, pp 147-69.
13. Wellens HJJ: The electrocardiogram in digitalis intoxication. In Yu PN, Goodwin JF, editors: *Progress in Cardiology*, vol 5, Philadelphia, 1976, Lea & Febiger, pp 271-90.
14. Rosenbaum MB, Lepeschkin E. Effects of ventricular systole on auricular rhythm in auriculo-ventricular block, *Circulation* 11:240-61, 1955.
15. Pick A, Dominguez P: Nonparoxysmal AV nodal tachycardia, *Circulation* 16:1022-32, 1957.
16. Vanagt EJ, Wellens HJJ: The electrocardiogram in digitalis intoxication. In Wellens HJJ, Kulbertus HE, editors: *What's New in Electrocardiography?* The Hague, 1981, Martinus Nijhof, pp 315-43.
17. Heininger-Rothbucher D, Bischinger S, Ulmer H, et al: Incidence and risk of potential adverse drug interactions in the emergency room, *Resuscitation* 49:283-8, 2001.
18. Marcus FI: Pharmacokinetic interactions between digoxin and other drugs, *J Am Coll Cardiol* 5:82A-90A, 1985.
19. Klein HO, Lang R, Weiss E, et al: The influence of verapamil on serum digoxin concentration, *Circulation* 65:998-1003, 1982.
20. Ma G, Brady WJ, Pollack M, et al: Electrocardiographic manifestations: digitalis toxicity, *J Emerg Med* 20:145-52, 2001.
21. Crockroft DW, Gault MH: Prediction of creatinine clearance from serum creatinine, *Nephron* 16:31-41, 1976.

CHAPTER
7
Drug-Induced Arrhythmic Emergencies

EMERGENCY TREATMENT

Torsades de Pointes
1. Stop the offending drug.
2. Establish continuous ECG monitoring.
3. Give magnesium (as MgCl or MgSO$_4$) as a 1- to 2-g intravenous bolus over a 5-minute period.
4. Start infusion, 1 to 2 g/hr for 4 to 6 hours.
5. If intravenous magnesium is unsuccessful, increase the heart rate with isoproterenol or by pacing.

Sustained (Incessant) Monomorphic VT
1. Stop the offending drug.
2. In case of hemodynamic compromise, give inotropic support with isoproterenol or epinephrine, which will also counteract slowing in conduction velocity induced by class IA or class IC drugs.
3. If VT persists and is poorly tolerated, pace the atrium at the rate of the VT. Use an AV interval that will provide maximal contribution of atrial contraction to ventricular filling.

Drug-Induced Bradycardia
1. Stop the offending drug.
2. Give atropine or start temporary transvenous pacing in case of Adams-Stokes attacks, a low ventricular rate leading to hypotension, or bradycardia-dependent ventricular arrhythmias.

Drug-induced arrhythmic emergencies can be caused by antiarrhythmic agents, noncardiac drugs, and even non-prescription drugs. These arrhythmic complications may result in sudden death.[1]

MECHANISMS OF DRUG-INDUCED ARRHYTHMIAS

The different mechanisms playing a role in the genesis of cardiac arrhythmias are reentry, abnormal automaticity, and afterdepolarizations (Figure 7-1). When arrhythmias are drug induced, afterdepolarizations and reentry have been described as the probable mechanisms.

AFTERDEPOLARIZATIONS

Afterdepolarizations are the result of two distinct mechanisms designated as "late" (delayed) and "early." Certain drugs, cardiac and noncardiac, are capable of creating cellular conditions that prolong the QT interval and are favorable for the generation of afterdepolarizations.

As shown in Figure 7-1, a tachycardia may be initiated when either type of afterdepolarization reaches threshold potential for certain membrane channels.[2,3]

Delayed Afterdepolarizations

Delayed afterdepolarizations are the result of interference with the sodium-potassium–adenosine triphosphatase pump and intracellular calcium overload. This mechanism is associated with digitalis toxicity and is discussed in Chapter 6.

Early Afterdepolarizations

Early afterdepolarizations usually result from a disruption of transmembrane potassium channels caused by either genetic mutation, discussed in Chapter 11, or QT-prolonging drugs. The unique tachycardia spawned by this cellular disruption and supported by reentry is

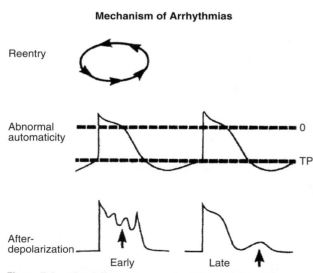

Mechanism of Arrhythmias

Reentry

Abnormal automaticity

After-depolarization

Early   Late

Figure 7-1 The different causes of cardiac arrhythmias: reentry, abnormal automaticity, and afterdepolarizations. The role of abnormal automaticity in drug-induced arrhythmias is not currently clear. *TP,* Threshold potential.

known by the French term *torsades de pointes* (TdP)[4,5] and usually occurs against a background of QT prolongation and pauses in rhythm.

QT PROLONGATION

Drugs that prolong the QT interval favor the development of early afterdepolarizations in phases 2 and 3 of the ventricular membrane action potential (see Figure 7-1). On reaching threshold potential for the slow calcium channel, the early afterdepolarization may result in ectopic impulse formation.[2,3] The ectopic impulses thus formed may in turn trigger reentrant excitation of the ventricle, resulting in TdP.

In cases in which QT-prolonging drugs are being used, the tachycardia itself and the unique ECG characteristics of TdP are the results of the electrophysiologic actions of those drugs, in that they may induce heterogeneity in action potential duration at neighboring ventricular sites.[4,5] Susceptibility for this mechanism is genetically determined by and based on the ability of the different QT-prolonging drugs to induce repolarization currents, especially in Purkinje fibers and midmyocardial cells.[6,7]

TORSADES DE POINTES
ECG Findings

- Polymorphic VT with beat-to-beat changes in the QRS axis ("twisting of the points") is a characterization of TdP.[4]
- QT prolongation typically precedes TdP along with a pause-dependent (long-short cycle) initiation of the arrhythmia (Figure 7-2).
- Bradycardia facilitates the occurrence of TdP.
- Alternation of the QT configuration may precede the initiation of the arrhythmia (Figure 7-3).

Causes

There is a long and ever-expanding list of drugs that prolong the QT interval and may promote the occurrence of early afterdepolarizations and TdP, including antiarrhythmic drugs, structurally diverse noncardiac drugs, nonprescription drugs, and in some cases herbal medications (Box 7-1).[8]

Risk Factors

As shown in Box 7-2 several factors increase the risk of drug-induced TdP because of QT prolongation. Progressive lengthening of the QT interval and the development of a prominent U wave are seen as markers of an increased risk for serious adverse drug effects, syncope, or death from TdP. Prolongation of the absolute QT interval beyond 500 msec is regarded as a value that requires prompt critical reevaluation of the risks and

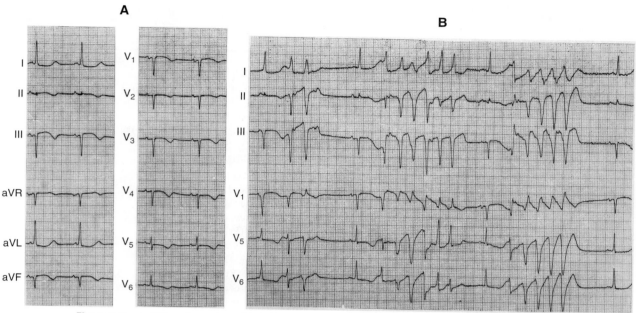

Figure 7-2 **A,** QT prolongation after quinidine administration. **B,** Torsades de pointes. Note the prolonged QT interval, the long-short cycles preceding the onset of the tachycardia, and the typical oscillating morphologic features of the ventricular complexes.

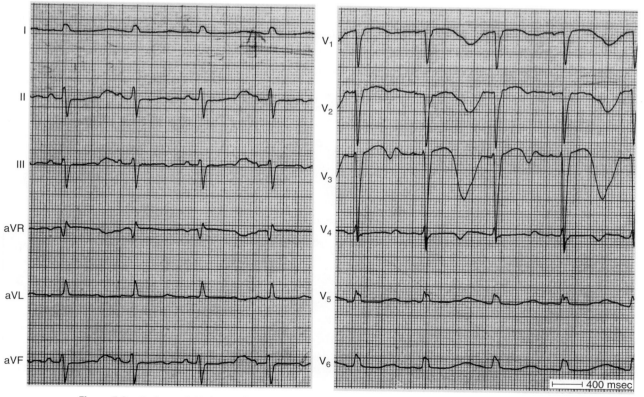

Figure 7-3 Prolonged QT interval and U waves, with alternation of the QT configuration after the administration of sotalol.

BOX 7-1

Drugs That Prolong the QT Interval

Acrivastine* (Semprex-D)
Ajmaline
Almokalant
Amantadine (Symmetrel)
Amiodarone (Cordarone)
Amitriptyline (Elavil, Endep, Etrafon, Limbitrol, Triavil)
Amoxapine (Asendin)
Ampicillin (Omnipen, Polycillin, Principen)
Amrinone (Inocor)
Aprinidine
Astemizole† (Hismanal)
Azimilide
Bepridil (Vascor)
Bretylium (Bretylate, Bretylol)
Budipine
Cetirizine* (Zyrtec)
Chloral hydrate
Chloroquine (Aralen)
Chlorpromazine (Largactil; Thorazine)
Cisapride‡ (Propulsid)
Citalopram (Celexa)
Clarithromycin (Biaxin)
Clemastine (Tavist)
Clofilium
Clomipramine (Anafranil)
Co-trimoxazole (Septra, Bactrim, SMX-TMP)
Droperidol (Inopsine)
Desipramine (Norpramin)
Diphenhydramine (Benadryl)
Disopyramide (Norpace)
Dofetilide (Tikosyn)
Doxepin (Sinequan, Zonalon)
Droperidol (Inapsine)
Ebastine (Ebastel)
Erythrocin (Erythrostatin, Ilotycin, PCE, Staticin)
Erythromycin (Akne-Mycin, EES, E-Mycin, Eryderm, Erygel, Ery-Tab, Eryc, EryPed)
Fexofenadine* (Allegra)
Flecainide (Tambocor)
Fludrocortisone (Florinef)
Fluphenazine (Permitil, Prolixin)
Gatifloxacin
Grepafloxacin
Halofantrine (Halfan)
Haloperidol (Haldol)
Hydroxyzine (Atarax, Atazine, Dovaril, Hypam, Vistacot, Vistaril, Vistawin)
Ibutilide (Corvert)
Imidazole (Lotrimin)
Imipramine (Tofranil)
Indapamide (Lozol)

Ipecac
Itraconazole (Sporanox)
Ketanserin (Aserinox, Ketensin, Perketan, Serepress, Sufrexal)
Ketoconazole (Nizoral)
Lidoflazine (Clinium, Ordiflazine)
Lithium
Loratidine* (Claritin)
Lubeluzole (Prosynap)
Maprotiline (Ludiomil)
Mefloquine (Lariam)
Mesoridazine (Serentil)
Milrinone (Primacor)
Mibefradil (Posicor)
Mizolastine* (Mistamine)
Moricizine (Ethmozine)
N-acetyl-procainamide
Nortriptyline (Pamelor)
Papaverine, intracoronary
Pentamidine (Nebupent, Pentam, Pentacarinat)
Pericycline
Perphenazine (Trilafon)
Phenothiazines (chlorpromazine, Compazine, Mellaril, Permitil, Prolixin, pinacidil, Serentil, Stelazine, Thorazine, Trilafon, Vesprin)
Pimozide (Orap)
Pinacidil (Pindac anhydrous)
Prenylamine† (Prenylamin)
Probucol (Lorelco)
Procainamide (Procan, Procanbid, Pronestyl)
Prochlorperazine (Compazine)
Propafenone (Rythmol)
Protriptyline (Vivactil)
Quetiapine (Seroquel)
Quinidine (Cardioquin, Duraquin, Quinaglute, Quinidex)
Quinine
Risperidone (Risperdal)
Sematilide
Sertindole† (Serdolect)
DL-Sotalol (Betapace)
Sparfloxacine
Spiramycin
Sultopride (Cloridrato)
Tamoxifen (Nolvadex)
Terikalant
Terfenadine‡ (Seldane)
Terodiline†
Thioridazine (Mellaril)
Thiothixene (Navane)
Timiperone
Trifluoperazine (Stelazine)

BOX 7-1—cont'd
Drugs That Prolong the QT Interval
Trimethoprim sulfamethoxazole (Bactrim, Septra)
Troleandomycin (Tao)
Vasopressin (Pitressin)
Zimeldine (Zelmid)
Ziprasidone (Geodon)

See also www.torsades.org.
*New nonsedating antihistamine; effect on IKr needs confirmation.
†Off the market.
‡Off the market in some countries.

BOX 7-2
Risk Factors for Drug-Induced Torsades de Pointes
Baseline QT prolongation
Bradycardia
Cardiac hypertrophy
Congestive heart failure
Diabetes mellitus
Diet:
■ Liquid protein
■ Starvation
■ Anorexia nervosa
■ Hunger strike
Female sex
Hyperaldosteronism
Hyperparathyroidism
Hypocalcemia
Hypokalemia
Hypomagnesemia
Hypothyroidism
Intracranial trauma
Liver diseases
Mitral valve prolapse
Myocardial ischemia
Myocarditis
Pheochromocytoma
Recent conversion from atrial fibrillation, especially after a QT-prolonging drug
Renal diseases
Right neck dissection or hematoma

benefits of the drug given and consideration of therapeutic alternatives, together with a search for underlying predisposing factors (see Box 7-2).

Progressive QT prolongation and arrhythmias may occur shortly after the initiation of drug therapy, such as with quinidine or sotalol, but may also occur later, such as when CYP3A4 inhibitors are used, a second QT-prolonging drug is taken, or when risk factors occur. As recently reported by Zeltser et al,[9] both cardiac and non-cardiac drugs do cause QT-related arrhythmias after several days of use. They also found that most of the patients taking these drugs had one or more risk factors.

TdP is especially common in the outpatient setting, particularly in women, in the elderly, and when other risks factors, such as those shown in Box 7-2, are present.

Cytochrome P-450 3A4 Inhibitors

TdP may be facilitated when cytochrome P-450, especially P450 3A4 (CYP3A4) inhibitors, is given with QT-prolonging drugs,[10] generally by interfering with the hepatic metabolism of the QT-prolonging drug. Many drugs are known to be inhibitors of cytochrome P450 enzymes, such as calcium channel blockers, macrolide antibiotics, antifungal agents, antiretroviral drugs, tranquilizers, statins, and antidepressants (Box 7-3). As recently shown by Ray et al,[11] this fact may have important consequences.

In patients taking the QT-prolonging drug erythromycin, the already doubled incidence of sudden death from cardiac causes increased to 5 times as high when patients were also taking verapamil.[11] Grapefruit is an important CYP3A4 inhibitor and may cause TdP in susceptible patients when taken with clinical doses of QT-prolonging drugs. Grapefruit also may impair the metabolism of the major metabolite of amiodarone, N-desethylamiodarone, for at least 3 days after ingestion of the fruit or its juice (processed or fresh). The effects of grapefruit juice on amiodarone are reflected on the ECG by lengthening the PR and QTc intervals.

Risks to Women

The longer QT interval present in women makes them more susceptible to TdP development.[12-14] In fact, 70% of TdP episodes occur in women. The longer QT interval associated with women may be further prolonged in response to a variety of commonly used drugs (see Box 7-1). In women, quinidine and sotalol cause greater QT prolongation than in men at equivalent serum concentrations.[15,16] Although the proarrhythmia risk is low with amiodarone (less than 1%), women have a prevalence of TdP twice that of men. Also, in studies with the newly developed potassium channel blockers dofetilide and azimilide, of those who did have TdP develop, the majority were women.[17,18] After exercise, the greater QT prolongation in women

---

BOX 7-3

Cytochrome P-450 Inhibitors

Amiodarone
Clarithromycin (Biaxin)
Cyclosporine (Neoral)
Danazol (Danocrine)
Delavirdine (Rescriptor)
Diltiazem (Cardizem)
Erythromycin (E-Mycin)
Ethinyl estradiol
Fluconazole (Diflucan; weak inhibitor)
Fluvoxamine (Luvox)
Grapefruit and grapefruit juice (active only in the small
    bowel mucosa)
Imidazole (Lotrimin)
Indinavir (Crixivan)
Isoniazid (INH)
Itraconazole (Sporanox)
Ketoconazole (Nizoral)
Methylprednisone
Metronidazole (Flagyl)
Mibefradil (Posicor)
Miconazole (Monistat)
Nefazodone (Serzone)
Nelfinavir (Viracept)
Nicardipine (Cardene)
Norethindrone
Norfloxacin (Norflox)
Oxiconazole (Oxistat)
Prednisone (Deltasone, Liquid Pred, Metocorten, Orasone,
    Panasol, Prednicen-M)
Quinine
Red wine (in some individuals)
Ritonavir (Norvir)
Saquinavir (Invirase)
Troleandomycin (Tao)
Verapamil (Calan)
Zafirlukast (Accolate)

---

during the decelerating heart rate may play a role in increasing proarrhythmic risk.[19]

Prevention

The most important preventive measure to avoid TdP is to make certain that the following do not occur:

■ Concurrent administration of two or more drugs that prolong the QT interval

■ Concurrent administration of a QT-prolonging drug plus another drug that inhibits its clearance

Emergency Treatment

In the event of drug-induced TdP, the following five steps should be taken:

1. Discontinue the offending drug.
2. Establish continuous ECG monitoring.
3. Correct electrolyte abnormalities with potassium and magnesium.
4. Give MgCl or $MgSO_4$ as a 1- to 2-g intravenous bolus over a 5-minute period.
5. Start an infusion of MgCl or $MgSO_4$ 1 to 2 g/hr for 4 to 6 hours. MgCl is preferred to $MgSO_4$ because sulfate binds calcium and chloride does not.
6. If intravenous magnesium is unsuccessful, an increase in basic heart rate with isoproterenol or by ventricular pacing may be necessary.

REENTRY

Reentry is another drug-induced mechanism of cardiac arrhythmias in which the drug slows conduction velocity in myocardial fibers to such an extent that the occurrence of reentrant arrhythmias is facilitated. This finding is typical with class IC drugs (flecainide and propafenone), especially during rate increase, because the slowing in conduction velocity is inversely related to heart rate.

The reentry circuit requires slow conduction somewhere in the circuit and one-way conduction. This common arrhythmogenic mechanism, in addition to its role in drug-induced tachycardias, is also capable of supporting both SVTs and VTs.

Drug-induced reentrant arrhythmias are facilitated when the drug in question slows conduction velocity in some myocardial fibers to such an extent that reentry of the impulse into unaffected fibers becomes possible. The mechanism of reentry is illustrated and described in Figure 7-4. Note the anterograde block because of a difference in refractory periods, which permits one-way conduction and perpetuation of the reentry circuit.

CLASS IC DRUG-RELATED EMERGENCIES

Class IC drugs include flecainide and propafenone. The emergence of a sustained VT after starting such a drug or after an increase in drug dose indicates an adverse drug effect. The drug dose does not have to be toxic, but merely large enough to slow conduction velocity sufficiently to facilitate circulation of the impulse within the reentry circuit. In contrast to the occurrence of TdP, which is promoted by a slow heart rate, induction of VT by a class IC drug is promoted by a fast heart rate (Figure 7-5) because slowing in conduction velocity after the administration of class IC

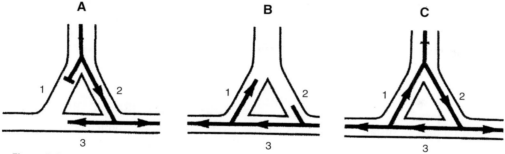

Figure 7-4   Mechanism of reentry. **A,** Arrival of an impulse at the site of division into two pathways. Because of differences in the duration of the refractory period of the two pathways, the impulse is blocked in one pathway and not the other (pathway 1 has the longer refractory period). **B,** The impulse emerging from pathway 2 can reenter pathway 1 (through 3). If the proximal portion of pathway 1 has recovered, the impulse is able to return to the site of origin. **C,** If this mechanism perpetuates, a regular tachycardia results because of reentry. Drugs that accentuate differences in duration of refractory periods and slow conduction velocity of the impulse facilitate this mechanism.

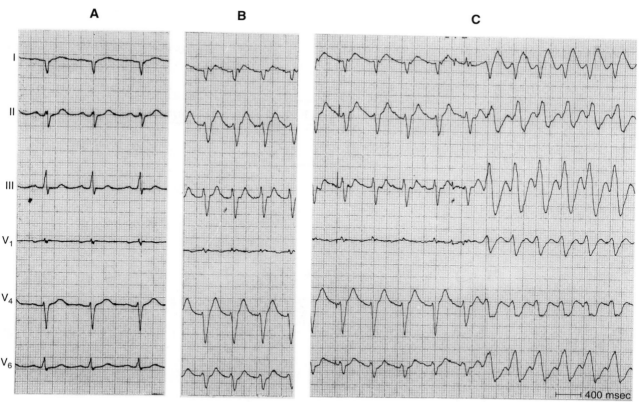

Figure 7-5   Initiation of a sustained VT during exercise testing in a patient receiving flecainide. **A,** Before exercise. The heart rate is 80 beats/min and the QRS width measures 100 msec. **B,** During exercise. The heart rate is 130 beats/min, QRS width is 160 msec, and left-axis deviation is present. **C,** Shortly thereafter a ventricular tachycardia begins with a rate of 150 beats/min.

drugs becomes more marked when the heart rate is increased.

Characteristics

The VT caused by class IC drugs has the following four clinical signs:

1. Spontaneous onset occurs after starting the drug or increasing the dose.
2. The tachycardia has a sustained or persistent nature.
3. The QRS complexes are quite wide because the class IC drug causes intramyocardial slowing in conduction velocity.
4. The VT can frequently not be terminated by cardioversion or programmed ventricular stimulation, or it resumes after only one or two sinus beats.

Emergency Treatment

1. Stop the offending drug.
2. Establish continuous ECG monitoring.
3. In case of hemodynamic compromise, give inotropic support with isoproterenol or epinephrine, which will counteract slowing in conduction velocity induced by class IA or class IC drugs.
4. In case of persistence of VT, pace the atrium at the rate of the VT by using an AV interval that allows for maximal contribution of atrial contraction to the ventricular filling.

DRUG-INDUCED BRADYCARDIA

Several drugs may produce bradycardia in the form of sinus bradycardia, SA block, AV nodal block, or sub–AV nodal block (Table 7-1):

Sinus bradycardia may be caused by beta-blocking agents such as propranolol and metoprolol.

SA block may be the result of treatment with class IA drugs (e.g., quinidine, procainamide, disopyramide), class IC drugs (e.g., flecainide, propafenone), beta-blocking agents, class III drugs (e.g., sotalol, amiodarone), and digitalis. The ECGs shown in Figure 7-6 are examples of atrial tachycardia and drug-induced bradycardia. The patient was given intravenous DL-sotalol for the treatment of atrial tachycardia, which resulted in the suppression of the tachycardia. However, it also caused

TABLE 7-1	Possible Sites of Block in Relation to Different Types (Classes) of Antiarrhythmic Drugs		
	Site of Block		
Class	SA	AV Nodal	His-Bundle Branches
IA Quinidine Procainamide Disopyramide Ajmaline	+	n/e	+
IB Tocainide Mexiletine	n/e	n/e	+
IC Flecainide Propafenone	+ +	n/e +	+ +
II Beta-blocking drugs	+	+	n/e
III Azimilide Dofetilide	n/e	n/e	+
IV Verapamil Diltiazem	+	+	n/e
Drugs with combined class effects Amiodarone DL-sotalol	+	+	+
Digitalis	+	+	n/e

n/e, No effect.

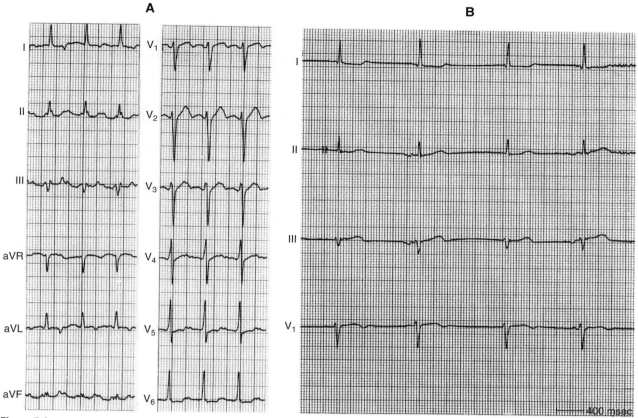

Figure 7-6   A severe bradycardia (**B**) after termination of an atrial tachycardia (**A**) by intravenous DL-sotalol. **B** shows complete sinoatrial block with escape beats arising in the low atrium and AV junction.

complete SA block and resulting in bradycardia (46 beats/min).

AV nodal block may occur after the administration of beta-blocking agents, class III drugs, calcium antagonists (e.g., verapamil, diltiazem), and digitalis.

Sub–AV nodal (His-Purkinje) block may be induced by class IA drugs, class IB drugs (e.g., mexiletine, tocainide), class IC drugs, and class III drugs.

Emergency Treatment

1. Stop the offending drug.
2. Establish continuous ECG monitoring.
3. Give atropine or start temporary intravenous pacing in case of Adams-Stokes attacks, a low ventricular rate leading to hypotension or congestive failure, or bradycardia-dependent ventricular arrhythmias.

SUMMARY

Cardiac and noncardiac drugs may induce or worsen cardiac arrhythmias. This possibility should always be

suspected when a patient reports worsening of his or her condition after the start of drug therapy.

REFERENCES

1. Lasser KE, Allen PD, Woolhandler SJ, et al: Timing of new black box warnings and withdrawals for prescription medications, *JAMA* 287:2215-20, 2002.
2. Roden DM, Hoffman BF: Action potential prolongation and induction of abnormal automaticity by low quinidine concentrations in canine Purkinje fibers: relationship to potassium and cycle length, *Circ Research* 56:857-67, 1984.
3. Brachmann J, Scherlag BJ, Rosenshtraukh LV, et al: Bradycardia-dependent triggered activity: relevance to drug-induced multiform ventricular tachycardia, *Circulation* 68:846-56, 1983.
4. Dessertenne F: La tachycardie ventriculaire a deux foyers opposes variables, *Arch Mal Coeur* 59:263-72, 1966.
5. Roden DM: Drug-induced prolongation of the QT interval, *N Engl J Med* 350:1013-22, 2004.
6. Sicouri S, Antzelevitsch C: Drug-induced afterdepolarizations and triggered activity occur in a discrete subpopulation of ventricular muscle cells (M cells) in the canine heart: quinidine and digitalis, *J Cardiovasc Electrophysiol* 4:48-58, 1993.
7. Akar FG, Yan GX, Antzelevitsch C, et al: Unique topographical distribution of M cells underlies re-entrant mechanism of torsades de pointes in the long QT syndrome, *Circulation* 105:1247-53, 2002.

8. Nattel S: The molecular and ionic specificity of antiarrhythmic drug actions, *J Cardiovasc Electrophysiol* 10:272-82, 1999.

9. Zeltser D, Justo D, Halkin A, et al: Torsade de pointes due to non-cardiac drugs: most patients have easily identifiable risk factors, *Medicine (Baltimore)* 82:282-90, 2003.

10. Dresser GK, Spence JD, Bailey DG: Pharmacokinetic-pharmacodynamic consequences and clinical relevance of cytochrome P450 3A4 inhibition, *Clin Pharmacokinet* 38:41-57, 2000.

11. Ray WA, Murray KT, Meredith S, et al: Oral erythromycin and the risk of sudden death from cardiac causes, *New Engl J Med* 351:1089-96, 2004.

12. Makkar RR, Fromm BS, Steinman RT, et al: Female gender as a risk factor for torsades de pointes associated with cardiovascular drugs, *JAMA* 270:2590-7, 1993.

13. Ebert SN, Liu XK, Woosley RL: Female gender as a risk factor for drug-induced cardiac arrhythmias: evaluation of clinical and experimental evidence, *J Womens Health* 7:547-57, 1998.

14. Wolbrette D, Naccarelli G, Curtis A, et al: Gender differences in arrhythmias, *Clin Cardiol* 2549-56, 2002.

15. Lehmann MH, Hardy S, Archibald D, et al: Sex difference in risk of torsades de pointes with d,l-sotalol, *Circulation* 94:2535-41, 1996.

16. Benton RE, Sale M, Flockhart DA, et al: Greater quinidine-induced QTc interval prolongation in women, *Clin Pharmacol Ther* 67:413-18, 2000.

17. Torp-Pedersen C, Moller M, Bloch-Thomsen PE, et al: Dofetilide in patients with congestive heart failure and left ventricular dysfunction, *N Engl J Med* 341:857-65, 1999.

18. Page RL, Connolly SJ, Wilkinson WE, et al: Azimilide supraventricular arrhythmia program (ASAP) Investigators: Antiarrhythmic effects of azimilide in paroxysmal supraventricular tachycardia: efficacy and dose-response, *Am Heart J* 143:643-9, 2002.

19. Chauhan VS, Krahn AD, Walker BD, et al: Sex differences in QT interval and QT dispersion: dynamics during exercise and recovery in healthy subjects, *Am Heart J* 144:858-64, 2002.

CHAPTER
8
Potassium-Related Emergencies

EMERGENCY APPROACH

ECG Recognition of Severe or Progressive Hyperkalemia

- Slow heart rate
- P-wave widening with low voltage, followed by loss of P wave
- Broad QRS
- Frequently, left-axis deviation
- Loss of ST segment (S wave merges with T wave)
- Tall, tented T waves
- QTc interval normal or shortened

Treatment

1. Give calcium gluconate (10%) 10 to 30 ml intravenously over a 1- to 5-minute period with constant ECG monitoring.
2. Administer 10 U of insulin in 500 ml 10% glucose intravenously in a 30-minute period.
3. Add salbutamol 5 µg/kg body weight in 15 ml glucose 5% intravenously in a 15-minute period.
4. Add sodium bicarbonate (2 to 3 ampules) to 1 L 5% dextrose in 0.9% saline.
5. Administer cation exchange resins (sodium polystyrene sulfonate) by retention enema; this may be repeated until potassium levels are within safe limits. Oral doses of 20 g are given three or four times a day with 20 ml of 70% sorbitol solution.
6. If renal failure occurs, institute hemodialysis or peritoneal dialysis with one of the treatments above.

ECG Recognition of Severe Hypokalemia (Serum Level Less than 2.5 mEq/L)

- ST depression
- Decrease in T-wave amplitude
- Increase in U-wave amplitude
- QT prolongation

Treatment

1. Give potassium chloride intravenously, not to exceed 40 mEq/L at an infusion rate not to exceed 20 mEq/hr (approximately 200 to 250 mEq/day).
2. Give oral potassium chloride.

POTASSIUM

The potassium ion plays a key role in the normal function of the cells of the human body.[1] In the heart, specific levels of intracellular and extracellular potassium are essential for normal impulse generation and conduction. Potassium is excreted by the body in the urine, feces, and perspiration. Diuretics, vomiting, perspiration, and diarrhea can rapidly deplete the body of this vital ion (hypokalemia). Conversely, anuria can cause a potassium buildup (hyperkalemia). Both conditions may produce serious arrhythmias and even death.[2]

The potassium gradient across the cell membrane, along with the intracellular negativity generated by the sodium-potassium adenosine triphosphatase (ATPase) pump, determines the resting membrane potential and thus conduction velocity and helps confine pacing activity to the sinus node. In the resting state, approximately 30 times as much potassium is within the cell as is in the extracellular fluid. A normal gradient and normal sodium-potassium pump activity create a resting membrane potential of −90 mV, which in turn permits rapid depolarization (phase 0 of the membrane action potential), leading to optimal stimulation of neighboring cells.

HYPERKALEMIA

An elevated serum potassium level is one of the more common acute, life-threatening metabolic emergencies and is found in 5% to 10% of hospitalized patients.[3] The incidence of hyperkalemia is increasing because of the increasing use of angiotensin-converting enzyme (ACE) inhibitors and angiotensin receptor blockers. These drugs impair urinary potassium excretion by interfering with the renin-angiotensin-aldosterone system.[4] The occurrence of hyperkalemia in patients taking ACE inhibitors or angiotensin receptor blockers is further increased when other risk factors are present (Box 8-1).

Another factor increasing the incidence of hyperkalemia is the use of aldosterone antagonists in heart failure.[5-7] Spirolactone, an aldosterone antagonist that has been increasingly prescribed in patients with heart failure after the Randomized Aldactone Evaluation Study[6] was published, resulted in a higher incidence of hospitalization for hyperkalemia, especially when patients were also treated with an ACE inhibitor.[5]

Electrophysiologic Consequences

An increase in extracellular potassium decreases the gradient of potassium across the cell membrane, thereby reducing the resting membrane potential. This, in turn, reduces the height and steepness of phase 0 of the action potential and slows conduction. Furthermore, the

velocity of phase 3 (terminal repolarization) accelerates and the action potential duration shortens, resulting in a typical ECG pattern when the serum potassium level reaches 6 mEq/L.

ECG Changes in Progressive Hyperkalemia

Figure 8-1 is a schematic representation of ECG changes as the serum potassium concentration goes from normal to 8 mEq/L.[8,9] The following ECG signs will help the clinician differentiate mild from severe degrees of hyperkalemia.

ECG Changes in Mild Hyperkalemia (Less Than 6.0 mEq/L)

The following ECG signs are the result of slowing of conduction in the atria and ventricles:

■ The P wave widens with a loss in height.
■ The PR interval prolongs.
■ The QRS complex widens.
■ The T wave becomes tall without prolongation of the QTc.

ECG Changes in Severe Hyperkalemia (Greater Than 6.0 mEq/L)

■ The QRS complex continues to broaden. At more than 6 mEq/L, the additional widening of the QRS complex takes place primarily in its second portion, which shows marked notching or slurring (Figures 8-1 and 8-2). Interestingly, little delay occurs in the initial portion of the QRS complex because hyperkalemia has less slowing effect on conduction in the Purkinje fibers than in muscle cells.

■ The frontal plane QRS axis usually shifts to the left because of the delay in LV activation unless marked RV enlargement is present.

■ The ST segment disappears into the upsweep of the T wave with further broadening of the QRS complex. The slow activation of the ventricles leads to repolarization of earlier activated areas while other parts of the ventricles are still being depolarized. This results in merging of the wide QRS with the tall peaked T waves and obliteration of the ST segment.

■ The PR interval continues to lengthen and the P wave flattens (see Figure 8-2) because of a decrease in conduction velocity in the atria. Figure 8-3 shows that ultimately the P wave disappears because of a further increase in potassium.

Treatment of Mild Hyperkalemia

1. Determine the cause (usually renal disease).
2. If possible, correct the underlying disease.

Treatment of Severe Hyperkalemia

1. Start an intravenous infusion of 10 to 30 ml of calcium gluconate (10%) over a 1- to 5-minute period

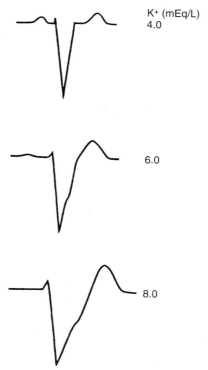

Figure 8-1 The ECG changes during progressive hyperkalemia (as seen in lead V_1).

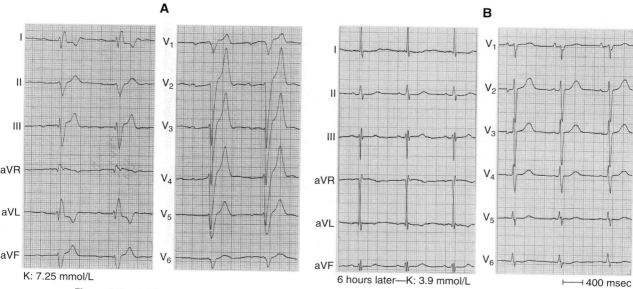

Figure 8-2 **A,** The ECG during hyperkalemia. Note bradycardia; wide, low-voltage P waves with a prolonged PR interval; widened QRS with left-axis deviation; loss of the ST segment because of merging of the S and T waves; and peaked, tented T waves. **B,** The ECG after dialysis.

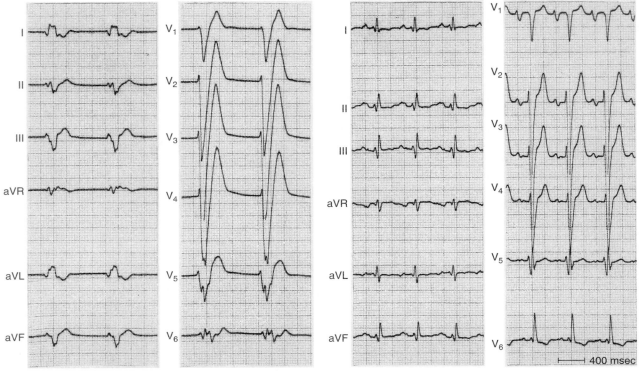

Figure 8-3   The ECG on the *left* shows severe hyperkalemia with a serum potassium level of 8.6 mEq/L. The ECG on the *right* was obtained after treatment. The P wave has returned, the QRS duration is shorter, and the QRS complex and T wave are separated.

with constant ECG monitoring. Although the calcium infusion may not lower plasma potassium concentration, it will, however, immediately but transiently alter the effect of potassium on the cell membrane.

2. Give 10 U of insulin in 500 ml of hypertonic glucose solution (10%) intravenously over a 30-minute period. Glucose decreases the effect of potassium toxicity by shifting potassium into the cell.

3. Give salbutamol 5 mcg/kg body weight in 15 ml glucose 5% intravenously in a 15-minute period to promote potassium shifting into the cell.

4. Add sodium bicarbonate (2 to 3 ampules) to 1 L of 5% dextrose in 0.9% saline. Sodium bicarbonate helps shift potassium into the cell even in patients who are not acidotic.

5. Give cation exchange resins (sodium polystyrene sulfonate) by retention enema; this may be repeated until potassium levels are within safe limits. Give oral doses of 20 g three or four times a day with 20 ml of 70% sorbitol solution.

In cases of renal failure, initiate hemodialysis or peritoneal dialysis along with one of the treatments above.

Figure 8-3 illustrates the 12-lead ECG before and after treatment of severe hyperkalemia.

HYPOKALEMIA

Hypokalemia, defined by a serum potassium level of less than 3.5 mEq/L, has been estimated to occur in 20% of hospitalized patients. However, severe hypokalemia (less than 2.5 mEq/L) is relatively uncommon.

Mechanism

Hypokalemia promotes the occurrence of early afterdepolarizations (see Chapter 7), which may lead to torsades de pointes arrhythmias. It also causes arrhythmias by enhanced automaticity.

In progressive hypokalemia the cell membrane becomes less and less negative until the cell is eventually nonexcitable. Moreover, if digitalis is administered when the extracellular potassium level is low, arrhythmogenicity is likely to be promoted.[6]

Digitalis and potassium compete for membrane binding sites, and with lower potassium in the extracellular fluid, more digitalis binds to the potassium position on the membrane sodium-potassium–ATPase, augmenting digitalis toxicity.

ECG Changes in Progressive Hypokalemia

- Progressive ST depression
- Decrease in T-wave amplitude
- Increase in U-wave amplitude; in advanced stages the T and U waves are fused
- In advanced hypokalemia the QRS amplitude and duration increase
- P-wave amplitude and duration are usually increased
- PR interval is usually slightly prolonged

Figure 8-4 is a schematic representation of the typical T- and U-wave changes associated with progressive hypokalemia. Figure 8-5 shows a tracing from a patient with severe hypokalemia. Note that the U wave has fused with the T wave (best seen in leads V_2 to V_6) and is larger than the T wave.

Cause

The underlying cause of hypokalemia should be determined. Fluid and potassium loss induced by severe diarrhea or potassium loss from diuretics is usually responsible. Occasionally other causes can be found, such as use of a liquid protein diet (to lose weight) or frequent ingestion of licorice.

Treatment of Severe Potassium Deficiency

1. Give intravenous potassium chloride (40 to 60 mEq/L at 20 mEq/hr, approximately 200 to 250 mEq/day).
2. Perform continuous ECG monitoring.
3. If torsades de pointes arrhythmias are present, in addition to potassium supplements give magnesium intravenously (MgCl or $MgSO_4$ 1 to 2 g over a 5-minute period, followed by an infusion with 1 to 2 g MgCl per hour for 4 to 6 hours).
4. If intravenous magnesium is unsuccessful, an increase in heart rate with isoproterenol or ventricular pacing may be necessary. Figure 8-5 shows the 12-lead ECG of a patient during severe hypokalemia and after treatment.

Treatment of Moderate Hypokalemia

Moderate hypokalemia can be treated by giving potassium salts by mouth.

SUMMARY

Severe hyperkalemia is characterized by bradycardia, loss of the P wave, a broad QRS, left-axis deviation, merging

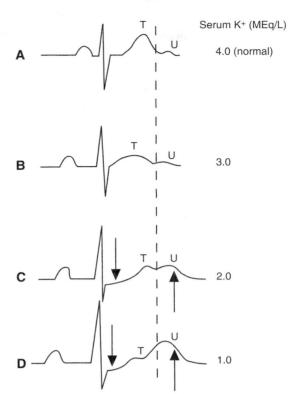

Hypokalemia

Figure 8-4   The progressive T-wave, U-wave, and ST segment changes in progressive hypokalemia. **A,** At a normal serum concentration of 4 to 5.5 mEq/L, the amplitude of the T wave is appreciably greater than that of the U wave. **B,** By the time the serum potassium level has dropped to 3 mEq/L, the T-wave amplitude has decreased and the U-wave amplitude has increased. The U-wave amplitude is, in fact, approaching the height of the T wave. **C** and **D,** With a further drop in the level of potassium, the amplitude and duration of the QRS and the P wave have increased, the P wave may lengthen slightly, the ST segment becomes depressed *(down arrow)*, and the U wave begins to tower over *(up arrow)* and fuse with the T wave. (Reprinted from Conover M: *Understanding electrocardiography,* St Louis, 2003, Mosby.)

of the QRS and T wave, and tall, tented T waves. The emergency treatment of hyperkalemia includes calcium gluconate, hypertonic glucose solution, sodium bicarbonate, and cation exchange resins.

Severe hypokalemia is marked by ST segment depression, a decrease in T-wave amplitude, and an increase in U-wave amplitude. The emergency treatment is intravenous and oral potassium chloride.

A   **B**

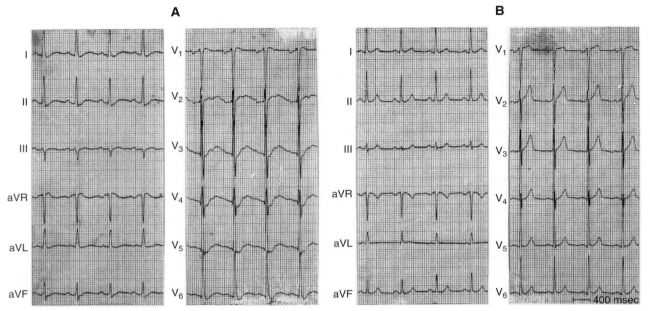

Figure 8-5   **A,** A 12-lead ECG from a patient with hypokalemia (serum potassium of 1.47 mEq/L). Note the giant U wave, which is best seen in the precordial leads V_2 to V_6. **B,** ECG from the same patient after correction of hypokalemia.

REFERENCES

1. Rose BD, Post TW: *Clinical physiology of acid-base and electrolyte disorders,* ed 5, New York, 2001, McGraw-Hill.
2. Weiner ID, Wingo CS: Hyperkalemia: a potential silent killer, *J Am Soc Nephrol* 9:1535-43, 1998.
3. Paice B, Gray JMB, McBride D, et al: Hyperkalemia in patients in hospital, *BMJ* 286:1189-92, 1983.
4. Palmer BF: Managing hyperkalemia caused by inhibitors of the renin-angiotensin-aldosterone system, *N Engl J Med* 351:585-92, 2004.
5. Juurlink DN, Mamdani MM, Lee DS, et al: Rates of hyperkalemia after publication of the randomized aldactone evaluation study, *N Engl J Med* 351:543-51, 2004.
6. Pitt B, Zannad F, Remme WJ, et al: The effect of spirolactone on morbidity and mortality in patients with severe heart failure, *N Engl J Med* 341:709-17, 1999.
7. Pitt B, Remme WJ, Zannad F, et al: Eplerenone, a selective aldosterone blocker in patients with left ventricular dysfunction after myocardial infarction, *N Engl J Med* 348:1309-21, 2003.
8. Bryant GM: Effect of potassium on ventricular deflections of the electrocardiogram in hypertensive cardiovascular disease, *Proc Soc Exp Biol Med* 7:557-8, 1948.
9. Suki WN, Jackson D: Hypokalemia: cause and treatment, *Heart Lung* 7:854-60, 1978.

9

ECG Recognition of Acute Pulmonary Embolism

EMERGENCY APPROACH

Examine the ECG For

- Rhythm disturbances
- A shift in the axis to the right compared with the ECG prior to the acute event (need not be outside the normal range of +90 to −30 degrees)
- Appearance of an RBBB pattern
- Pseudoinfarction patterns

If Changes in the ECG Occur That Suggest Pulmonary Embolism, Call For

- Emergency echocardiogram
- Arterial oxygen saturation
- D-Dimer measurement

Therapy

- Oxygen
- Analgesics
- Full-dose heparin
- Thrombolytic therapy

Prevention

1. Avoid venous stasis
   - Early mobilization and ambulation when possible
   - External compression of the legs for patients on complete bed rest
2. Anticoagulants
   - If heart failure is present or the patient is on long-term bed rest

---

Pulmonary embolism is commonly overlooked and often fatal. If the acute phase is recognized and treated appropriately, death can be prevented in 75% of patients who otherwise would have died.

VALUE OF THE ECG

When acute pulmonary embolism is suspected, serial ECG tracings are necessary because, although sudden dilation of the RV and elevated right-sided pressures are usually accompanied by dynamic ECG changes, a single ECG may show no obvious signs of pulmonary embolism, whereas the changes may be apparent on subsequent tracings.

The ECG signs of acute pulmonary embolism are not 100% diagnostic, and prior cardiac disease may make these ECG signs even less specific and less obvious.[1] However, certain ECG findings can cause the informed clinician to have a high degree of suspicion, in which case the diagnosis can be confirmed by an emergency echocardiogram.

VALUE OF THE ECHOCARDIOGRAM

The echocardiogram sensitively reflects the RV pressure and volume overload of acute pulmonary embolism and is quite useful for this often difficult diagnosis.[2,3] A D-dimer measurement can also be helpful in making the correct diagnosis.[4]

ECG FINDINGS DURING THE ACUTE PHASE

The common ECG findings in the acute phase of pulmonary embolism consist of arrhythmias and abnormalities of the P wave, QRS complex, ST segment, and T wave (Box 9-1).

Arrhythmias

The following arrhythmias are associated with acute pulmonary embolism and are the result of RV failure and acute dilation of the right atrium and RV:

- Sinus tachycardia
- Atrial fibrillation
- Atrial flutter
- Right APBs
- Right VPBs

P-Wave Abnormalities

P-wave changes, when present in acute pulmonary embolism, are those of right-axis deviation and right atrial enlargement (P pulmonale). The ECG signs of P pulmonale are tall P waves (more than 2.5 mm) in leads II, III, and aVF.

> **BOX 9-1**
>
> **ECG Findings in Acute Pulmonary Embolism**
>
> **Arrhythmias**
> - Sinus tachycardia
> - Atrial fibrillation
> - Atrial flutter
> - Right APBs
> - Right VPBs
>
> **P Waves**
> - Right-axis deviation
> - >2.5 mm in leads II, III, and aVF (P pulmonale)
>
> **QRS Complexes**
> - Axis shifts to the right
> - Late R wave in V_1 with abrupt appearance and growth, especially with ST elevation and positive T wave (ominous sign)
> - S waves in leads I and aVL
> - Transitional zone to the left (clockwise rotation of the heart)
> - Q waves in leads III and aVF (if also QS complex in V_1, high degree of suspicion)
> - QS may appear in lead V_1 (if also Q waves in III and aVF, high degree of suspicion)
>
> **ST Segments and T Waves**
> - ST segment elevation in V_1 (early sign)
> - T waves symmetrically negative in precordial leads (at 24 to 48 hours)

QRS Complex Abnormalities

Axis. In the frontal plane, the QRS axis usually shifts to the right of the axis in the preembolic state. Such an axis shift does not have to be in the abnormal range, although on occasion frank right-axis deviation of more than +90 degrees occurs.

RV conduction delay. In acute pulmonary embolism an abrupt appearance of an RBBB pattern often occurs because of acute stretching of that bundle branch when the right heart abruptly dilates. This is reflected by an ECG pattern of incomplete or complete RBBB. Normally, the RV contributes little to the QRS complex so that the sudden appearance and growth of a late R wave in lead V_1 is an important sign of acute pulmonary embolism, especially when combined with ST elevation and a positive T wave in that lead.

In patients with no preexisting heart disease, the completeness of the RBBB pattern correlates with the percentage of pulmonary blood flow blocked by the embolus. When the pattern is that of complete RBBB

(QRS more than 0.11 seconds), 50% or more occlusion of the pulmonary circulation is present.

The appearance of S waves in leads I and aVL reflects the delayed activation of the RV.

Because of clockwise rotation of the heart, Q waves appear in leads III and aVF, a finding that is often misdiagnosed as acute inferior wall MI.

ST Segment Elevation

ST segment elevation may be seen in leads V_1 and aVR; both leads reflect right-sided dilation. The ST segment elevation in lead V_1 is an early sign, and when associated with an RBBB pattern and a positive T wave in that lead, it should immediately raise the suspicion of pulmonary embolism. Such a pattern differs from that of uncomplicated RBBB, in which the ST segment is not elevated and the T wave is opposite in polarity to the QRS.

T-Wave Abnormalities

Symmetrical T-wave negativity in the precordial leads usually develops within 24 to 48 hours of the acute event and may persist for several weeks.

Clockwise Rotation

The clockwise rotation of the heart seen in acute pulmonary embolism is the result of the sudden right-sided dilation and pressure elevation. This is reflected in the precordial ECG leads by a shift in the transitional zone (equiphasic complex) to the left.

Normally in the precordial leads the transition from mostly negative to mostly positive occurs at lead V_3 or V_4. In acute pulmonary embolism, this transition takes place more to the left at lead V_5 and sometimes even at lead V_6. When this occurs, clockwise rotation of the heart is said to be present. Normal and abnormal transitional zones are illustrated in Figure 9-1.

Abnormal Q or S Waves

Because in acute pulmonary embolism the right precordial leads record an intracavitary complex over a dilated right atrium and displaced interventricular septum, QS complexes may appear in lead V_1. When this pattern is associated with Q waves in leads III and aVF, pulmonary embolism should be carefully ruled out.

In Figure 9-2, the preembolic ECG should be compared with the ECG in the acute phase of pulmonary embolism. Note the development of sinus tachycardia and all the signs of acute dilation of the right heart (RBBB pattern, slight ST elevation in leads V_1 and aVR, a shift of the QRS axis from −45 degrees to +90 degrees,

the development of Q waves in lead III, the development of S waves in leads I and aVL, and clockwise rotation of the heart). T-wave inversion occurs in leads II, aVF, and V_1 to V_5.

Other examples from patients in the acute phase of pulmonary embolism are given in Figures 9-3 and 9-4. All show the typical ECG pattern of acute pulmonary embolism.

ECG DURING THE SUBACUTE PHASE

The ECG pattern in the subacute phase of pulmonary embolism after resolution of the clot spontaneously or with thrombolytic therapy depends on the moment when the tracing is recorded in the evolving course of the pathology. Serial ECG recordings may show resolution of the RV conduction delay, resolution of the axis shift, and development of deep T-wave inversion in the precordial leads up to leads V_5 and V_6 and in leads III and aVF. These T-wave changes may persist for weeks. The ECG changes in subacute pulmonary embolism are shown in Figure 9-5 and are summarized in Box 9-2.

ECG DURING THE CHRONIC PHASE

The ECG during the chronic phase of pulmonary embolism depends on the dissolution of the clot. Residual evidence of right atrial and RV hypertrophy may be present, such as P pulmonale and an RBBB pattern in lead V_1.

PATHOPHYSIOLOGY

Acute pulmonary embolism is the sudden obstruction of a central or peripheral pulmonary artery. Postmortem studies have shown that the majority of patients with pulmonary embolism also have thromboembolism in the leg veins.[5]

If the pulmonary artery obstruction is significant, it results in the following:
- Hemodynamic decompensation
- Acute pulmonary hypertension

BOX 9-2

ECG Findings in Subacute Pulmonary Embolism

- Resolution of RBBB
- Resolution of axis shift
- Development of deep T-wave inversion in precordial leads
- Development of deep T-wave inversion in leads III and aVF

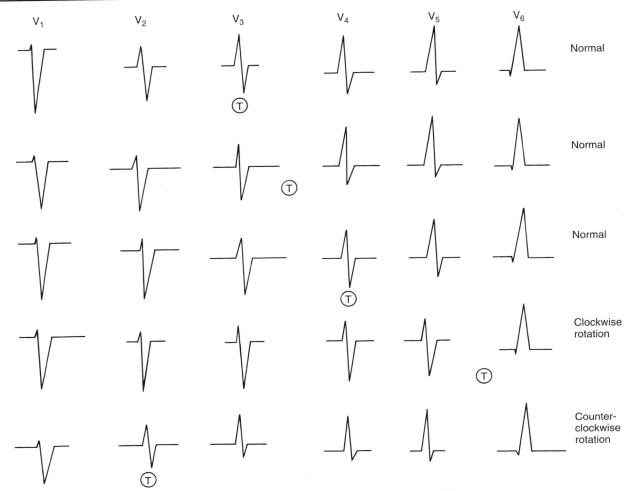

Figure 9-1 Normal and abnormal transitional zones (T).

- Right-sided dilation
- Clockwise cardiac rotation
- Marked ventilation-perfusion disturbance
- Acute lowering of the cardiac output
- RV failure (ultimately)

SIGNS AND SYMPTOMS

Patients with acute pulmonary embolism usually have dyspnea, pleuritic chest pain, and sometimes syncope. The following symptoms relate to a decrease in pulmonary blood flow with its attendant decrease in oxygen exchange in the affected zone and eventual decrease in cardiac output:

- Hypoxemia
- Hyperventilation
- Dyspnea
- Apprehension
- Confusion
- Syncope or shock (if the decrease in cardiac output is severe)

If pulmonary infarction is present, hemoptysis may be present and the patient may have pleuritic chest pain.

Special Consideration

Patients on bed rest. Clinicians should be alerted to the possibility of pulmonary embolism when a patient on bed rest is exhibiting unexplained fever, dyspnea, tachypnea, and tachycardia.

The elderly. Collapse, even in the absence of chest pain, cyanosis, and hypoxia, is an important symptom of acute pulmonary embolism in the elderly.

Older patients with acute pulmonary embolism do not often have a classic presentation, so much so that the diagnosis and initiation of treatment may be delayed.

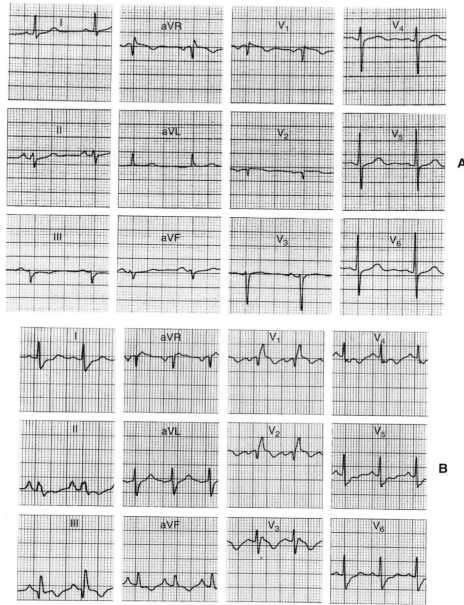

Figure 9-2   The preembolic ECG (**A**) compared with the postembolic ECG (**B**). Note the development of sinus tachycardia, RBBB pattern, a shift in the QRS axis from −45 degrees to +90 degrees, S waves in leads I and aVL, and Q waves in lead III. ST segment elevation is shown in leads V_1 and aVR and T-wave inversion in leads V_1 to V_5.

When comparing older and younger patients with acute pulmonary embolism, Timmons et al[6] have shown that the elderly are much more likely to present with collapse (24% versus 3%) and less likely to report chest pain and show signs of cyanosis and hypoxia.

PHYSICAL FINDINGS

Physical findings are related to RV hypertension, RV failure, and the increase in pulmonary artery pressure. The physical signs of right heart failure are particularly useful in young patients who may be asymptomatic in the face

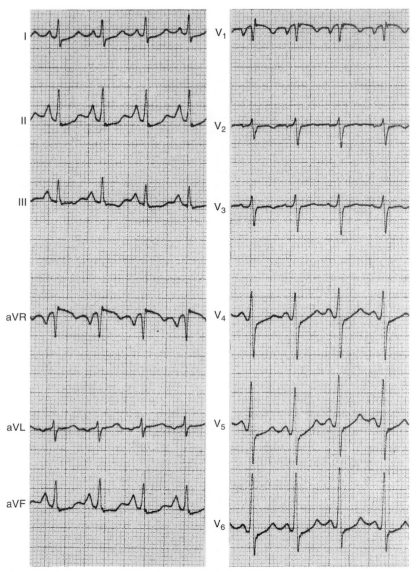

Figure 9-3 A 12-lead ECG in acute pulmonary embolism. Note sinus tachycardia, an incomplete RBBB pattern, and S waves in leads I and aVL. The ST segment in leads V_1 and aVR is elevated. Clockwise rotation of the heart is present, indicated by the location of the ECG transitional zone between leads V_4 and V_5.

of an acute massive pulmonary embolism and right heart failure.[7]

Possible Results of RV Hypertension

- Palpable RV impulses
- Increase in "a" waves in the jugular venous pulse
- Audible RV S4 heart sound

Possible Results of RV Failure

- Tachycardia
- Increase in jugular venous distention
- Tricuspid regurgitation murmur
- S3 heart sound
- Hepatomegaly

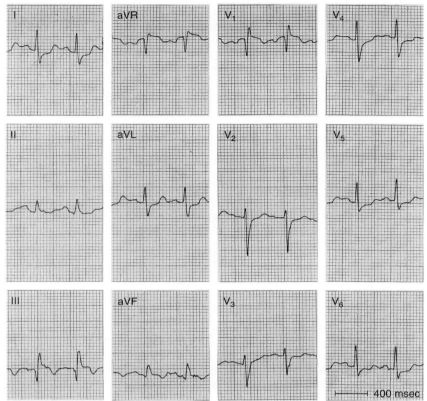

Figure 9-4   Another ECG in acute pulmonary embolism illustrating the pseudoinferior MI pattern (leads III and aVF). Note also sinus tachycardia, an RBBB pattern, and elevated ST segment in leads V_1 and aVR.

Possible Results of Increased Pulmonary Artery Pressure

- Palpable pulmonary artery pulsations
- Splitting of S2 with an exaggerated P2
- Pulmonary ejection murmur

INCIDENCE

In the United States alone, pulmonary embolism leads to more than 90,000 hospitalizations per year, with close to a 15% mortality rate.[8-11] As many as 85% of patients with pulmonary emboli are undiagnosed, and of those with fatal emboli, only 15% received appropriate treatment before they died.[12,13]

DIFFERENTIAL DIAGNOSIS
MI

Acute massive pulmonary embolism involving the main pulmonary arteries may simulate MI, especially because both conditions are associated with a fall in cardiac out-

put, abnormal Q waves, ST segment elevation, and T-wave changes. For example, right-axis deviation, with Q waves and T-wave changes in the inferior leads, may mimic inferior wall MI. Although the RBBB pattern and ST segment elevation in lead V_1 should raise the suspicion of pulmonary embolism, this pattern is also seen when acute anteroseptal infarction is complicated by RBBB.

The following differences help in the diagnosis, although none is truly specific:

- Acute shortness of breath is more pronounced in acute pulmonary embolism than would be expected in MI.
- The ECG in acute pulmonary embolism, although abnormal, is not typical for MI. For example, one 12-lead ECG may suggest the presence of both inferior wall and anterior wall MI (Q waves may be seen in leads III and aVF, but not in lead II, and these may be associated with a QR pattern in lead V_1).

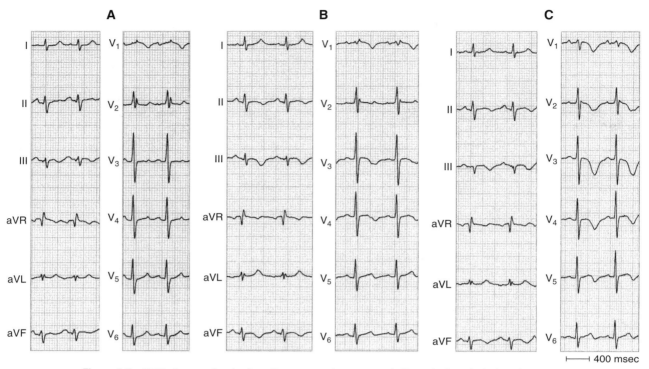

Figure 9-5 ECG changes developing after acute pulmonary embolism. **A,** On admission sinus tachycardia, an S1-S2-S3 pattern and an incomplete RBBB are shown. **B,** Twenty-four hours later T-wave inversion has developed in the precordial leads. **C,** Three days later deep T-wave inversion and QT prolongation are shown in several leads.

■ The chest x-ray in acute pulmonary embolism does not show pulmonary congestion, although severe dyspnea is present.

The diagnostic usefulness of the ECG is enhanced when combined with echocardiography, arterial oxygen saturation, and D-dimer measurement.

EMERGENCY TREATMENT

1. Oxygen
2. Analgesics
3. Full-dose heparin[14]
4. Thrombolytic therapy[15,16]

In patients with acute pulmonary embolism who are hemodynamically unstable, thrombolytic therapy is necessary to reduce the thrombus rapidly and restore RV function.

PREVENTION

Early ambulation. Every effort should be made to prevent acute pulmonary embolism by encouraging early ambulation or mobilization when possible. Other preventative measures include graduated compression stockings and intermittent pneumatic compression, a device that, along with direct physical stimulation of venous blood flow, also stimulates endogenous fibrinolytic activity. Placement of a temporary or permanent inferior vena caval filter may also be considered.

High-risk patients. Graduated compression stockings plus intermittent pneumatic compression boots may be combined with low-molecular-weight heparin.

SUMMARY

The ECG changes associated with acute pulmonary embolism are the result of acute RV dilation. Recognition of these changes, which begin abruptly, requires serial ECG tracings. Rhythm disturbances, axis shifts, the sudden appearance of an RV conduction delay, a Q wave in lead III, an S wave in lead I, and pseudoinfarction patterns may develop.

REFERENCES

1. Brugada P, Gorgels AP, Wellens HJJ: The electrocardiogram in pulmonary embolism. In Wellens HJJ, Kulbertus HE: *What's new in electrocardiography,* The Hague, 1981, Martinus Nijhoff, pp 366-80.

2. Come PC: Echocardiographic recognition of pulmonary arterial disease and determination of its cause, *Am J Med* 84:384-94, 1988.

3. Jardin F, Dubourg O, Guret P, et al: Quantitive two-dimensional echocardiography in massive pulmonary embolism: emphasis on ventricular interdependence and leftward septal displacement, *J Am Coll Cardiol* 10:1201-6, 1987.

4. Wells PS, Anderson DR, Roger M: Excluding pulmonary embolism at the bedside without diagnostic imaging: management of patients with suspected pulmonary embolism presenting to the emergency department by using a simple clinical model and D-dimer, *Ann Intern Med* 135:98-107, 2001.

5. Colman W, Hirsh J, Marder VJ, et al, editors: Epidemiology, pathogenesis, and natural history of venous thrombosis. In *Hemostasis and thrombosis, basic principles and clinical practice,* ed 4, Philadelphia, 2001, Lippincott Williams & Wilkins, pp 1153-7.

6. Timmons S, Kingston M, Hussain M, et al: Pulmonary embolism: differences in presentation between older and younger patients, *Aging* 32:601-5, 2003.

7. Goldhaber SZ, Elliott CG: Acute pulmonary embolism. Part II: Risk stratification, treatment and prevention, *Circulation* 108:2834-8, 2003.

8. Goldhaber SZ: Pulmonary embolism, *N Engl J Med* 339:93-104, 1998.

9. Silverstein MD, Heit JA, Mohr DN, et al: Trends in the incidence of deep vein thrombosis and pulmonary embolism: a 25 year population-based study, *Arch Intern Med* 158:585-93, 1998.

10. Siddique RM, Siddique MI, Connors AF Jr, et al: Thirty-day case fatality rates for pulmonary embolism in the elderly, *Arch Intern Med* 156:2343-7, 1996.

11. The PIOPED Investigators: Value of the ventilation/perfusion scan in acute pulmonary embolism. Results of the prospective investigation of pulmonary embolism diagnosis (PIOPED), *JAMA* 263:2753-9, 1990.

12. Walden R, Bass A, Modan R, et al: Pulmonary embolism in postmortem material with clinical correlation in 425 cases, *Int Angiol* 4:469-73, 1985.

13. Mandelli V, Schmid C, Zogno C, et al: "False negatives" and "false positives" in acute pulmonary embolism: a clinical postmortem comparison, *Cardiologia* 42:205-210, 1979.

14. Raskob GE, Carter CJ, Hull RD: Heparin therapy for venous thrombosis and pulmonary embolism, *Blood Rev* 2:251-8, 1988.

15. Tissue plasminogen activator for the treatment of acute pulmonary embolism. A collaborative study by the PIOPED Investigators, *Chest* 97:528-33, 1990.

16. Verstraete M, Miller GA, Bounameaux H, et al: Intravenous and intrapulmonary recombinant tissue-type-plasminogen activator in the treatment of acute massive pulmonary embolism, *Circulation* 77:353-60, 1988.

10

Hypothermia

EMERGENCY APPROACH

ECG Recognition
- Slow heart rate
- Widened P waves
- Widened QRS
- Osborn waves
- Prolonged QT

Treatment
1. Gradually rewarm the patient in cases of exposure to cold environment.
2. Identify the cause and treat accordingly because hypothermia may not be caused by exposure to cold.

HYPOTHERMIA

Hypothermia is usually caused by exposure to a cold environment. Figure 10-1 shows the ECG of a man who fell asleep outdoors during cold weather after the consumption of a considerable amount of alcohol. His body temperature at the time of the recording was 29.6° C.

Typical ECG Features

- Sinus bradycardia of fewer than 50 beats/min is present.
- P waves widen (because of slowing of intraatrial conduction velocity).
- QRS complexes widen (because of slowing of intraventricular conduction velocity).
- QT intervals are prolonged.
- Osborn waves[1-4] (J waves) appear in many leads.

The body temperature is inversely related to the amplitude of the Osborn wave, a concave elevation of the segment between the end of the QRS and the beginning of the ST segment.

The electrophysiologic mechanism of Osborn waves on the ECG in cases of hypothermia is unclear. Various explanations have been given, such as delay of depolarization, a current of injury, and early repolarization.

Clinical Implications

Hypothermia may lead to the following conditions:
- Myocardial damage (usually reversible)
- Hypotension

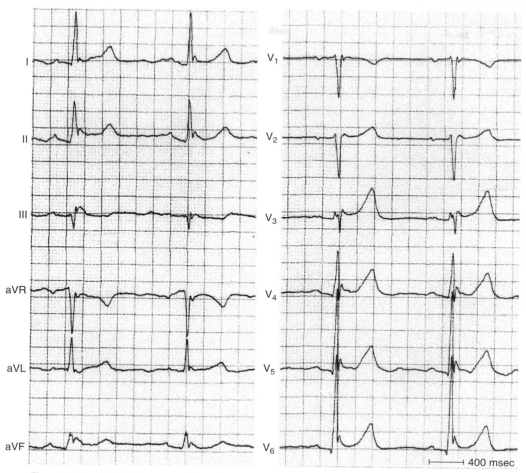

Figure 10-1   ECG during severe hypothermia. Shown are sinus bradycardia, widening of the P wave and QRS complex, QT prolongation, and Osborn waves. (Courtesy Dr. Anton Gorgels.)

- Atrial fibrillation
- Ventricular fibrillation (occasionally)
- Pulmonary, hematologic, and renal complications

Treatment

- Gradual core warming
- Management of pulmonary, hematologic, and renal complications

HYPOTHERMIA NOT CAUSED BY EXPOSURE TO COLD

As recently reviewed by Sheikh and Hurst,[5] a number of nonenvironmental conditions may produce hypothermia (Box 10-1). These conditions have the same ECG

BOX 10-1

Nonenvironmental Causes of Hypothermia

Endocrine dysfunction
Hypothyroidism
- Hypopituitarism
- Hypoglycemia
- Diabetic ketoacidosis
Neurologic dysfunction
Cerebrovascular accidents
Infections
Antipsychotic medications
Alcohol

findings as those seen in hypothermia caused by exposure to cold. Familiarization with these possible nonenvironmental causes is essential because they require an approach directed toward the causal mechanism.

REFERENCES

1. Osborn JJ: Experimental hypothermia. Respiratory and blood pH changes in relation to cardiac function, *Am J Physiol* 175:389-97, 1953.

2. Clements SD, Hurst JW: Diagnostic value of electrocardiographic abnormalities observed in subjects accidentally exposed to cold, *Am J Cardiol* 29:729-34, 1972.

3. Okada M, Nishimura F, Yoshino H: The J wave in accidental hypothermia, *J Electrocardiol* 16:23-8, 1983.

4. Weinberg AD: Hypothermia, *Ann Emerg Med* 22:104-10, 1993.

5. Sheikh AM, Hurst JW: Osborn waves in the electrocardiogram. Hypothermia not due to exposure, and death due to diabetic ketoacidosis, *Clin Cardiol* 26:555-60, 2003.

11

Emergency Decisions in Monogenic Arrhythmic Diseases

EMERGENCY APPROACH

When the patient presents with a broad QRS tachycardia, either monomorphic or polymorphic VT or ventricular fibrillation (VF), proceed as follows:

If Hemodynamically Unstable

- Cardiovert.
- Obtain a history.
- Examine the preconversion and postconversion ECG to determine the possibility and type of monogenic disease.

If Hemodynamically Stable

- Evaluate the 12-lead ECG.
- In case of a long QT interval with torsades de pointes (TdP), see the section on emergency management of TdP (p. 177). In the absence of QT prolongation, give intravenous procainamide. If not successful:
  1. Cardiovert.
  2. Obtain a history.
  3. Examine the preconversion and postconversion ECG to determine the possibility and type of monogenic disease.

During the last decade genetic diagnosis of cardiac disorders became possible in a number of patients because of certain ECG features. This has been helpful in the risk stratification and management of carriers of monogenic diseases prone to cardiac arrhythmias and sudden death. Box 11-1 lists currently known arrhythmic familial diseases with a monogenic basis. The most common are discussed in this chapter. However, it is important to stress that the ECG of patients with monogenic diseases has a high specificity but a low sensitivity because of marked differences in phenotypic expression, and the characteristic ECG changes may only be present intermittently.[1]

As pointed out by Behr et al,[2] screening is important in first-degree relatives of young individuals who die suddenly and unexpectedly and in whom postmortem pathoanatomic investigations do not reveal abnormalities.

<table>
<tr><td colspan="1">

BOX 11-1

Familial Diseases with a Monogenic Basis for Cardiac Arrhythmias and Sudden Death

Hypertrophic cardiomyopathy
Arrhythmogenic RV dysplasia/cardiomyopathy
Long QT syndrome
Brugada syndrome
Catecholaminergic polymorphic VT
Short QT syndrome
Dilated cardiomyopathy
Wolff-Parkinson-White syndrome
Sick sinus syndrome
Lev-Lenègre AV block
Atrial fibrillation
Myotonic dystrophy

</td></tr>
</table>

Hypertrophic Cardiomyopathy

Hypertrophic cardiomyopathy (HCM) is the most common monogenic cardiac disorder. Together with arrhythmogenic RV dysplasia/cardiomyopathy (ARVD/C), it is the most frequent cause of exertion-related sudden cardiac death in individuals younger than 25 years.[3]

HCM has an incidence of approximately 2 in every 1000 young adults.[4] This disorder, which is more prevalent in men than in women (0.26% versus 0.09%), and in blacks than in whites (0.24% versus 0.10%),[4] is transmitted in an autosomal-dominant pattern involving 200 mutations in genes encoding proteins for the myocardial contractile process.[5]

ECG FINDINGS

The ECG of the patient with HCM should be evaluated together with the clinical, echocardiographic, and magnetic resonance imaging findings.

Figures 11-1 and 11-2 demonstrate that the ECG in HCM may vary considerably and include the following findings:

During Sinus Rhythm

P wave. The P wave shows left atrial or biatrial enlargement.

QRS complex
- Widening, often with a slurred upstroke (pseudo pre-excitation), or a typical bundle branch block pattern
- Left- or right-axis deviation
- Q waves
- Signs of left, right, or biventricular hypertrophy

ST-T segment
- ST depression in the left precordial leads
- T-wave inversion

Arrhythmias
Atrial level: Atrial fibrillation
Ventricular level: VPBs, VT, VF

DIFFERENTIATION BETWEEN HYPERTROPHIC CARDIOMYOPATHY AND ATHLETE'S HEART SYNDROME

The ventricular hypertrophy in HCM occurs in the absence of LV cavity dilation, which is unusual in the physiologic changes occurring in the athlete's heart.[6] The best way to differentiate HCM from athlete's heart syndrome is to check for the decrease in LV cavity size and wall thickness after the interruption of training for at least 3 months.[7] That decrease is not seen in the patient with HCM.

RISK FACTORS FOR SUDDEN DEATH

The long list of risk factors for sudden death in HCM includes the following:
- Unexplained syncope
- A familial history of sudden death at a young age
- LV hypertrophy greater than 3 cm
- Abnormal blood pressure response during exercise
- Nonsustained VT
- Genotype

Each factor has a low positive predictive accuracy, although risk increases with the presence of two or more factors.

EMERGENCY RESPONSE

An emergency response is required when the patient presents with a serious ventricular arrhythmia. The correct response is determined by the hemodynamic effects of the arrhythmia, as noted on p. 205.

LONG-TERM MANAGEMENT

Long-term management of patients with HCM includes the following:
- Treatment of symptoms
- Evaluation of family members and their genetic profile
- Prevention of sudden death
- Beta-blockers or verapamil as the first therapeutic choices for all symptomatic patients

Other considerations include the following:
- Transcoronary alcohol ablation of septal hypertrophy or surgical septal myectomy, which is effective

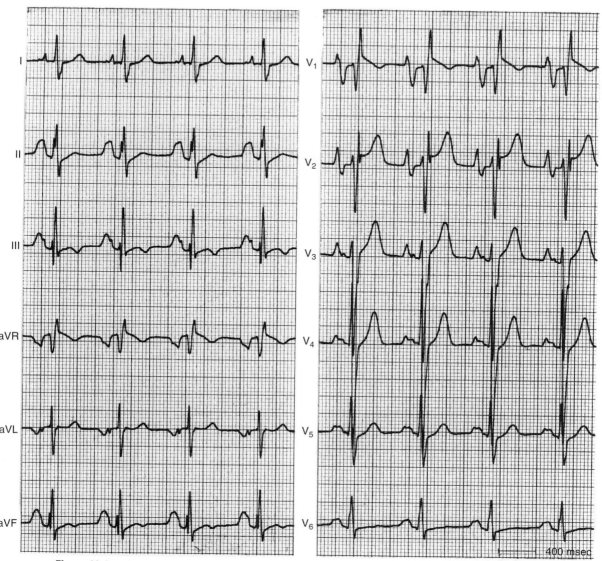

Figure 11-1 The ECG during sinus rhythm in a patient with hypertrophic cardiomyopathy. Shown are biatrial enlargement (large biphasic P waves in lead V_1 and wide, tall, notched P waves in the limb leads), QRS widening with an atypical RBBB pattern, and ST-T segment changes.

in reducing symptoms. Transcoronary ablation results in 50% of cases in complete RBBB, whereas surgical septal myectomy frequently results in LBBB. Both procedures have a 3% to 5% incidence of complete AV block.

■ An implantable cardioverter-defibrillator (ICD) with or without amiodarone is justified for patients successfully resuscitated from cardiac arrest or sustained VT. However, selection of candidates for an ICD who have the clinical features associated with increased risk for sudden death depends on the

individual risk profile and requires further refinement.[8,9]

Arrhythmogenic RV Dysplasia/Cardiomyopathy

ARVD/C is a myocardial disease that primarily affects the RV and is histologically characterized by the replacement of muscle cells by adipose and fibrous tissue.[10] Patients with ARVD/C often have nonsustained or sustained VT and may die suddenly.

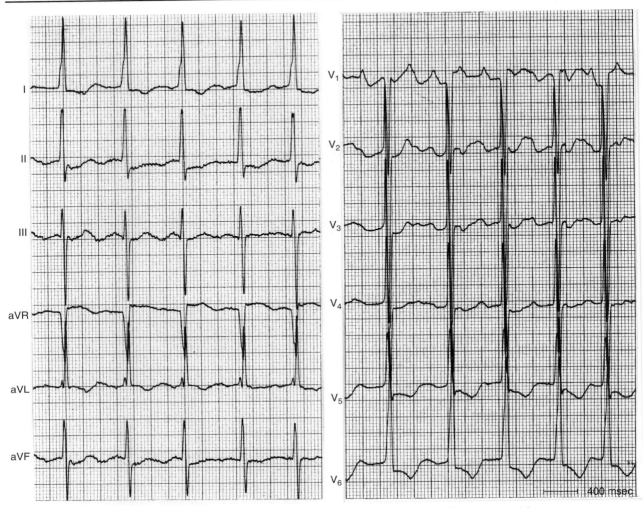

Figure 11-2   Atrial fibrillation in a patient with hypertrophic cardiomyopathy. Coarse atrial fibrillation is present, suggesting atrial enlargement. A slurred upstroke of the QRS is present in lead I, and signs of biventricular hypertrophy in the ST-T segment are abnormal.

ECG RECOGNITION

ECG features of the disease were initially described by Marcus et al[10] and were recently reviewed and extended by Nasir et al (Box 11-2 and Figures 11-3 and 11-4).[11]

Nasir et al[11] called attention to a new finding: *a prolonged S-wave upstroke (more than 55 msec) in leads V_1 to V_3 was found to be the most frequent ECG finding in ARVD/C*. The sign correlated with disease severity and inducibility of VT on electrophysiologic study. This ECG feature may be difficult to recognize. Therefore, to increase the accuracy of measurement, Nasir et al enlarged the ECG two times.

ARVD/C may be localized (inflow RV, outflow RV, or apex RV) or diffuse. A correlation exists between the number of the different ECG changes during sinus rhythm listed in Box 11-2 and the extent of the disease.[11]

Not mentioned in Box 11-2 but of clinical value in diagnosing diffuse RV involvement in ARVD/C is the finding of *low voltage in the extremity leads during sinus rhythm*.

THE ECG DURING NONSUSTAINED AND SUSTAINED VT

LBBB pattern: Because the tachycardia usually originates in the RV, the VT has an LBBB shape.

BOX 11-2

ECG Characteristics of Arrhythmogenic RV Dysplasia/Cardiomyopathy

Epsilon wave in lead V_1
RBBB
QRS duration >110 msec in leads V_1 to V_3
QRS duration:

$$\frac{V_1 + V_2 + V_3}{V_4 + V_5 + V_6} = >1.2$$

QRS dispersion >40 msec
S-wave upstroke >55 msec in leads V_1 to V_3
QT dispersion >65 msec
T-wave inversion in leads V_1 to V_3

QRS width: Depends on the site of origin of the VT and the extent of the disease.

QRS axis: Depends on the extent of the disease and the site of origin of the VT in the RV.

■ **Outflow tract of the RV:** Vertical axis.
■ **Inflow tract of the RV:** Intermediate axis.
■ **Apex of the RV:** Leftward axis.

DIFFERENTIATING ARRHYTHMOGENIC RV DYSPLASIA/CARDIOMYOPATHY VT FROM IDIOPATHIC VT

The QRS axis is important in differentiating ARVD/C VT from idiopathic VT. Idiopathic VT arises in the outflow tract of the RV, resulting in a QRS axis between +60 and +120 degrees. **Therefore, whenever an**

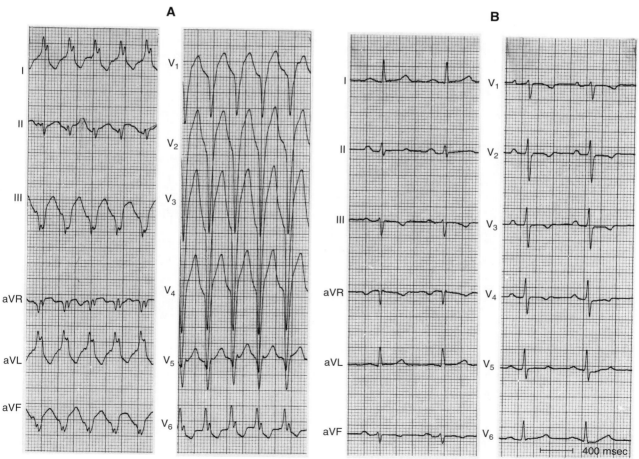

A   **B**

Figure 11-3 A 20-year-old patient with localized arrhythmogenic RV dysplasia/cardiomyopathy in the apex of the RV. **A,** VT with an LBBB shape is present. Note the AV dissociation (best seen in lead II) and left-axis deviation. **B,** During sinus rhythm T-wave inversion is present in leads V_1 to V_4. The S-wave upstroke duration is 60 msec in lead V_2.

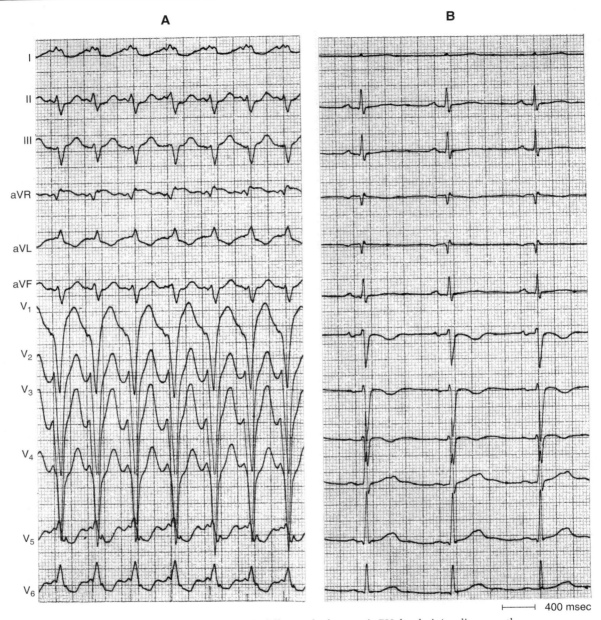

Figure 11-4   A 26-year-old patient with diffuse arrhythmogenic RV dysplasia/cardiomyopathy. **A,** VT with an LBBB shape and a QRS axis of −60 degrees. The QRS width is 200 msec. **B,** During sinus rhythm T-wave inversion occurs in leads V_1 to V_3. The QRS width is 120 msec in leads V_1 and V_2 and 90 msec in V_6.

LBBB-shaped VT shows left-axis deviation in the absence of coronary heart disease, ARVD/C should be the first suspicion.

This probability also holds true when isolated VPBs with an LBBB shape and left-axis deviation are present. Of course, when the LBBB-shaped VT has an intermediate or vertical axis, both ARVD/C and idiopathic VT are possible.

INCIDENCE

The incidence of ARVD/C has been estimated to be from 1 in 3000 to 1 in 10,000. Gemayel et al[12] found an incidence of 1 in 5000.

DIAGNOSIS

Major and minor diagnostic criteria for ARVD/C have been proposed by an international task force for

ARVD/C. For a diagnosis, one should have from the lists below: two major criteria, one major plus two minor criteria, or four of the five listed minor criteria.[13]

Major Diagnostic Criteria

■ Severe segmental or diffuse RV dilation
■ Reduction of RV ejection fraction with no, or only mild, LV enlargement
■ Localized RV aneurysms
■ Fibro-fatty replacement of myocardium (on endomyocardial biopsy)
■ Epsilon waves or prolongation of the QRS by more than 110 msec in leads V_1 to V_3
■ Familial disease confirmed at necropsy or surgery

Minor Diagnostic Criteria

■ Global or regional dysfunction and structural alterations (mild global RV dilation or ejection fraction reduction with normal LV, mild segmental dilation of the RV or regional RV hypokinesia)
■ Inverted T waves in leads V_2 and V_3 in those older than 12 years and without RBBB
■ Late potentials on signal-averaged ECG
■ V_1-negative VT, sustained or nonsustained (by ECG, Holter, or during exercise testing)
■ Family history (premature sudden death before age 35 years because of suspected RV cardiomyopathy or clinical diagnosis of ARVD/C in family members based on this criteria)

Magnetic Resonance Imaging

Magnetic resonance imaging is an optimal technique for the detection and follow-up of patients with VT with an LBBB-like pattern because, compared with other imaging modalities, MRI provides the clearest visualization of functional and structural abnormalities such as[14-16]:

■ Global RV dilation
■ Global systolic and diastolic dysfunction
■ RV wall thinning
■ Localized aneurysms of the RV and its outflow tract
■ Fatty infiltration
■ Regional wall motion abnormalities of the inferior and anterior RV free wall and the RV outflow tract
■ Severe alteration of the RV with decreased ejection fraction and possible involvement of the LV

Electrophysiologic Study

Niroomand et al[17] found that a diagnosis of ARVD/C can be reliably made on the basis of clinical presentation,

imaging techniques, and an electrophysiologic study. In their study of 55 patients with an RV arrhythmia, the following results identified patients with ARVD/C:

■ Inducibility of VT by programmed electrical stimulation with ventricular extrastimuli (idiopathic right VT [IRVT] at 3% versus ARVD/C at 93%; $P < 0.0001$)
■ Presence of more than one ECG morphology during VT (IRVT at 0% versus ARVD/C at 73%; $P < 0.0001$)
■ Fragmented diastolic potentials during the ventricular arrhythmia (IRVT at 0% versus ARVD/C at 93%; $P < 0.0001$)

SYMPTOMS

Symptoms are usually related to episodes of VT, such as palpitations, vertigo, presyncope, syncope, dyspnea, chest pain, or abrupt extreme weakness, in an individual who is apparently in good health. However, sudden death in association with *exercise* is not uncommon and may be the first clinical manifestation of this disease. ARVD/C is a leading cause of sudden death during athletic activity because the VT associated with this condition is provoked by exercise-induced catecholamine discharge.[18]

PROGNOSIS

ARVD/C progresses from a silent course to the appearance of arrhythmias, structural changes, and heart failure, in that order, if sudden death does not occur first.

The annual mortality rate for ARVD/C is approximately 2.5%.[19] Recently, Hulot et al,[20] using natural history findings in a large series of patients with ARVD/C, found that a history of VT, syncope, and clinical signs of RV failure and LV dysfunction were the strongest predictors of cardiovascular death during follow-up.

CAUSE

Both ARVD/C and catecholaminergic polymorphic VT, which can cause sudden death in children, have been shown to result from mutations in the cardiac ryanodine receptor (hRYR2), which is the cardiac sarcoplasmic reticulum calcium release channel and a key component in cardiac excitation-contraction coupling. A mutation of the gene for this channel results in heart failure and life-threatening VT.[21]

MANAGEMENT
Emergency Response

Appropriate management is dictated by the hemodynamic tolerance of the arrhythmia (see p. 207).

Long-Term Management

No cure is available for ARVD/C. When the diagnosis of ARVD/C is made, *the patient should refrain from intense exertion.*

Treatment is related to the presence or absence of heart failure and is directed at identifying patients at high risk and preventing life-threatening cardiac arrhythmias with options that include:

- Antiarrhythmic drugs (amiodarone, sotalol, vera-pamil, beta-blockers, flecainide)
- Diuretics
- Angiotensin-converting enzyme inhibitors
- Anticoagulants
- Catheter ablation if the VT is refractory to drugs, especially when the pathologic condition is localized
- An ICD, also indicated in primary prevention if the patient has ARVD/C and a family history of sudden death at young age is present[22]
- Cardiac transplantation in cases of progressive biventricular failure

Congenital Long QT Syndrome

The congenital LQTS is a hereditary disorder characterized by a prolonged QT interval, is commonly associated with a polymorphic VT known as TdP, which often leads to severe symptoms such as syncope and sudden cardiac death. Genetic studies have so far identified seven forms of congenital LQTS caused by mutations in genes of the potassium and sodium channels or the membrane adapter located on chromosomes 3, 4, 7, 11, 17, and 21.[23]

The congenital LQTS may be precipitated by a variety of circumstances such as exercise, emotion, rest, sleep, or sudden noise (Figures 11-5 and 11-6), depending on the affected gene. In most adults with congenital LQTS, TdP is preceded by a pause (pause dependent) that exacerbates the already prolonged QT interval. In children, who often have a more severe form of the disease, the onset of TdP is less often pause dependent.[24]

Additionally, it is believed that susceptible individuals with a prolonged QT interval or TdP after the administration of one of a variety of drugs (acquired LQTS) may have a subclinical variant of the congenital LQTS exacerbated by the administration of a drug from an ever-expanding list of prescription and nonprescription drugs that block potassium channels (see Chapter 7).

Sympathomimetic drugs are best avoided by patients with congenital LQTS. If their administration becomes unavoidable, careful ECG monitoring is necessary.

LONG QT SYNDROME MANAGEMENT
Emergency Management of Torsades de Pointes in Acquired or Congenital Long QT Syndrome
1. Stop the offending drug when drug related.
2. Establish continuous ECG monitoring.
3. Give magnesium as MgCl or $MgSO_4$, 1 to 2 g intravenous bolus over a 5-minute period, followed by infusion with 1 to 2 g/hr for 4 to 6 hours.
4. If intravenous magnesium is unsuccessful, increase heart rate with isoproterenol or by pacing.

Long-Term Management of Patients with Long QT Syndrome
1. Treat all patients with long QT syndrome (LQTS) with beta-blockers unless contraindicated. Note that the following facts apply:
   - LQT1 patients have a low incidence of cardiac events and should be treated with a beta-blocker as first-line therapy.
   - LQT2 and LQT3 patients have a higher risk of cardiac events while on beta-blocker therapy.
   - Prophylactic use of the ICD is recommended in patients with LQT2 with a QTc interval more than 500 msec on therapy and in all patients with LQT3.
2. Beta-blocking therapy should also be given when the patient has been treated with a pacemaker, left cardiac sympathetic denervation, or an ICD.
3. Educate patients and family members regarding potential risks associated with strenuous exercise and interruption of beta-blocker therapy.
4. Keep in mind that some LQTS gene carriers will have a normal QTc interval.
5. Screen for LQTS in family members of the proband.

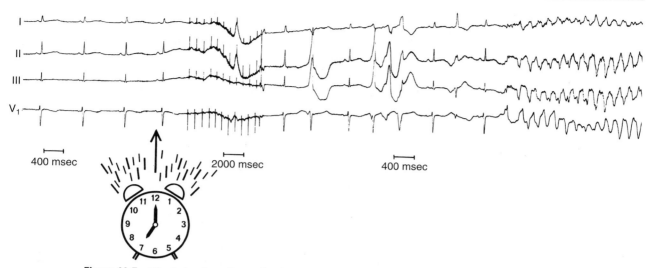

Figure 11-5   The induction of torsades de pointes by arousal from sleep by an alarm clock. Note that after the alarm goes off the QT prolongs, ventricular ectopic activity develops, and torsades de pointes is initiated. This mode of initiation is especially seen in long QT syndrome type 2.

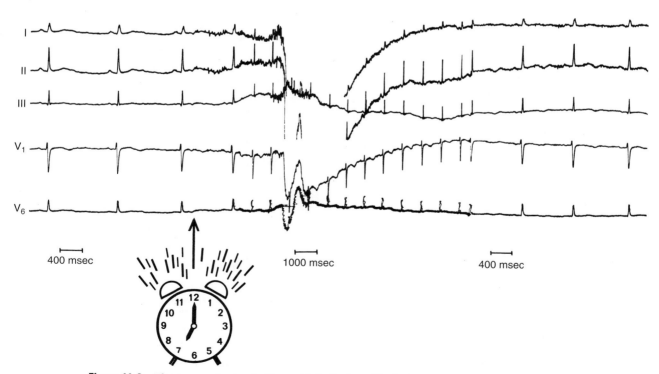

Figure 11-6   The same patient as in Figure 11-5 after beta-blockade. No arrhythmias are initiated during arousal.

See Box 11-3 (p. 210) for the long list of drugs that should be avoided in patients with congenital LQTS.

INCIDENCE

One in 10,000 persons is believed to be a gene carrier for LQTS. Congenital LQTS causes as many as 3000 sudden deaths in children and young adults each year in the United States alone.[25]

ECG SIGNS

The ECG signs of LQTS are prolongation of the QT interval and morphologic abnormalities of the T wave. However, in contrast to the acquired form of LQTS, approximately 12% of long QT gene carriers have a normal QTc (0.44 seconds or less).[26] For this reason, although the QTc intervals of nonsymptomatic family members may not be diagnostic, congenital LQTS cannot be excluded on this basis alone. However, the shape of the T wave may be an additional helpful diagnostic clue.

QT Interval

QT prolongation is evaluated in light of age, sex, and heart rate; it is longer in women than in men and children and lengthens with bradycardia and shortens with tachycardia. To determine the QTc, divide the QT interval by the square root of the RR interval (Bazett's formula).

The range of QTc intervals in congenital LQTS is from 0.41 seconds to more than 0.60 seconds. In LQT1 and LQT2 the QTc averages 0.49 seconds, with 500 msec or more being an independent predictor of risk among patients with LQT1 and LQT2 but not among those with a mutation at the LQT3 locus.[27,28] In LQT3 this value may be longer, with a mean of 0.51 seconds.

Thus the diagnosis of LQTS is likely with a QTc of 0.48 seconds or more in women and 0.47 seconds in men. When the QTc is between 0.41 and 0.46 seconds, the diagnosis is uncertain and additional tests are required.

The T Wave

The T-wave morphologic features are relatively characteristic for each genotype. The characteristic ECG patterns seen in the three distinct forms of LQTS are shown in Figure 11-7.

The T wave does not always have the same configuration in the same patient. It is influenced by sympathetic stimulation such as anxiety and exercise (see Figure 11-5).

Figure 11-8 shows three ECGs from the same patient with LQT1 at intervals of 2 years (the last two with the patient taking beta-blocking drugs). Note the changes in the QT configuration. The possibility of these changes should be kept in mind when trying to classify the patient with LQTS.

QT Interval in Women

Women are more commonly affected by both the congenital form and the drug-induced form of LQTS and are particularly at risk during the postpartum period.[29,30]

TORSADES DE POINTES

TdP is a life-threatening polymorphic VT of more than 170 beats/min with a unique undulating QRS pattern. It occurs against a background of prolonged QT intervals, ventricular ectopic beats, T- and U-wave abnormalities, and pauses. TdP is generally believed to be initiated by an early afterdepolarization. A reentrant mechanism has been suggested for the maintenance of TdP,[31] which may spontaneously terminate or deteriorate into ventricular fibrillation.

RISK FACTORS: AGE AND SEX

Zareba et al[29] of the International Long QT Syndrome Registry recently demonstrated that age and sex have different genotype-specific modulating effects on the risk of cardiac events in patients with LQTS. The risk factors for LQT1, LQT2, and LQT3 are discussed.

Long QT Syndrome Type 1

During childhood, the risk of cardiac events is significantly higher in male patients with LQT1 than in female patients with LQT1.

During adulthood, females with LQT1, because of their longer QT intervals, have a significantly higher risk of cardiac events than males. However, the yearly mortality rate of individuals with cardiac events is higher in male patients with LQT1 (5%) than in female patients with LQT1 (2%).

Long QT Syndrome Type 2

During childhood, no significant sex-related difference in the risk of cardiac events among LQT2 carriers is present.

During adulthood, women with LQT2 have a significantly higher risk of cardiac events than men with LQT2. However, as in LQT1, the yearly mortality rate of individuals with cardiac events is higher in men with LQT2 (6%) than in women with LQT2 (2%).

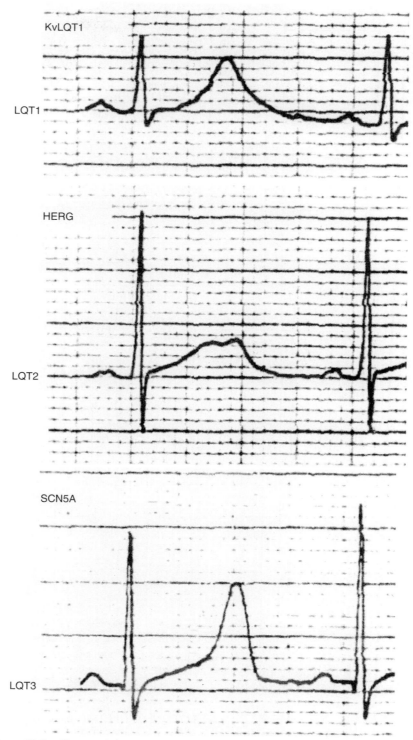

Figure 11-7 Characteristic ECG patterns in three distinct forms of long QT syndrome (*LQT1, LQT2, LQT3*). Note that in LQT1 a broad T wave is present; LQT2 demonstrates a bifid T wave, and a prolonged QT with a normal T wave are present in LQT3. (Reprinted from Keating MT, Sanguinetti MC: Familial cardiac arrhythmias. In Scriver CR, Beaudet AL, Sly WS, et al, editors: *The metabolic and molecular bases of inherited disease,* ed 8, New York, 2001, McGraw-Hill.)

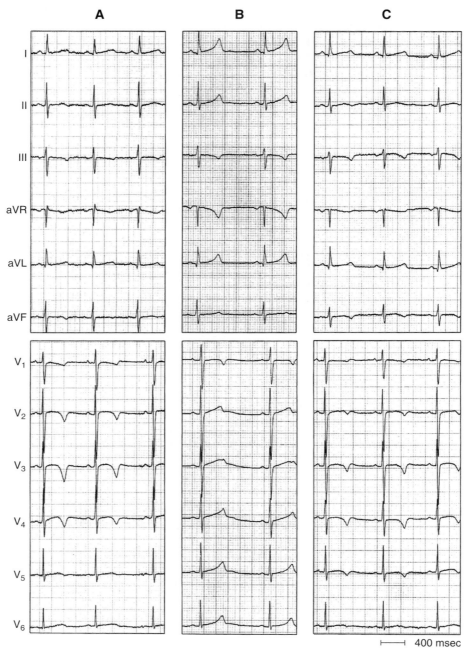

Figure 11-8 Three 12-lead ECGs at 2-year intervals in a patient with long QT syndrome type 1. **A,** An ECG when the boy was 8 years old and 2 days after he was resuscitated from cardiac arrest during swimming. **B** and **C** were recorded during beta-blockade.

Long QT Syndrome Type 3

During childhood, no significant sex-related difference in the risk of cardiac events among LQT3 carriers is present.

During adulthood, the mortality rate of individuals with cardiac events is highest in men and women with LQT3 (19% and 18%, respectively) compared with men and women with LQT1 and LQT2.

CLINICAL CHARACTERISTICS

Within LQTS families, 50% of the first patients (proband) to be diagnosed have had at least one syncopal episode or have died by age 12 years, and 90% have had at least one syncopal episode or have died by age 40 years. Probands are usually brought to medical attention because of a syncopal episode during childhood or the teenage years. Syncope occurs in approximately two thirds of gene carriers, with sudden death in 10% to 15% of untreated patients.

Other clinical characteristics are:

- Female sex
- Congenital deafness (Jervell and Lange-Nielsen syndrome)
- Resting heart rate less than 60 beats/min
- QTc of 0.50 seconds or more

EMERGENCY RESPONSE TO TORSADES DE POINTES IN CONGENITAL LONG QT SYNDROME

The current treatment for congenital LQTS–mediated TdP and VF is the same as for acquired LQTS (see p. 177).

LONG-TERM MANAGEMENT
Checklist

1. Measure QTc intervals. Risk is related to the length of the QTc interval.
2. Treat patients with LQTS with beta-blockers unless contraindicated.
3. Educate patients and family members regarding potential risks associated with strenuous exercise and interruption of beta-blocker therapy.
4. Screen for LQTS in family members of the proband.

Beta-Blockers

The incidence of cardiac events in LQTS patients can be significantly reduced by beta-blockers, although such therapy may not be sufficient for cardiac arrest survivors and for those with LQT3.[32] To prevent sudden death, beta-blockers should be prescribed prophylactically in patients with asymptomatic congenital LQTS.

Pacemakers

Permanent cardiac pacemakers have been recommended as an adjuvant to beta-blockers in patients with congenital LQTS associated with sinus bradycardia, pauses during sinus rhythm, or AV conduction block and particularly patients with LQT3, who usually have slow heart rates. Prolongation of the QT interval is exacerbated following pauses or during bradycardia, increasing the risk for TdP. Pacemakers are always used in combination with beta-blocker therapy because even rapid pacing does not mitigate the effects of sympathetic stimulation.[33] Practical recommendations on programming pacemakers for pause-dependent arrhythmias, which differs from the standard pacemaker programming, have been compiled by Viskin et al.[33]

Left Cardiac Sympathetic Denervation

The rationale for the therapeutic value of left cardiac sympathetic denervation is based on the recognition of the arrhythmogenic potential of the left stellate ganglion and the antifibrillatory effect of left stellectomy.[34,35] The intervention is performed in symptomatic patients who have arrhythmic recurrences despite beta-blocking therapy.[36] Left cardiac sympathetic denervation is a useful intervention for the management of high-risk teenagers, who are frequently less compliant with beta-blocking therapy.[36]

Implantable Cardioverter-Defibrillators

ICDs with dual-chamber pacing capability are indicated for patients at high risk. The most frequent indications are aborted sudden cardiac death and recurrent symptoms despite combined beta-blocker and pacemaker therapy. An ICD should especially be considered in LQT2 with a QTc of more than 500 msec and in patients with LQT3.[32]

IMPORTANCE OF COUNSELING

Noncompliance places patients at increased risk for life-threatening cardiac events. Thus frequent counseling of young patients and their parents is critical. Counseling includes warnings regarding the role of physical and emotional stress as triggers for cardiac events, the necessity of taking a beta-blocker, drugs to be avoided, and the prevention of electrolyte loss.

Physical and Emotional Stress

Vigorous exercise should be avoided, especially swimming and exposure to significant emotional stimuli. These warnings are especially true for patients with LQT1. Life-threatening arrhythmias tend to occur under specific circumstances in a gene-specific manner. Patients with LQT1 have 62% of their events during exercise and only 3% during rest or sleep. Patients with LQT2 or LQT3 are less likely to have events during exercise (13%) and more likely to have events during rest or sleep (29% and 39%, respectively).[36] In LQT2 arousal from sleep may initiate TdP (see Figure 11-5).

Drugs to Avoid

A growing number of cardiac and noncardiac drugs have been found to block potassium ion (K^+) channels, prolonging the QT interval and causing TdP when administered alone, with another drug that also blocks K⁺ channels, or to an individual whose K⁺ channels are already genetically blocked (Box 11-3). Box 11-4 lists additional drugs that patients with LQTS should avoid. Patients with LQTS (and their parents) should be warned about the dangers of recreational drugs such as ecstasy (methylenedioxymethamphetamine) and cocaine.

BOX 11-3

Drugs That Prolong the QT Interval or Induce Torsades de Pointes

Acrivastine* (Semprex-D)
Ajmaline
Almokalant
Amantadine (Symmetrel)
Amiodarone (Cordarone)
Amitriptyline (Elavil, Endep, Etrafon, Limbitrol, Triavil)
Amoxapine (Asendin)
Ampicillin (Omnipen, Polycillin, Principen)
Amrinone (Inocor)
Aprindine
Astemizole† (Hismanal)
Azimilide
Bepridil (Vasocor)
Bretylium (Bretylate, Bretylol)
Budipine
Cetirizine* (Zyrtec)
Chloral hydrate
Chloroquine (Aralen)
Chlorpromazine (Largactil, Thorazine)
Cisapride‡ (Propulsid)
Citalopram (Celexa)
Clarithromycin (Biaxin)
Clemastine (Tavist)
Clofilium
Clomipramine (Anafranil)
Co-trimoxazole (Septra, Bactrim, SMX-TMP)
Desipramine (Norpramin)
Diphenhydramine (Benadryl)
Disopyramide (Norpace)
Dofetilide (Tikosyn)
Doxepin (Sinequan, Zonalon)
Droperidol (Inapsine)
Ebastine (Ebastel)
Erythrocin (Erythrostatin, Ilotycin, PCE, Staticin)
Erythromycin (Akne-Mycin, EES, E-Mycin, Eryderm, Erygel, Ery-Tab, Eryc, EryPed)
Fexofenadine* (Allegra)
Flecainide (Tambocor)
Fludrocortisone (Florinef)
Fluphenazine (Permitil, Prolixin)
Gatifloxacin
Grepafloxacin
Halofantrine (Halfan)
Haloperidol (Haldol)

Hydroxyzine (Atarax, Atazine, Dovaril, Hypam, Vistacot, Vistaril, Vistawin)
Ibutilide (Corvert)
Imidazole (Lotrimin)
Imipramine (Tofranil)
Indapamide (Lozol)
Ipecac
Itraconazole (Sporanox)
Ketanserin (Aserinox, Ketensin, Perketan, Serepress, Sufrexal)
Ketoconazole (Nizoral)
Lidoflazine
Lithium
Loratadine* (Claritin)
Maprotiline (Ludiomil)
Mefloquine (Lariam)
Mesoridazine (Serentil)
Milrinone (Primacor)
Mizolastine* (Mistamine)
Moricizine (Ethmozine)
N-acetyl-procainamide
Nortriptyline (Pamelor)
Papaverine, intracoronary
Pentamidine (Nebupent, Pentacarinat, Pentam)
Pericycline
Perphenazine (Trilafon)
Phenothiazines (chlorpromazine, Compazine, Mellaril, Permitil, Prolixin, Serentil, Stelazine, Thorazine, Trilafon, Vesprin)
Pimozide (Orap)
Prenylamine†
Probucol (Lorelco)
Procainamide (Procan, Procanbid, Pronestyl)
Prochlorperazine (Compazine)
Propafenone (Rythmol)
Protriptyline (Vivactil)
Quetiapine (Seroquel)
Quinidine (Cardioquin, Duraquin, Quinaglute, Quinidex)
Quinine
Risperidone (Risperdal)
Sematilide
Sertindole† (Serdolect)
Sotalol (Betapace)
d,l-sotalol, d-sotalol

BOX 11-3—cont'd
Drugs That Prolong the QT Interval or Induce Torsades de Pointes
Sparfloxacine
Spiramycin
Sultopride (Cloridrato)
Tamoxifen (Nolvadex)
Terfenadine‡ (Seldane)
Terodiline†
Thioridazine (Mellaril)
Thiothixene (Navane)
Timiperone
Trifluoperazine (Stelazine)
Trimethoprim sulfamethoxazole (Bactrim, Septra)
Troleandomycin (Tao)
Vasopressin (Pitressin)
Zimelidine (Zelmid)
*New nonsedating antihistamine; effect on IKr needs confirmation. †Off the market. ‡Off the market in some countries.

BOX 11-4
Additional Drugs to Be Avoided by Patients with Long QT Syndrome
Asthma and Allergy Medications Ephedrine (adrenaline) Epinephrine Isoproterenol (Isuprel, Medinhaler-Iso) **Decongestants** Phenyldrine Phenylephrine Phenylpropanolamine **Drugs to Prevent Hypotension** Midodrine (Proamatine) Norepinephrine (Levophed) **Asthma Medications** Albuterol Metaproterenol Salmeterol Terbutaline **Diet Pills** Fenfluramine (Pondimin) Phentermine (Adipex, Fastin, Ionamin, Obe-Nix, Obephen, Obermine, Obestin, T-Diet) Sibutramine (Meridia) **Drug to Prevent Preterm Labor** Ritodrine (Yutopar)

Electrolyte Loss

Patients are instructed to replace electrolytes with fluids that contain potassium in case of diaphoresis, diarrhea, or vomiting.

SUMMARY OF INHERITED LQTS

Table 11-1 summarizes important characteristics of the inherited LQTS, concentrating on the most common types.

Brugada Syndrome

Brugada syndrome is an autosomal dominant disease caused by a mutation of *SCN5A*, the same gene responsible for LQT3 that also codes for the cardiac voltage–

dependent sodium ion (Na$^+$) channels.[37] The syndrome consists of the risk of sudden death and a peculiar ECG pattern showing an incomplete RBBB configuration with an elevated J point, ST-segment elevation in leads V$_1$ to V$_3$, and a normal QT interval.

The ECG pattern itself was first reported in 1953 by Osher and Wolff[38] and in 1954 by Edeiken.[39] It was first associated with sudden death in 1989 by Martini et al[40] and again in 1990 by Aihara et al.[41] In 1992 Brugada

---

TABLE 11-1	ECG, Effect of Beta-Blockade, and Circumstances Favoring Arrhythmic Events in Long QT Syndrome Types 1, 2, and 3		
	Type 1	Type 2	Type 3
QTc	Prolonged	More prolonged	More prolonged
T wave	Normal	Widened; or, bifid	Delayed onset
Beta-blockade	Effective	Less effective	Less effective (implantable cardioverter-defibrillator)
Emotional stress	+	±	−
Physical stress	+	±	−
Auditory stimuli	−	+	−
Rest, sleep	−	−	+

> **EMERGENCY RESPONSE**
> Appropriate management of Brugada syndrome is dictated by the patient's risk profile.
> In case of an arrhythmia, treatment should be as outlined in Chapter 4 (SVT) and
> Chapter 5 (VT).

and Brugada[42] described the ECG findings in leads V_1 to V_3 of "RBBB and persistent ST elevation" as a distinct clinical and ECG syndrome in eight patients who died suddenly or whose sudden death had been aborted. All but Edeiken called the ECG pattern in leads V_1 to V_3 RBBB. Recognition of this ECG pattern is important because it permits early identification and treatment of those at risk for sudden death.

ECG DIAGNOSIS

Figure 11-9 is an example of Brugada syndrome during sinus rhythm. The ECG signs are limited to the right precordial leads V_1, V_2, and V_3. Originally, two ECG patterns were described: "coved" and "saddlebacked."[43]

In the *coved ECG pattern (also called type 1 Brugada)*, the ST segment in leads V_1 to V_3 shows an upward convex shape, dipping in to a negative T wave without an isoelectric line (see Figure 11-9). Figure 11-10 shows a pseudo-Brugada pattern.

In the *saddleback ECG pattern (also called type 2 Brugada)*, ST elevation in V_1 and V_2 is followed by a positive or biphasic T wave (Figure 11-11).

Currently only the coved shape is accepted as a diagnostic criterion for Brugada syndrome.[44,45] Discussion

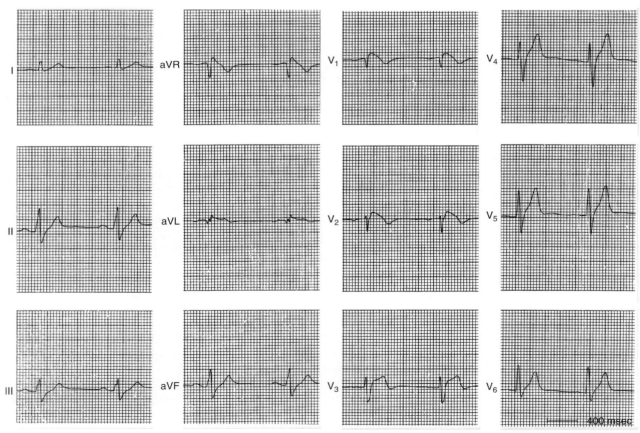

Figure 11-9 Brugada syndrome. The ECG was recorded in a 42-year-old man who was resuscitated from cardiac arrest 3 days previously. Note the typical ECG changes in leads V_1 to V_3 with the coved ST segment followed by a negative T wave.

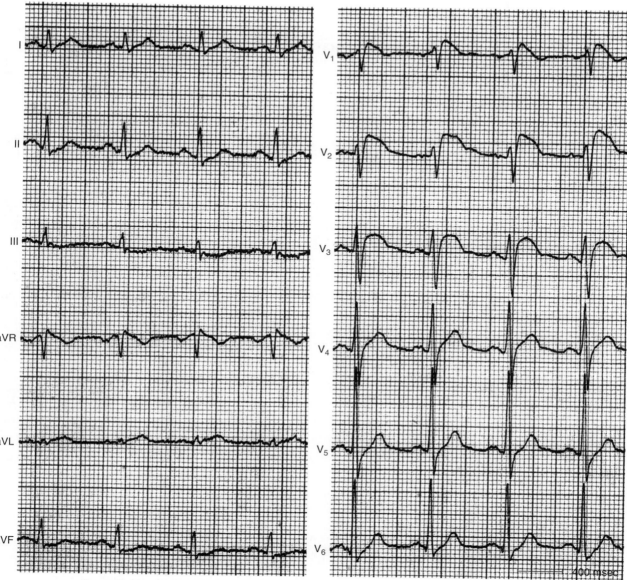

Figure 11-10 Pseudo-Brugada syndrome, in which a 12-lead ECG with a coved ST segment in leads V_1 to V_3 suggests Brugada syndrome. However, the T wave does not become negative in those leads. The ECG is from an asymptomatic 22-year-old man with no family history of syncope and sudden death.

is ongoing about how much ST segment elevation (more than 1 mm or 2 mm) is required to make a positive diagnosis.

Pseudo-Brugada Pattern

Figures 11-9, 11-10, and 11-11 compare Brugada and pseudo-Brugada patterns. Figure 11-10 (a pseudo-

Brugada) has a coved ST segment that fits the description for Brugada syndrome, but the T wave is positive. Figure 11-11 shows a saddleback configuration that fits the original description of the Brugada pattern, type 2 Brugada. However, the patient whose ECG is seen in Figure 11-11 was a trained asymptomatic athlete with LV hypertrophy and early repolarization, changes often seen

A   B

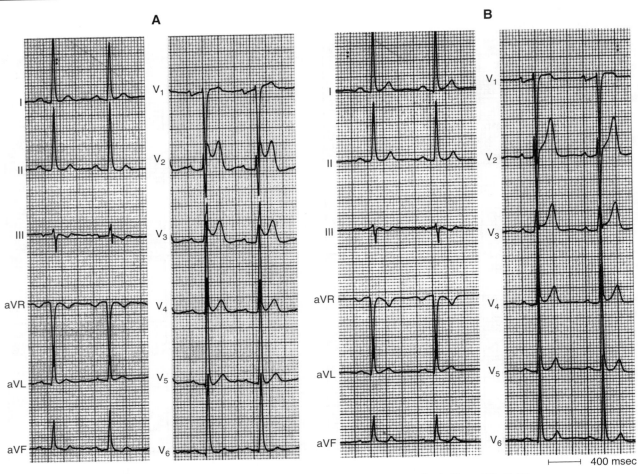

Figure 11-11   **A,** A 12-lead ECG showing a saddleback pattern in leads V$_2$ and V$_3$. **B,** The same patient 1 week later. The patient is an asymptomatic endurance athlete with LV hypertrophy without a family history of syncope or sudden death.

in the athlete's ECG and that disappear on cessation of intense training.

UNMASKING CONCEALED AND INTERMITTENT FORMS

Although the diagnosis of overt Brugada syndrome is easily made by the ECG, it can be missed in concealed and intermittent forms. In suspicious cases, the presence of an *SCN5A* mutation can be revealed on the ECG by modulating changes in autonomic balance and administering antiarrhythmic drugs. Beta-adrenergic stimulation normalizes the ECG, whereas intravenous ajmaline, flecainide, or procainamide accentuates the elevated J wave and are capable of unmasking the concealed and intermittent forms. These drugs are helpful in identifying the risk of sudden death.[46]

The Flecainide Test

The flecainide test is widely used in Brugada syndrome. During the test intravenous flecainide, 2 mg/kg, is given over a 10-minute period while a 12-lead ECG is continuously recorded. Because the occurrence of major ventricular arrhythmias has been shown to be significantly higher in both symptomatic and asymptomatic patients with a documented *SCN5A* gene mutation, the test should be performed in an optimal setting for electrical cardioversion and defibrillation and under experienced medical supervision.[43]

The test is considered positive if the coved type of ST segment elevation appears or when a J-point elevation of more than 2 mm is seen in a patient with a previously normal ECG. Administration of flecainide is stopped when the test is positive or when ventricular arrhythmias appear.

Patients undergoing the test should be monitored until the drug is metabolized and excreted.

In cases of ventricular arrhythmias during or after the test, intravenous isoprenaline (1 to 3 μg/kg per minute) can be therapeutic. In countries where ajmaline is available, this sodium channel blocker (1 mg/kg intravenously over a 5-minute period) is preferred as a test drug because of its short half-life.

Beta-Adrenergic Stimulation

When the ECG signs are overt, beta-adrenergic stimulation (exercise, intravenous isuprel) normalizes the ECG,[47] whereas beta-blockade may exaggerate the J wave.[48]

PATHOPHYSIOLOGIC CHARACTERISTICS

J-point elevation may be caused by a more prominent epicardial manifestation of the spike-and-dome action potential morphologic feature, mediated by a transient outward potassium current.[46] Conditions that enhance the current predispose to dispersion of repolarization, which may in turn lead to arrhythmias based on phase 2 reentry. This phenomenon is most pronounced in the free wall and outflow tract of the RV. Those places have therefore been suggested as the site of origin of the arrhythmias.[46,49]

INCIDENCE

The incidence of Brugada syndrome is difficult to estimate because some people are carriers and exhibit no symptoms. In the United States Brugada syndrome occurs in approximately 1 in 40,000 individuals, but worldwide it is more prevalent in southeast Asia, especially in Thailand and Laos.[50] In these countries the disease represents the most frequent cause of death in young adults. Death usually occurs at night during sleep.

RISK STRATIFICATION

The clinical presentation of Brugada syndrome may vary considerably. Some asymptomatic individuals have never had a serious ventricular arrhythmia, and some die suddenly from a polymorphic VT or VF.

According to Brugada et al,[51] at the highest risk for life-threatening arrhythmias and sudden death is the patient who has the typical ECG (a coved ST segment in leads V_1 to V_3) with a history of syncope and in whom a polymorphic VT or VF can be induced during programmed ventricular stimulation. Other investigators have questioned the value of inducibility of VT or VF during electrophysiologic study.[52,53] They believe that high-risk recognition should be based on a history of

syncope in the presence of a spontaneously typical ECG. The high-risk patient should be protected by an ICD.

A recent study from Finland has shown that a J-point elevation with a saddleback ST segment in the right precordial leads can be found in asymptomatic subjects without a family history of sudden death.[45] In those individuals the ECG pattern is a normal variant rather than a specific predictor of life-threatening arrhythmias.

TREATMENT
Emergency Approach

The emergency approach to arrhythmias in the Brugada syndrome is directed by the type and hemodynamic tolerance of the arrhythmia.

Long-Term Treatment

Implantable cardioverter-defibrillator. The ICD is the only proven effective treatment to provide protection from sudden death in patients with high-risk Brugada syndrome.[54]

Quinidine. Belhassen et al[55] recently reported that quinidine prevented VF induction in patients with Brugada syndrome. They also suggested that quinidine suppressed spontaneous ventricular arrhythmias in their patients and that quinidine could be a safe alternative to ICD therapy. Randomized studies comparing these two therapies will be necessary to give a definite answer.

SUMMARY OF BRUGADA SYNDROME

Brugada syndrome may cause sudden death in patients with "normal" hearts. It is observed worldwide but is more common in southeast Asia. The syndrome is more common in men. Ventricular arrhythmic events may occur at a young age but usually appear in patients in their early 40s and at rest. The coved ST segment pattern in leads V_1 to V_3, followed by a negative T wave, is required for the diagnosis. The ECG characteristics may be intermittent and unmasked by sodium channel blockers.

Brugada syndrome is inherited in an autosomal dominant manner with incomplete penetrance and wide genetic heterogeneity. Mutations in the cardiac sodium channel are found in 15% of patients. High-risk patients should receive an ICD.

Catecholaminergic Polymorphic VT

Catecholaminergic polymorphic VT (CPVT) was described by Coumel et al[56] in 1978 and more extensively by

Leenhardt et al[57] in 1995. These patients have polymorphic VT during sympathetic stimulation, such as exercise, and may die suddenly. Often the polymorphic VT is preceded by a bidirectional VT showing alternating morphologic features of the QRS complex. The arrhythmias start at a young age, and in approximately one third of the cases a family history of juvenile sudden death or stress-related syncope is present. An example of the arrhythmia is given in Figure 11-12. The disease usually shows an autosomal dominant pattern of inheritance, although it may also be a recessively inherited trait.[58,59] Mutations in the cardiac ryanodine receptor gene have been found to underlie CPVT.[59]

MANAGEMENT

Beta-blockers. The availability of genetic analysis allows for the presymptomatic diagnosis of CPVT. Early diagnosis identifies individuals at risk who are likely to benefit from long-term treatment with a beta-blocker. In symptomatic patients, the effectiveness of beta-blocking therapy should be evaluated by exercise testing, which will allow the physician to identify those patients in whom complex arrhythmias are not controlled and who may benefit from an ICD.[60]

Short QT Syndrome

This recently described disease, characterized by exceptionally short QT intervals, has a high rate of sudden death, even at a very young age. At invasive electrophysiologic study the ventricular refractory periods are very short, and malignant ventricular arrhythmias can be reproducibly induced.[61,62] The causal gene for this syndrome has been identified.[63] Short QT syndrome resembles patients described by Coumel et al[64] and Leenhardt et al,[65] showing TdP initiated by very shortly coupled VPBs. In those patients, the QT interval was normal and no structural heart disease could be demonstrated. An example of the arrhythmia is shown in Figure 11-13. In 30% of these patients a family history of sudden cardiac death was present. No adequate prevention of TdP was possible by pharmacologic means, and ICD seems to be the correct therapy. It would be of interest to study the genetics of patients with shortly coupled TdP to see whether a relation exists with the short QT syndrome.

Recently, Gaita et al[66] showed that in patients with the short QT syndrome, quinidine prolonged the QT interval, suggesting potential effective therapy for these

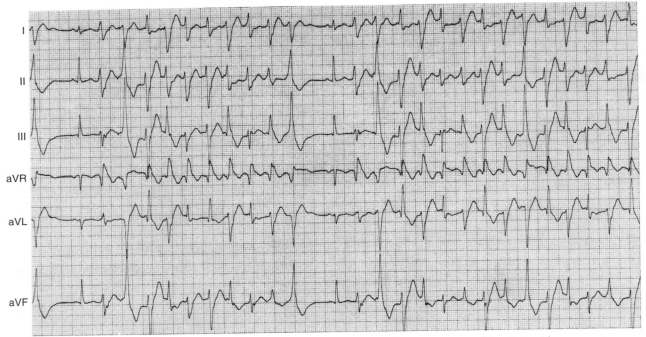

Figure 11-12 An ECG taken during exercise shows polymorphic VT in a 12-year-old patient with catecholaminergic polymorphic tachycardia.

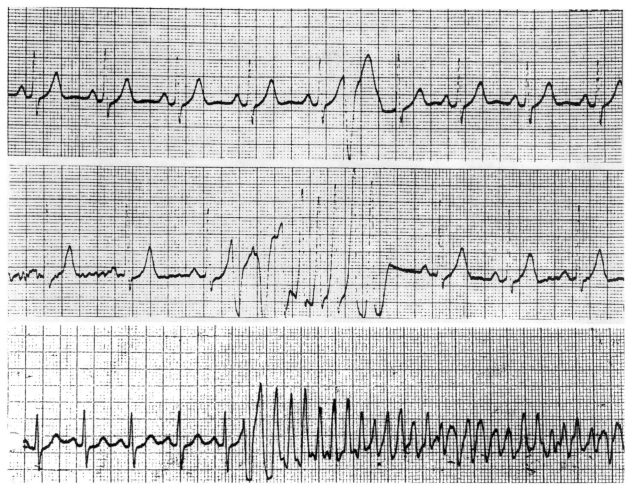

Figure 11-13   Shortly coupled torsades de pointes. Note the extremely short coupling interval of the arrhythmia in initiating VPB.

patients. Effective therapy is needed because these patients are at risk of sudden death from birth, and ICD implant is not feasible in very young children.

REFERENCES

1. Roden DM: The problem, challenge and the opportunity of genetic heterogeneity in monogenic diseases predisposing to sudden death, *J Am Coll Cardiol* 40:357-9, 2002.
2. Behr E, Wood DA, Wright M, et al: Cardiological assessment of first degree relatives in sudden arrhythmic death syndrome, *Lancet* 362:1457-9, 2003.
3. Maron BJ, Casey SA, Hurrell DG, et al: Relation of left ventricular thickness to age and gender in hypertrophic cardiomyopathy, *Am J Cardiol* 91:1195-8, 2003.
4. Maron BJ, Gardin JM, Flack JM, et al: Prevalence of hypertrophic cardiomyopathy in a general population of young adults. Echocardiographic analysis of 4111 subjects in the CARDIA study, *Circulation* 92:785-9, 1995.
5. Seidman JG, Seidman C: The genetic basis for cardiomyopathy from mutation identification to mechanistic paradigms, *Cell* 104:557-67, 2002.
6. Maron BJ, Pelliccia A, Spirito P: Cardiac disease in young trained athletes. Insights into methods to distinguish athlete's heart from structural heart disease, with particular emphasis on hypertrophic cardiomyopathy, *Circulation* 91:1596-601, 1995.
7. Maron BJ, Pelliccia A, Spataro A, et al: Reduction in left ventricular wall thickness after deconditioning in highly trained Olympic athletes, *Br Heart J* 69:125-8, 1999.
8. Begley DA, Mohiddin SA, Tripodi D, et al: Efficacy of implantable cardioverter defibrillator therapy for primary and secondary prevention of sudden cardiac death in hypertrophic cardiomyopathy, *Pacing Clin Electrophysiol* 26:1887-96, 2003.
9. Reith S, Klues HG: Therapy and risk stratification in hypertrophic cardiomyopathy—a current survey, *Z Kardiol* 92:283-93, 2003.

10. Marcus FI, Fontaine GH, Guiraudon G, et al: Right ventricular dysplasia: a report of 24 adult cases, *Circulation* 65:384-98, 1982.

11. Nasir K, Bomma C, Harikrisna T, et al: Electrocardiographic features of arrhythmogenic right ventricular dysplasia/cardiomyopathy according to disease severity. A need to broaden diagnostic criteria, *Circulation* 110:1527-34, 2004.

12. Gemayel C, Pelliccia A, Thompson PD: Arrhythmogenic right ventricular cardiomyopathy, *J Am Coll Cardiol* 38:1773-81, 2001.

13. McKenna WJ, Thiene G, Nava A, et al: Diagnosis of arrhythmogenic right ventricular dysplasia/cardiomyopathy: task force of the working group myocardial and pericardial disease of the European Society of Cardiology and of the Scientific Council on Cardiomyopathies of the International Society and Federation of Cardiology, *Br Heart J* 71:215-8, 1994.

14. Kaiser HW, De Roos A, Schalij MJ, et al: Usefulness of magnetic resonance imaging in diagnosis of arrhythmogenic right ventricular dysplasia and agreement with electrocardiographic criteria, *Am J Cardiol* 91:356-7, 2003.

15. Tandri H, Calkins H, Nasir K, et al: Magnetic resonance imaging findings in patients meeting task force criteria for arrhythmogenic right ventricular dysplasia, *J Cardiovasc Electrophysiol* 14:476-82, 2003.

16. di Cesare E: MRI assessment of right ventricular dysplasia, *Eur Radiol* 13:1387-93, 2003.

17. Niroomand F, Carbucicchio C, Tondo C, et al: Electrophysiological characteristics and outcome in patients with idiopathic right ventricular arrhythmia compared with arrhythmogenic right ventricular dysplasia, *Heart* 87:41-7, 2002.

18. Turrini P, Corrado D, Basso C, et al: Non-invasive risk stratification in arrhythmogenic right ventricular cardiomyopathy, *Ann Noninvasive Electrocardiol* 8:61-9, 2003.

19. Fontaine G, Gontalaliran F, Hebert J, et al: Arrhythmogenic right ventricular dysplasia, *Ann Rev Med* 50:17-35, 1999.

20. Hulot J, Jouven X, Empana JP, et al: Natural history and risk stratification of arrhythmogenic right ventricular dysplasia/cardiomyopathy, *Circulation* 110:1879-84, 2004.

21. Scoote M, Williams AJ: The cardiac ryanodine receptor (calcium release channel): emerging role in heart failure and arrhythmia pathogenesis, *Cardiovasc Res* 56:359-72, 2002.

22. Corrado D, Leoni L, Link M, et al: Implantable cardioverter-defibrillator therapy for prevention of sudden death in patients with arrhythmogenic right ventricular cardiomyopathy/dysplasia, *Circulation* 108:3084-91, 2003.

23. Priori SG, Napolitano C, Vicentini A: Inherited arrhythmia syndromes. Applying the molecular biology and genetics to the clinical management, *J Intervent Cardiac Electrophysiol* 9:93-101, 2003.

24. Viskin S, Fish R, Zeltser D, et al: Arrhythmias in the congenital long QT syndrome: how often is torsades de pointes paused dependent? *Heart* 83:661-6, 2000.

25. Napolitano C, Schwartz PJ, Brown AM, et al: Evidence for a cardiac ion channel mutation underlying drug-induced QT prolongation and life threatening arrhythmias, *J Cardiovasc Electrophysiol* 11:691-6, 2000.

26. Vincent GM: Ventricular arrhythmias. Long QT syndrome, *Cardiol Clin* 18:309-25, 2000.

27. Vincent GM, Timothy K, Fox J, et al: The inherited long QT syndrome: from ion channel to bedside, *Cardiol Rev* 7:44-55, 1999.

28. Priori SG, Schwartz PJ, Napolitano C, et al: Risk stratification in the long QT syndrome, *N Engl J Med* 348:1866-74, 2003.

29. Zareba W, Moss AJ, Locati EH, et al: International long QT syndrome registry: modulating effects of age and gender on the clinical course of long QT syndrome by genotype, *J Am Coll Cardiol* 42:103-9, 2003.

30. Rashba EJ, Zareba W, Moss AJ: Influence of pregnancy on risk for cardiac events in patients with hereditary long QT syndrome, *Circulation* 97:451-6, 1998.

31. Antzelevitch C, Yan GX, Shimizu W, et al: Electrical heterogeneity, the ECG, and cardiac arrhythmias. In Zipes DP, Jalife J, editors: *Cardiac electrophysiology: from cell to bedside,* ed 3, Philadelphia, 2000, WB Saunders.

32. Priori SG, Napolitano C, Schwartz PJ, et al: Association of long QT syndrome loci and cardiac events among patients treated with beta blockers, *JAMA* 292:1341-4, 2004.

33. Viskin S: Cardiac pacing in the long QT syndrome: review of available data and practical recommendations, *J Cardiovasc Electrophysiol* 11:593-600, 2000.

34. Moss AJ, McDonald J: Unilateral cervicothoracic sympathetic ganglionectomy for the treatment of long QT interval syndrome, *N Engl J Med* 285:903-4, 1971.

35. Schwartz PJ: The rationale and the role of left stellectomy for the prevention of malignant arrhythmias, *Ann NY Acad Sci* 427:199-221, 1984.

36. Schwartz PJ, Priori SG, Cerrone M, et al: Left cardiac sympathetic denervation in the management of high risk patients affected by the long QT syndrome, *Circulation* 109:1826-1833, 2004.

37. Gussak I, Antzelevitch C, Bjerregaard P, et al: The Brugada syndrome: clinical, electrophysiological, and genetic considerations, *J Am Coll Cardiol* 33:5-15, 1999.

38. Osher HL, Wolff L: Electrocardiographic pattern simulating acute myocardial injury, *Am J Med Sci* 226:541-5, 1953.

39. Edeiken J: Elevation of RS-T segment, apparent or real in right precordial leads as probable normal variant, *Am Heart J* 48:331-9, 1954.

40. Martini B, Nava A, Thiene G, et al: Ventricular fibrillation without apparent heart disease. Description of six cases, *Am Heart J* 118:1203-9, 1989.

41. Aihara N, Ohe T, Kamakura S: Clinical and electrophysiologic characteristics of idiopathic ventricular fibrillation, *Shinzo* 22:80-6, 1990.

42. Brugada P, Brugada J: Right bundle branch block, persistent ST segment elevation and sudden cardiac death: a distinct clinical and electrocardiographic syndrome: a multicenter report, *J Am Coll Cardiol* 20:391-6, 1992.

43. Wilde A, Antzelevitch C, Borggrefe M, et al: Proposed diagnostic criteria for the Brugada syndrome. Consensus report, *Circulation* 106:2515-9, 2002.

44. Littmann L, Monroe MH, Kerns WP, et al: Brugada syndrome and "Brugada sign": clinical spectrum with a guide for the clinician, *Am Heart J* 145:768-78, 2003.

45. Junttila MJ, Raatikainen MJP, Karjalainen J, et al: Prevalence and prognosis of subjects with Brugada type ECG pattern in young and middle-aged Finnish population, *Eur Heart J* 25:874-8, 2004.

46. Brugada R, Brugada J, Antzeleitch C, et al: Sodium channel blockers identify risk for sudden death in patients with ST segment elevation and RBBB but structurally normal hearts, *Circulation* 101:1510-5, 2000.

47. Brugada J, Brugada P, Brugada R: The syndrome of RBBB ST segment elevation in V$_1$-V$_3$ and sudden death—the Brugada syndrome, *Europace* 1:156-66, 1999.

48. Kasanuki H, Ohnishi S, Ohtuka M, et al: Idiopathic ventricular fibrillation induced with vagal activity in patients without obvious heart disease, *Circulation* 95:2277-85, 1997.

49. Alings M, Wilde A: "Brugada" syndrome: clinical data and suggested pathophysiological mechanism, *Circulation* 99:666-73, 1999.

50. Nademanee K, Veerakul G, Nimmannit S, et al: Arrhythmogenic marker for the sudden unexplained death syndrome in Thai men, *Circulation* 96:2595-2600, 1997.

51. Brugada P, Brugada R, Mont L, et al: Natural history of Brugada syndrome: the prognostic value of programmed electrical stimulation of the heart, *J Cardiovasc Electrophysiol* 14:455-7, 2003.

52. Eckhardt L, Kirchhof P, Schulze-Bahr E, et al: Mode of induction of ventricular tachyarrhythmias in Brugada syndrome, *Pacing Clin Electrophysiol* 24:558-63, 2001.

53. Prior SG, Napolitano C, Gasparini M, et al: Natural history of Brugada syndrome. Insights for risk stratification and management, *Circulation* 105:1342-7, 2002.

54. Brugada J, Brugada R, Antzelevitch C, et al: Long-term follow up of individuals with the electrocardiographic pattern of RBBB and ST segment elevation in precordial leads V_1-V_3, *Circulation* 105:73-8, 2002.

55. Belhassen B, Glick A, Viskin S: Efficacy of quinidine in high-risk patients with Brugada syndrome, *Circulation* 110:1731-7, 2004.

56. Coumel P, Fidelle J, Luchet V, et al: Catecholaminergic induced severe ventricular arrhythmias with Adams-Stokes syndrome in children. Report of four cases, *Br Heart J* 40:28-37, 1978.

57. Leenhardt A, Lucet V, Denjoy I, et al: Catecholaminergic polymorphic ventricular tachycardia in children. A 7 year follow-up of 21 patients, *Circulation* 91:1512-9, 1995.

58. Lahat H, Eldar M, Levy-Nissenbaum E, et al: Autosomal recessive catecholamine- or exercise-induced polymorphic ventricular tachycardia, *Circulation* 103:2822-7, 2001.

59. Priori SG, Napolitano C, Tisso N, et al: Mutations in the cardiac ryanodine receptor gene (hRyR2) underlie catecholaminergic polymorphic ventricular tachycardia, *Circulation* 103:196-200, 2001.

60. Priori SG, Napolitano C, Memmi M, et al: Clinical and molecular characterization of patients with catecholaminergic polymorphic ventricular tachycardia, *Circulation* 106:69-74, 2002.

61. Gaita F, Giustetto C, Bianchi F, et al: Short QT syndrome. A familial cause of sudden death, *Circulation* 108:956-70, 2003.

62. Gussak I, Brugada P, Brugada J, et al: ECG phenomenon of idiopathic and paradoxical short QT intervals, *Card Electrophysiol Rev* 6:49-53, 2002.

63. Brugada R, Hong K, Dumaine R, et al: Sudden death associated with short QT syndrome linked to mutations in HERG, *Circulation* 109:30-5, 2004.

64. Coumel P, LeClercq JF, Rosengarten MD, et al: Unusual forms of severe ventricular tachyarrhythmias: their relationships with the QT interval and the vago-sympathetic balance. In Kulbertus H, Wellens H, editors: *Sudden death,* The Hague, 1980, Martinus Nijhoff, pp. 199-215.

65. Leenhardt A, Glaser E, Burguera M, et al: Short-coupled variant of torsades de pointes: a new electrocardiographic entity in the spectrum of idiopathic ventricular tachyarrhythmias, *Circulation* 89:206-15, 1994.

66. Gaita F, Giustetto C, Bianchi F, et al: Short QT syndrome: pharmacological treatment, *J Am Coll Cardiol* 43:1494-9, 2004.

CHAPTER
12
Pacemaker and Defibrillator Emergencies

Pacing Emergencies

EMERGENCY APPROACH

Failure to Capture and Sense

1. If unable to capture, increase the output (amplitude or pulse width).
2. If unsuccessful, reposition the electrode catheter.
3. If unable to sense, increase the sensitivity; when sensing is still inadequate, change to unipolar sensing.
4. If unsuccessful, reposition the catheter.

Pacing Failure

1. If no pacemaker spikes are present, suspect a break in the system anywhere from the pacing wire to the pulse generator.
2. If intermittent pacemaker spikes occur during bipolar pacing, only one electrode may be involved; convert to a unipolar system.

Pacemaker Syndrome

1. Prevent pacemaker syndrome by carefully selecting the pacing mode.
2. When VVI pacing is chosen, check for the presence of ventriculoatrial conduction during temporary pacemaker insertion.
3. If pacemaker syndrome is recognized after implantation, program the rate so that the majority of beats are spontaneous.
4. If unsuccessful, reoperation is necessary for conversion to an atrial pacing device in case of intact AV conduction or to a dual-chamber unit in case of AV block.

Myocardial Perforation

1. To confirm myocardial perforation during temporary pacing, record a unipolar electrogram from the pacing electrode(s); an ECG showing QRS and T waves similar to those recorded on precordial lead V_3 or V_4 indicates that the electrode is outside the heart.
2. Gently withdraw the pacing catheter while recording the electrogram from the electrode; in case of a bipolar catheter, *use the distal electrode.* When the QRS

complex and T wave are opposite to lead V_3 or V_4, the distal electrode is again inside the RV.

3. If pericardial tamponade is present, immediate pericardiocentesis and drainage are indicated.
4. Closely monitor the patient.
5. Discontinue anticoagulants.

Pacemaker-Mediated Tachycardia

1. Reprogram the atrial sensing refractory period so that retrograde atrial signals are not sensed.
2. Decrease atrial sensing sensitivity.
3. Program a short AV interval *or*
4. Switch to a DVI mode, which eliminates atrial sensing and terminates the tachycardia.

Managing Occasional Atrial Tachycardias

1. Limit the time available for atrial sensing to provide a fixed safety limit.
2. Limit the ventricular pacing rate to provide a fixed safety limit.
3. Switch temporarily to a nontracking mode with sensor rate during the tachycardia to provide a desirable sensor-controlled rate.

Burst-Type Antitachycardia Pacing

A variety of burst-pacing sequences are offered by modern devices. Pacing pulses are applied for several seconds at a rate faster than the tachycardia rate, with the intention to create refractoriness within the reentry circuit of the tachycardia. The procedure is as follows:

1. The device automatically selects optimal preprogrammed burst sequences and assesses the results.
2. If unsuccessful, another burst of the same or a different design is given.

Some units are preprogrammed to select the first burst rate automatically as a percentage above the tachycardia rate; other units select an increment or decrement rate, and some set the number of paces in the burst or the duration of the burst.

Thrombosis and Pulmonary Embolism

Heparin and thrombolytic therapy are usually sufficient for clinically important thrombosis.

Infection or Erosion of the Pulse Generator

When infection or erosion of the pulse generator is present:

1. A temporary pacemaker is inserted, the entire permanent pacing unit is removed, and a new unit is installed on the contralateral side.
2. The removal of the involved lead is usually difficult; laser-assisted removal is often the preferred method.
3. If removal fails thoracotomy may be necessary in cases of endocarditis.
4. The lead may be saved in the case of pacemaker erosion if the condition is detected early.

Electromyographic Inhibition

If electromyographic inhibition is present:

1. Decrease the sensitivity of the pacemaker. If unsuccessful:
2. Reprogram the pacemaker from a unipolar to a bipolar unit. If unsuccessful:
3. Reoperation may be necessary.

> **Emergency Temporary Pacing**
> Prepare for emergency temporary pacing if one of the following events occurs:
> 1. Complete AV block with a slow ventricular escape rhythm
> 2. Symptomatic sinus bradycardia, asystole, or prolonged sinus pauses
> 3. Acute anterior MI with complete heart block, acquired RBBB or LBBB with type II second-degree AV block or new hemiblock
> 4. Acute inferior MI with complete heart block leading to hypotension, congestive heart failure, or ventricular arrhythmias
> 5. Bradycardia-induced or drug-induced torsades de pointes
> 6. Malfunction of a permanent pacemaker
> 7. Digitalis toxicity–induced VT being treated with drugs (e.g., Dilantin) that suppress impulse formation

Consider the use of temporary pacing for tachycardias that do not respond to antiarrhythmic drug therapy, such as sustained VT, AV nodal tachycardia, and atrial flutter. In these patients the arrhythmia can frequently be terminated by pacing-induced premature stimuli or pacing above the tachycardia rate.

INTRODUCTION

The use and sophistication of permanent pacemakers have steadily increased after their first implantation in 1958.[1,2] Although pacemakers were initially indicated for the treatment of Adams-Stokes disease, advances in technology led to much broader indications, most recently resynchronization of ventricular activation by pacing.[3,4] More than 4 million pacemakers are currently in use worldwide.

Essential for the recognition of emergency situations in patients with pacemakers is an understanding of the principles of cardiac pacing and the different types of pacemakers currently in use. That information falls outside the aim of this chapter and can be found elsewhere.[5]

FAILURE TO CAPTURE OR SENSE

In a small percentage of patients, failure to capture or sense may occur during the first days following pacemaker implantation and may be corrected by adjusting the output amplitude, pulse width, or sensitivity. If adjustment is unsuccessful, reoperation with repositioning may be indicated.

Causes

Catheter dislodgement. The most common cause of failure to capture or sense is dislodgement of the catheter, which may not be seen on radiographs, depending on the degree of catheter displacement. When the magnitude of the pacemaker deflection is adequate, failure to capture usually indicates catheter dislodgement.

When a spontaneous rhythm is faster than the selected pacing rate, the intracardiac electrode transmits a signal of 2 mV or more to the generator's sensing circuit. This signal inhibits the output of the pacemaker and resets the pacing cycle. If the catheter displacement results in an intracardiac signal of less than 2 mV, premature ventricular complexes (VPBs) and the patient's own rhythm will no longer be sensed and the pacemaker no longer acts in the demand mode but performs like a fixed-rate pacemaker, discharging regardless of VPBs or the patient's own rhythm. This situation is dangerous in patients whose fibrillatory threshold is lowered because of acute myocardial ischemia, digitalis toxicity, or electrolyte imbalance.

Continuous subsensing. In continuous subsensing, no spontaneous QRS complexes are sensed, leading to fixed-rate pacing.

Intermittent sensing. If the catheter moves in the cardiac cavity, some spontaneous cardiac signals may generate sufficient voltage to be sensed and others not, which leads to intermittent sensing problems.

Oversensing. The T-wave or muscle-motion interference may occasionally generate sufficient voltage to be misinterpreted by the sensing system as a QRS complex. Oversensing results in suppression of pacemaker activity.

Undersensing. On rare occasions ectopic beats may not be sensed by a normally operating pacemaker. This undersensing occurs because currents generated from an ectopic focus may not take the same path as normal depolarizations and thus are not detected, causing the pacemaker spike to appear during or following the ectopic complex.

Sensing misinterpretation. In some cases, sensing failure is actually sensing misinterpretation. For example, the development of RBBB causes a delay in propagation of the impulse to the RV, where the electrode is located.

This delay is perceived by the electrode sensing unit as inactivity, and the pacemaker spike appears in the spontaneous QRS complex. This is known as a *paced fusion beat*. If the myocardium is already refractory because of the native beat, the pacing stimulus will have no effect. This situation is sometimes called *pseudofusion*.

Competitive pacing. When the sensing feature is switched off, as it would be during certain standard pacemaker tests, pacing is not inhibited by native beats. Pacing in the presence of native beats may result in *competitive pacing*, causing some fusion or pseudofusion beats (Figure 12-1).

ECG Recognition

Figure 12-2 is an example of intermittent failure to capture. Figure 12-3 illustrates failure to sense. In this tracing, the pacemaker fails to sense the patient's own rhythm and fires on the T waves of four complexes until it finally captures the heart.

Treatment

Because the threshold for capture can change with time, changes in body position, and minor shifts in electrode location, capture may be restored by simply increasing the output (amplitude or pulse width); failure to sense may be corrected by increasing the sensitivity.

If the sensing failure is caused by a dislodgement of the catheter, increasing the sensitivity may solve the problem. If this does not help, the permanent pacemaker should be converted from the demand mode to fixed-rate mode until the problem is corrected with reoperation and repositioning.

Summary

1. If unable to capture, increase the output (milliamperes or pulse width).
2. If unsuccessful, early reoperation is indicated, with repositioning of the permanent pacemaker.
3. If unable to sense, increase the sensitivity.

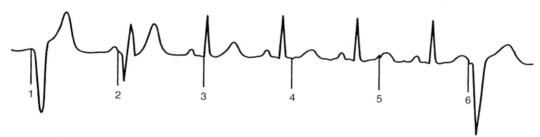

Figure 12-1 Competitive pacing (ventricular example). When the sensing function is turned off, stimuli occur without regard to native depolarizations. *Pace 1* results in a normal paced depolarization. *Pace 2* is a fusion. *Pace 3* is also a fusion, but the paced beat is hardly contributing to the QRS complex; only a slight variation in the T wave is noticeable. *Paces 4* and *5* fire when the ventricle is refractory. *Pace 6* occurs after the muscle around the electrode has recovered. The morphologic appearance shows that the QRS configuration was altered by the remaining refractory ventricular muscle.

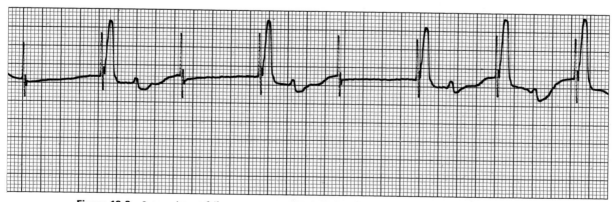

Figure 12-2 Intermittent failure to capture. Note pacemaker spikes 1, 3, and 5 are not followed by ventricular complexes, although the ventricles are nonrefractory.

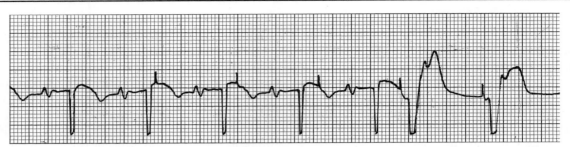

Figure 12-3   Failure to sense. The pacemaker fails to sense the patient's intrinsic rhythm and fires on T waves.

4. If unsuccessful in a patient with a permanent pacemaker, convert the demand mode to fixed-rate mode and prepare for reoperation.
5. If unsuccessful in a patient with a temporary pacemaker, reposition the catheter.

PACING FAILURE

Failure to pace may result in profound bradycardia and requires immediate intervention. Reoperation correcting the appropriate component is usually indicated.

Mechanism

Late failure to pace may be related to a change in myocardial threshold, battery depletion, or failure of the lead or pacemaker components. These conditions may require reoperation. Noninvasive diagnosis of the problem with information obtained by telemetry is possible with the newer pacemakers.

ECG Recognition and Treatment

Battery depletion. Special circuits in the generator monitor the battery status and report it to the programmer, giving advanced warning of the elective replacement time. However, some patients are lost to follow-up, requiring health care professionals to be alert to special warning rates. When the elective replacement time passes unattended, the pacemaker switches to a special rate called the elective replacement indicator (usually 65 beats/min). Additionally, to conserve energy most dual-chamber pacemakers (but not implantable cardioverter-defibrillators) convert to ventricular pacing only.

Break in the system. If no pacemaker spikes are present, a break in the system anywhere from the lead to the pulse generator is suspected. If the patient has a temporary pacemaker, all conducting wires and connections should be inspected and electrograms recorded from each electrode.

Wire fracture. Intermittent activity indicates wire fracture. Only one of the electrodes of a bipolar system may be involved. If so, conversion to unipolar pacing should be performed until the catheter can be replaced.

PACEMAKER SYNDROME

Pacemaker syndrome is a complex of symptoms related to adverse hemodynamic effects of single-chamber ventricular pacing.

Mechanism

Pacemaker syndrome is most common in patients with sick sinus syndrome who have intact ventriculoatrial (VA) conduction during ventricular pacing. Symptoms are the result of variations in cardiac output and blood pressure caused by nonsynchronization of atrial and ventricular contraction. Contraction of the atrium against a closed mitral valve leads to a decrease in LV filling, which in turn causes a lesser stroke volume and a lower blood pressure.[6]

ECG Recognition

The ECG typically shows independent beating of the atria and ventricles or VA conduction following the paced complexes.

Symptoms and Physical Findings

Symptoms include fatigue, dizziness, syncope, and pulmonary congestion. The diagnosis is made by the history alone or by observation of fluctuation in peripheral blood pressure and cannon A waves in the neck.

Treatment

1. During pacemaker insertion, prevent the syndrome by carefully checking for VA conduction. Select another pacing mode when necessary.
2. If pacemaker syndrome is first recognized after pacemaker implantation, lower the ventricular paced rate

so that the majority of beats are conducted sinus beats.

3. If unsuccessful, reoperation may be indicated for conversion to an atrial pacing device, with intact AV conduction or a dual-chamber unit, or with AV block.

PACEMAKER-MEDIATED TACHYCARDIA

Pacemaker-mediated tachycardia (also called pacemaker circus movement tachycardia) may occur in patients with intact VA conduction after implantation of an atrial synchronized, ventricular inhibited (VDD), or AV universal (DDD) pacemaker.[7]

Mechanism

The tachycardia begins following retrograde conduction of a P wave from a ventricular beat, either paced or spontaneous. The retrograde P wave is then sensed by the atrial electrode. The ventricular pacemaker waits for the programmed AV interval and then fires. Again, retrograde conduction occurs to the atria followed by paced ventricular activation. This repetitive tachycardia is comparable to that seen in patients with an accessory AV pathway. As long as the retrogradely conducted impulses reach the atrium after the pacemaker atrial refractory period has ended, tachycardia persists at a rate equal to or near the programmed atrial rate limit. Whether the retrograde P wave is sensed by the atrial circuit depends on the length of the refractory period of the atrial sensing amplifier.

Pacemaker-mediated tachycardia may also occur following failure to capture the atria with a paced beat, making VA conduction possible from the ventricular paced beat. This is possible even in the face of complete AV block because as many as one third of such patients have intact VA conduction at least intermittently.

ECG Recognition

- The tachycardia is paroxysmal.
- The P wave during the tachycardia is retrograde (negative in leads II, III, and aVF).
- The PR interval during tachycardia is the same as the PR interval during sinus rhythm because a programmed AV interval is present.
- The QRS complex of the tachycardia is a paced complex.

Figure 12-4 is an ECG tracing of a pacemaker-mediated tachycardia. A retrograde P wave follows the VPB. The atrial electrode senses this impulse and activates the ventricular pacemaker. Every subsequently paced ventricular beat is then retrogradely conducted to the atrium, leading to atrial sensing followed by ventricular

pacing. This repetitive sequence sustains the tachycardia until VA block occurs.

Treatment

1. Prolong the atrial sensing refractory period so that retrograde atrial signals fall within that refractory period.
2. Decrease atrial sensing sensitivity.
3. Program a short AV interval, thereby preventing VA conduction of the ventricular paced beat.
4. Or, switch to a DVI mode, which eliminates atrial sensing and terminates the tachycardia.

Prevention

In modes that allow tracking of the atria, verification that atrial depolarizations caused by VA conduction are not tracked is necessary. If tracked, each atrial depolarization would cause a ventricular pace that would produce another retrograde conduction in a self-sustained loop. To prevent tracking of retrograde beats after ventricular paced beats, an electronic atrial refractory period is programmed to be initiated by the ventricular event. It is programmed to be slightly longer than the time from the V-pace to the retrograded A-sense, so that the A-sense will not be responded to. Under these circumstances, pacemaker-mediated tachycardia cannot occur.

For patients in whom pacemaker-mediated tachycardia is unlikely, the post–ventricular atrial refractory period (PVARP) may be set short so as not to restrict the maximum atrial tracking rate. A special program is then provided for protection from pacemaker-mediated tachycardia by monitoring for this event and inserting a single long PVARP to terminate the tachycardia. Different methods are used by various manufacturers to handle fast rates.[8]

Not sensing any type of atrial event after a VPB is desirable; thus most pacemakers insert a PVARP after a VPB for one cycle. This PVARP is set long, usually 400 msec or more, because a VPB may originate at a distant location and have a long retrograde conduction time.

Another strategy for preventing pacemaker-mediated tachycardia is to pace the atria whenever a VPB is sensed, preventing retrograde conduction from entering the atria. When a pacemaker artifact is noted during a VPB, it should be determined if it is indeed an artifact or if some other explanation should be sought.

MYOCARDIAL PERFORATION AND TAMPONADE

Myocardial perforation by the pacing electrode may require gentle withdrawal of the pacing catheter. Pericardial tamponade is extremely rare and requires immediate pericardiocentesis and drainage.

DDD AV interval 150 msec Upper rate 150 bpm

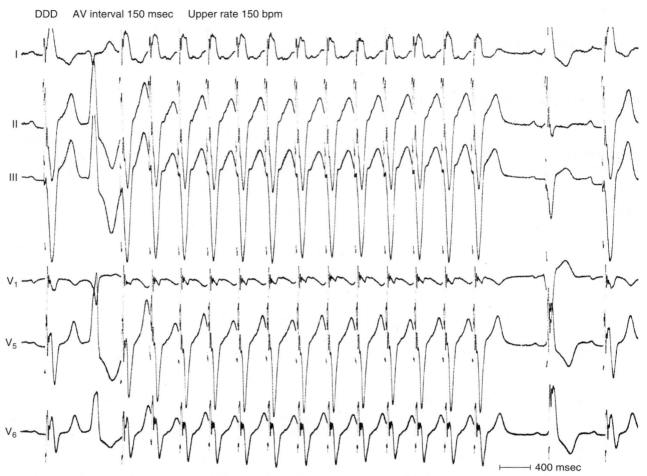

├─────┤ 400 msec

Figure 12-4 Pacemaker-mediated tachycardia. The ventricular premature complex is retrogradely conducted to the atria. The atrial electrode senses the retrograde P wave, which is followed by ventricular stimulation after the programmed AV delay. Every paced ventricular complex is followed by retrograde conduction to the atria. The tachycardia spontaneously terminates because of retrograde VA block.

ECG Recognition and Physical Findings

Myocardial perforation is suggested by:

- Loss of capture
- Intercostal or diaphragmatic stimulation
- Occurrence of a pericardial friction rub

Confirm perforation by recording a unipolar electrogram from the pacing electrode. With a bipolar electrode, record from the distal electrode. An electrogram with a positive R wave, mimicking lead V_3 or V_4, suggests perforation. A unipolar electrogram is recorded by connecting one of the V leads to the electrode of the catheter. If the electrode is situated in the RV apex, the QRS complex is negative and the ST segment elevated (Figure 12-5). If the myocardium has been perforated and the electrode is situated within the pericardial sac, the QRS is more positive and the T wave is opposite to the intracavitary T wave. If perforation has occurred, the ECG from the electrode is similar to the precordial lead V_3 or V_4. An *echocardiogram* may confirm the diagnosis.

Treatment

1. If myocardial perforation is the diagnosis, gently withdraw the pacing catheter.
2. If pericardial tamponade is present, immediate pericardiocentesis and drainage are indicated.
3. Closely monitor the patient.
4. Discontinue any anticoagulants.

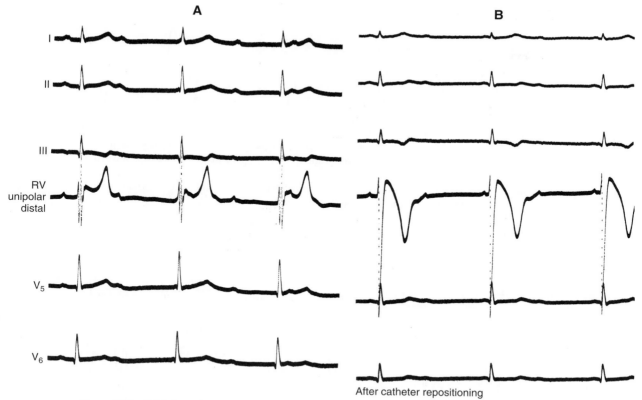

Figure 12-5   ECG from the electrode catheter in myocardial perforation. The distal unipolar recording from the RV electrode catheter in **A** shows an R/S ratio of the QRS of approximately one and T-wave polarity similar to the precordial leads V_5 and V_6. After withdrawal of the catheter (**B**) the electrogram shows the typical RV endocavitary complex (R/S ratio less than one, negative T wave).

MANAGING OCCASIONAL ATRIAL TACHYCARDIAS IN PATIENTS WITH PACEMAKERS

In modes that allow tracking of the atria, ensuring that occasional atrial tachyarrhythmias are not fully tracked to the ventricle is essential. The following three options are available:

1. Limit the time available for atrial sensing
2. Directly limit the ventricular pacing rate, *or*
3. Switch to a nontracking sensor mode during an atrial tachycardia

Limit the time available for atrial sensing. Limiting the time available for atrial sensing provides a fixed safety limit. The PVARP is used to program the pacemaker to not track any atrial events detected soon after the ventricular event. This interval lasts until the sense-initiated AV interval (SAV) and the PVARP have completed. Thus the SAV + PVARP is the shortest atrial cycle length that can be tracked and 60,000/(SAV + PVARP) defines the corresponding rate, known as the maximum atrial tracking rate (MATR). In patients with complete heart block,

at atrial rates higher than the MATR, the ventricular rate will be half the atrial rate, a condition known as pacemaker two-to-one block (Figure 12-6).

Directly limit the ventricular pacing rate. Limiting the ventricular pacing rate to a rate less than the MATR provides a fixed safety limit. A time interval corresponding to the interval of the rate limit, usually the ventricular upper rate limit, is set at each ventricular event. Any ventricular pace called for during this interval is delayed until the interval has expired. If the natural atrial rate is regular and slightly above the ventricular rate limit, the ventricular paces and associated PVARPs are progressively delayed until a PVARP prevents an atrial sense from being tracked, causing a skipped tracking cycle. This effect is called a pacemaker pseudo-Wenckebach (Figure 12-7).

Suspend tracking and use sensor rate during an atrial tachycardia. Depending on the manufacturer, one of several methods is used to switch to a nontracking sensor mode during an atrial tachycardia, a concept called *mode switch*. In the most common method, the atrial

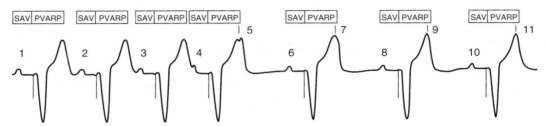

Figure 12-6   Limitation of tracking caused by the total of the atrial refractory period (sense-initiated AV interval *[SAV]* + postventricular atrial refractory period *[PVARP]*). The tracing shows what happens when the atrial rate increases in a patient with complete heart block. The P waves are numbered *1* through *11*. P waves *1* to *4* are tracked normally. As the length of the atrial cycle diminishes, each new P wave becomes closer to the previous PVARP. When further shortening of the atrial cycle length occurs *(5)*, the atrial sense occurs in the previous PVARP and is ignored; thus a cycle is skipped. The next P wave *(6)* is sensed, but the one that follows *(7)* is ignored. Likewise, *8* is sensed and *9* is ignored, and so forth. When the atrial cycle length becomes less than the SAV + PVARP, every other P wave is sensed and two-to-one pacemaker block occurs. (Courtesy John R. Buysman, PhD, Medtronic.)

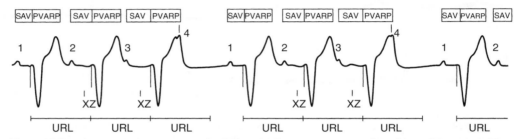

Figure 12-7   The ventricular upper rate limit *(URL)*. The P waves are numbered in each sequence. The atrial rate is slightly faster than the URL but less than the maximum atrial tracking rate. In the first sequence, P wave *1* is tracked normally. The second and third P waves are tracked, but the URL delays their ventricular paces from *X* to *Z* in each case. The fourth P wave occurs just before the end of the postventricular atrial refractory period *(PVARP)* and is ignored. On the next P wave the sequence repeats. In each sequence the first AV interval is in normal synchrony, the next few are lengthened, and the last is dropped (a Wenckebach-like rhythm). The ventricular rate within the sequence is at the URL, but because of dropped beats the average rate is less than the URL. *SAV,* Sense-initiated AV interval. (Courtesy John R. Buysman, PhD, Medtronic.)

sensing rate is constantly monitored. If it exceeds a given upper limit (the detection rate), tracking is temporarily suspended and the sensor rate is used to control the pacing rate instead. When the atrial rate returns to below the detection rate, tracking is resumed. Mode switch may take several seconds to activate, so an appropriate rate setting for either the upper rate limit or MATR is still required (Figure 12-8).

BURST-TYPE ANTITACHYCARDIA PACING

Antitachycardia pacing is based on the concept that a reentrant tachycardia has nonrefractory tissue in the circuit ahead of the circulating impulse.[9] If this were not so, the depolarizing wavefront would not be able to advance.

This nonrefractory section of the reentrant loop is the target for burst-type antitachycardia pacing.

Burst-type antitachycardia pacing is quite successful for terminating single-loop reentrant circuits with a consistent pathway. It is much less efficacious for multiloop or chaotic tachycardias and is never successful in terminating ventricular fibrillation.

The following are possible outcomes of burst-type antitachycardia pacing:

■ Type I break: The reentrant loop is interrupted and terminated when the paced beat invades and depolarizes the loop (Figure 12-9).

■ Type II break: The burst pacing does not invade and depolarize the reentrant loop; rather, it distorts

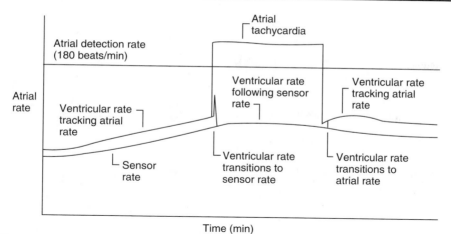

Figure 12-8 Mode switch. In this example of a patient at moderate activity, the natural atrial rate is a little faster than the sensor rate, so ventricular pacing is initially tracking the atria. The pacemaker constantly monitors the atrial rate. When an atrial tachycardia suddenly appears, the atrial rate is above the atrial tachycardia detection rate (programmed here at 180 beats/min), so tracking is suspended and ventricular pacing assumes the sensor rate. After the tachycardia ends, normal tracking is resumed. (Courtesy John R. Buysman, PhD, Medtronic.)

it and continues for several cycles before it terminates.

■ Failure to terminate the reentrant loop may occur if a reentrant loop has been distorted and then returns to its original cycle location.

Burst pacing, especially when applied to the atria, may initiate atrial fibrillation and is not an uncommon occurrence. The atrial fibrillation usually spontaneously terminates in a few seconds to several minutes, accomplishing the desired goal. When the target chambers are the ventricles, ventricular fibrillation may occur. Defibrillation must be immediately accomplished. Thus burst pacing in the ventricles must never be attempted without the proper equipment for high-energy ventricular defibrillation.

Procedure

A variety of burst-pacing sequences are offered by modern devices[9]:

1. The natural heart intervals are monitored and analyzed. The device then automatically selects optimal preprogrammed burst sequences and assesses the results.
2. If unsuccessful, another burst of the same or a different design is tried.

Pacing Options

Some units are preprogrammed to select the first burst rate automatically as a percentage above the tachycardia rate; other units select an increment or decrement rate, and some set the number of paces in the burst or the duration of the burst.

THROMBOSIS AND PULMONARY EMBOLISM

Evidence of mild venous thrombosis has been reported in up to 30% of patients with pacemakers. Serious thrombosis of the subclavian and axillary veins may occur in up to 2% of patients.

Pulmonary embolism caused by right atrial or RV thrombus on a pacing wire may occur. The ECG recognition of acute pulmonary embolism can be found in Chapter 9.

Treatment

Therapy with heparin and a thrombolytic agent is usually sufficient for clinically significant thrombosis.

INFECTION OR EROSION OF THE PULSE GENERATOR

Permanent pacemaker implantation may be complicated by early and late infections. *Staphylococcus aureus* is the most common organism in early infections, and *Staphylococcus epidermidis* is the most common in late infections. On rare occasions permanent pacemakers may erode through the skin. Reoperation is required to remove the pacemaker and insert a new one in a different location.[10,11]

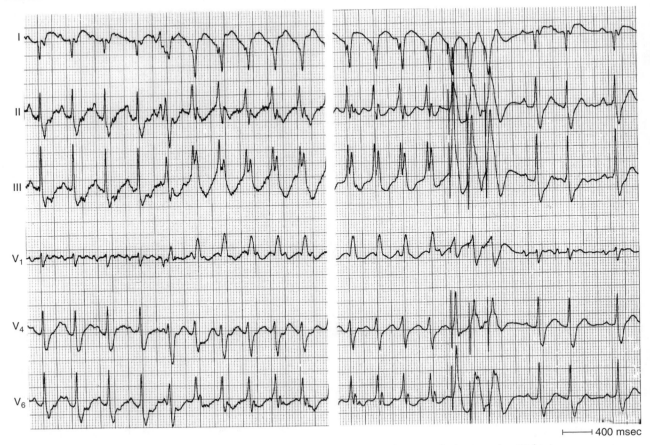

Figure 12-9 *Left*, A VT is initiated when the patient increases sinus rate during exercise. *Right*, A type 1 break of the VT by invasion of the ventricular reentry circuit by VPBs.

Treatment

When infection of the pulse generator pocket occurs, removal of the entire unit is almost always necessary. In general, medical therapy alone is unsatisfactory and surgical removal of the entire pacing system, interim use of a temporary pacemaker, and placement of a new unit on the contralateral side are recommended. In some cases without bacteremia, explantation and implantation of the new unit may be accomplished in the course of one operation. Removal of a lead that has been implanted for a long time is generally difficult and has been made more difficult by active fixation leads. The basic technique involves continuous careful traction applied to the lead once it is dissected from all its attachments. Currently, most leads can be removed by freeing the lead with a laser.[12]

If pacemaker erosion is detected early, the lead may be saved. Isolation of the lead in a relatively proximal position and attachment of a new coupling device are possible. The pacemaker generator is removed, the eroded pocket is closed, and the new pacemaker pack is placed in another location on the same side.

ELECTROMYOGRAPHIC INHIBITION
Mechanism

The electrical potentials generated by pectoral muscles around the pulse generator of a unipolar inhibitory pacemaker may be sensed as if they were a cardiac depolarization. Potentials are said to be *oversensed*; the result is inhibition of the pulse generator, which occurs in as many as one third of all unipolar pacemakers implanted. This inhibition causes symptoms in approximately half of those affected. Myopotentials may also cause false triggering in DDD units because of pacemaker interpretation of myopotentials as P waves. In current pacemakers, the electrical potentials from muscle activity are rejected because of improved filtering in the circuitry.[13]

ECG Recognition

Figure 12-10 shows a tracing from a Holter monitor lead that demonstrates myopotential inhibition of a demand pacemaker. The pectoral muscle potentials are picked up by the surface ECG and appear as an artifact. No pacemaker spikes are present.

Electromyopotential inhibition can be tested by having the patient raise a weight or press the hands together forcefully during ECG monitoring.

Treatment

Most pacemakers have an interference rate to which they revert if exposed to input signals greater than a rate determined by the manufacturer (usually 300 per minute). The interference rate is an asynchronous fixed-rate mode, which may be the same as the automatic rate but is usually faster. If this is not the case, the following steps may relieve the problem:

1. Decrease the sensitivity of the pacemaker.
2. Reprogram the unipolar unit to a bipolar unit.
3. If unsuccessful, reoperation may be necessary.

ARRHYTHMIAS DURING PACEMAKER INSERTION

During insertion of the pacing lead, atrial or ventricular arrhythmias may occur as a result of catheter manipulation. If ventricular fibrillation results, defibrillate immediately.

The Implantable Cardioverter-Defibrillator

The number of implanted cardioverter-defibrillators (ICD) placed in patients increases each year. In 2003, more than 170,000 ICDs were implanted worldwide. In 2006, close to 500,000 ICDs are expected to be in service around the world.

The growth in ICDs is, for the most part, the result of their use in the primary prevention of sudden arrhythmic death in high-risk patients. These patients frequently present in emergency situations because of frequent shocks in case of life-threatening arrhythmias or repeated shocks in the absence of ventricular arrhythmias, so-called *inappropriate shocks*. These patients may present challenging medical and psychologic management problems for health care providers.

Detailed management of ICD emergencies has been discussed elsewhere.[14-16] Treatment usually requires the expertise of health care providers familiar with the specifics of the particular type of ICD implanted. Discussion in this chapter is therefore limited to the

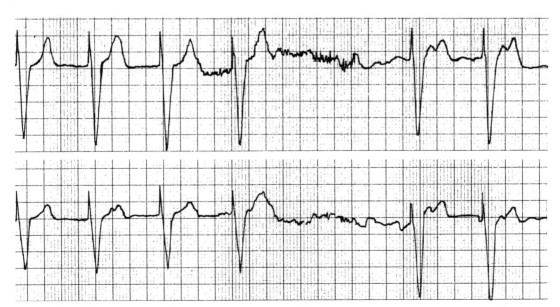

Figure 12-10 A Holter monitor lead demonstrating myopotential inhibition of a ventricular demand pacemaker. (Reprinted from Jacobs LJ, Kerzner JS, Diamond MA, et al: Pacemaker inhibition by myopotentials determined by Holter monitoring, *PACE* 5:30-33, 1982.)

EMERGENCY MANAGEMENT

1. Do not panic when confronted with a patient receiving implantable cardioverter-defibrillator shocks. These shocks cannot hurt medical personnel.
2. Evaluate whether a life-threatening arrhythmia is present and treatment modes are given appropriately.
3. If therapy is appropriate, especially during electrical storm, look for possible triggers such as cardiac ischemia, sedate the patient, administer beta-blockade, and consider additional antiarrhythmic therapy such as intravenous amiodarone.
4. When multiple shocks occur in the absence of a tachycardia, place a magnet on top of the device when the specific programmer is not readily available. A cardiologist or health care provider familiar with the device should search for the cause, such as oversensing, lead damage, a faulty connection between the lead and the header, or a faulty connection at the adapter site.

---

emergency situation, during which the patient with an ICD is initially seen by clinicians not familiar with the details of these complex devices.

Patients with an ICD should always carry an identification card with information about the manufacturer, model, and lead system of the ICD and a 24-hour emergency contact telephone number. Carrying an overpenetrated radiograph, including the generator, is also helpful because it permits the identification of the model by a radiopaque identifier.

IN CASE OF EMERGENCY

In emergency situations, the placement of a magnet on top of the device temporarily disables tachyarrhythmia recognition and treatment. The evaluation of patients with ICDs experiencing multiple shocks should be performed in a setting where ECG monitoring and advanced cardiac resuscitation are possible. There the electrophysiologist or a health care provider familiar with the device can interrogate the ICD by examining event logs, stored interval-by-interval cycle length data, and intracardiac electrograms.

ELECTRICAL STORM

Frequently recurring VT or ventricular fibrillation (VF), the so-called electrical storm, occurs in 5% to 10% of patients with ICDs and is an important marker for subsequent death, particularly in the first 3 months after its occurrence.[17,18] Electrical storm is defined as more than three separate episodes of VT or VF within a 24-hour period. A particular problem can be a short duration of sinus rhythm before reinitiation of VT or VF, which is not recognized by the device and therefore results in continuation of subsequent therapies. Exner et al[18] showed that patients with electrical storm had lower LV

ejection fractions, were more likely to have had VT than VF as their index arrhythmia, and were less likely to have received a revascularization procedure than patients with ICDs who did not have electrical storm.

TREATMENT

Control of electrical storm requires the following treatment:
- Sedation, usually intravenously
- Intravenous administration of a combination of a beta-blocker and amiodarone
- Hemodynamic support (when indicated)

After the storm, treatment should be directed toward optimizing cardiac function pharmacologically and by coronary artery revascularization in patients with ischemic LV dysfunction.[17,18]

PSYCHOSOCIAL CONSIDERATIONS

Multiple shocks and electrical storm usually lead to severe psychologic stress, anxiety, panic disorders, and a markedly diminished quality of life. Health care providers who have patients with ICDs should be aware of these side effects. Appropriate attention should be given to these problems, and psychosocial support should be advised and provided.[19]

In addition, therapeutic efforts such as antiarrhythmic drugs should aim at reducing the number of ICD discharges as much as possible.

REFERENCES

1. Furman S, Schwedel JB: An intracardiac pacemaker for Stokes-Adams seizures, *N Engl J Med* 261:943-8, 1959.
2. Greatbatch W, Schardack WM: A transistorized implantable pacemaker for the long-term correction of complete AV block, *NEREM Record* 1:8-9, 1959.

3. Glikson M, Espinosa RE, Hayes DL: Expanding indications for permanent pacemakers, *Ann Int Med* 123:443-51, 1995.

4. Cazeau S, Leclercq C, Lavergne T, et al: Effects of multisite biventricular pacing in patients with heart failure and intraventricular conduction delay, *N Engl J Med* 344:873-80, 2001.

5. Barold SS, Stroobandt R, Sinnave A: *Cardiac pacemakers, step by step: an illustrated guide,* Oxford, England, 2003, Blackwell Publishing.

6. Ausubel K, Furman S: The pacemaker syndrome, *Ann Intern Med* 103:420-9, 1985.

7. Den Dulk K, Lindemans F, Bar F, et al: Pacemaker related tachycardia, *PACE* 5:496-501, 1982.

8. Buysman JR: Pacemaker therapies for bradyarrhythmias. In Conover MB, editor: *Understanding electrocardiography,* ed 8, St Louis, 2003, Mosby.

9. Den Dulk K, Wellens HJJ: Antitachycardia pacing: clinical considerations. In Ellenbogen KA, Kay GN, Wilkoff BL, editors: *Clinical cardiac pacing,* Philadelphia, 1995, WB Saunders, pp. 735-43.

10. Choo MH, Holmes DR, Gersch B, et al: Permanent pacemakers infections: characterization and management, *Am J Cardiol* 48:559-64, 1981.

11. Lewis AB, Hayes DL, Holmes DR, et al: Update on infections involving permanent pacemakers: characterization and management, *J Thorac Cardiovasc Surg* 89:758-63, 1985.

12. Love CJ, Wilkoff BL, Byrd CL, et al: Recommendations for extraction of chronically implanted transvenous pacing and defibrillator leads: indications, facilities, training. North American Society of Pacing and Electrophysiology lead extraction conference faculty, *Pacing Clin Electrophysiol* 23:544-51, 2000.

13. Barold SS, Falkoff MD, Ong LS, et al: Diaphragmatic myopotential inhibition in multiprogrammable unipolar and bipolar pulse generators. In Steinbach K, editor: *Cardiac pacing,* Darmstadt, Germany, 1983, Steinkopf Verlag, pp. 537-40.

14. Pinski SL, Trohman RG: Implantable cardioverter-defibrillators: implications for the non-electrophysiologist, *Ann Intern Med* 122:770-7, 1995.

15. Wilbur SL, Marchlinski FE: Implantable cardioverter-defibrillator follow-up: what everyone needs to know, *Cardiol Rev* 7:176-90, 1999.

16. Pinski SL: Emergencies related to implantable antiarrhythmia devices, *Crit Care Med* 28(10 suppl):N174-80, 2000.

17. Credner SC, Klingenheben T, Mauss O, et al: Electrical storm in patients with transvenous implantable cardioverter-defibrillators. Incidence, management and prognostic implications, *J Am Coll Cardiol* 32:1909-15, 1998.

18. Exner DV, Pinski SL, Wyse G, et al: Electrical storm presages nonsudden death: the antiarrhythmics versus implantable defibrillators (AVID) trial, *Circulation* 103:2066-71, 2001.

19. Sears SF, Conti JB: Understanding implantable cardioverter defibrillator shocks and storms: medical and psychosocial considerations for research and clinical care, *Clin Cardiol* 26:107-11, 2003.

CHAPTER
13
Prehospital Cardiac Emergencies

The ability of paramedics and emergency medical technicians (EMTs) to obtain a 12-lead ECG in the field and transmit it to the hospital allows early physician consultation and rapid institution of treatment. To that end, the American College of Cardiology/American Heart Association Task Force on Practice Guidelines has included recommendations for prehospital health care providers in their guidelines for the management of acute MI.[1]

Of the approximately 800,000 persons with acute MI each year in the United States, approximately one fourth die, usually because of a fatal arrhythmia. At least half of those die within the first hour and before reaching the hospital. The survival rate can be significantly increased, infarct size reduced, and LV function improved with the following:

- Access to an emergency service such as 911
- An informed patient and family who recognize signs of MI
- Urgent response from an emergency medical service
- Early defibrillation in cases of ventricular fibrillation
- Advanced cardiac life support
- Prompt assessment, initial treatment, and speedy transport to a hospital with a 24-hour emergency cardiac catheterization laboratory and staff experienced in angiography and revascularization[1]

Reasons for Delay

The three main reasons for delay from the onset of symptoms to treatment lie in the spheres of patient and family awareness, training of the emergency response team, and in-hospital response. Thus the patient and family members should be instructed regarding the importance of acting promptly, and emergency medical service personnel should be well trained and share a sense of urgency. The hospital emergency department is the final link to expedient management of patients with angina or ischemia-like pain. As stated in Chapter 1, the ECG is of great value in decision making, such as in relation to the necessity and type of reperfusion therapy.

PATIENT AND FAMILY EDUCATION

The most important factor in a successful outcome for patients with ischemia-related chest discomfort is the early action of the patient, supported by family, and the critical education provided by health care providers. When the patient and family do not recognize the symptoms and seriousness of the situation and are unsure of what action to take, chances of the early opening of an occluded coronary artery and the best possible outcome decrease as minutes and hours tick by.

Patients at high risk for MI. Patients who are at high risk of MI should be given simple instructions regarding the common symptoms of acute MI and the action to be taken to respond effectively and eliminate or at least minimize the factor of patient delay.[2] The nature of chest discomfort should be explained, as well as the associated symptoms such as diaphoresis, shortness of breath, and a sense of impending doom. The patient and family should be made aware that chest discomfort may seem more like pressure than frank pain, and, although the retrosternal area is the most specific and the arms and mandible the most characteristic locations, the discomfort may be referred to any region above the waist, with an epigastric location being most likely to confuse the diagnosis. Knowing the words others have used to describe angina may be helpful for the patient (Box 13-1).[3]

How to proceed. Patients should be given instructions on how to proceed once they recognize the symptoms. These instructions should impress on the patient a sense of urgency and should include the prompt use of aspirin and nitroglycerin if available. The physician or nurse should confirm that the patient and family know how to summon emergency services, know the location of the nearest hospital with emergency cardiac care, and understand that the hospital, not the physician's office, should be their destination.

TRAINING OF THE EMERGENCY RESPONSE TEAM

Paramedics and EMTs trained and experienced in the recognition of the signs and symptoms of cardiac ischemia-like discomfort or pain and skilled in advanced cardiac life support, defibrillation, and the recording and evaluation of the ECG can decrease the delay in initiating definitive care and transporting to centers with capabilities for emergency cardiac catheterization and revascularization.

The chances for survival may be further improved when the emergency medical services team members have a sense of urgency and are skilled in identifying

---

BOX 11-1

Patient Descriptions of Angina[3]

- A red hot poker
- A shoe box in my chest
- A toothache
- Hot flame in the upper part of my mouth
- An elephant on my chest
- Jaw pain
- Arthritis (shoulder, elbow, or wrists)
- A "bad feeling" in the upper portion of my back
- Tracheitis
- A "good feeling" in the chest—like that in the side while running as a child
- Sternal whisper
- Dryness in the throat produced by effort or emotional stress
- Smoke in my chest
- Someone choking me from behind
- A large fish hook stuck under my jaw

---

patients requiring reperfusion therapy (see Chapters 1 and 2). Also, the correct identification and early treatment of patients with acute pulmonary embolism (see Chapter 9) or a tachycardia can be lifesaving (see Chapters 4 and 5).[1,4]

When considering such a program, an examination of the actual time it takes a highly trained emergency medical services team to deliver patients to the appropriate hospital in the local community is prudent. The advantage of prehospital thrombolytic therapy by nonphysicians may be offset by rapid transport and an efficient hospital response with a "door to needle" time of 30 minutes or less or a "door to percutaneous coronary intervention" time of fewer than 150 minutes.

INHOSPITAL RESPONSE

The base hospital should preferably have facilities for emergency cardiac catheterization, angioplasty, and cardiac surgery. If such facilities are not available and the patient's condition requires emergency intervention, the emergency response unit should be redirected to a hospital with facilities for an acute coronary intervention. At that hospital the emergency team should have been alerted by the mobile unit and be ready to respond.

Prehospital Assessment of High-Risk Patients with Chest Pain

Prehospital trials have shown that the best prehospital care should be based on a correct diagnosis.[1] Correct diagnosis requires a highly skilled prehospital assessment by the paramedic or EMT and presupposes the ability to complete the physical examination, record a 12-lead ECG, evaluate for high-risk MI, take a history aimed at excluding inappropriate candidates for thrombolysis, and be en route to the hospital, all within 20 minutes or less. A checklist may be helpful in expediting the history and physical examination and avoiding excessive evaluation times that delay the initiation of appropriate therapy. Prehospital thrombolysis should be considered for appropriate candidates when an informed physician agrees or when transport time will be more than 1 hour.[1]

HISTORY

The following questions should be included when taking the patient's history:

- Please point to where your pain is located: sternal, precordial, left chest, right chest, epigastrium/lower chest, or mid chest?
- How would you describe your pain? (If possible, this should be in the patient's own words without

suggestions from the examiner.) The pain may be described as sharp, dull, aching, like a weight on or in the chest, burning, tightness, or ripping.

- What eases your pain? What makes it worse (sitting up, leaning forward, lying flat, belching, vomiting, walking, nothing)?
- Does your pain radiate to another area (shoulder, jaw, neck, one arm, or both arms)?
- Have you been sweating?
- Are you short of breath?
- Did you use nitroglycerin (sublingual or patch)?
- Have you been nauseated or vomiting?
- Do you have a history of prior MI, angina, or coronary bypass surgery?
- Do you smoke or have high blood pressure, diabetes mellitus, high blood cholesterol, or a family history of MI or sudden death?

PHYSICAL EXAMINATION

The physical examination evaluates the pump function of the heart and the blood supply to the extremities. The following assessments should be made:

- Describe the patient's general appearance (pale, cyanotic, sweating, hemiparetic, lethargic, status of peripheral perfusion).
- Is jugular venous distention present?
- Can bruits be heard over the carotids?
- Are the lungs clear? Any rales?
- Describe the heart rhythm and sounds (regular, irregular, murmurs, S3 gallop, pericardial friction rub).
- Describe findings on abdominal palpation (tender, tense, pulsatile mass).
- Evaluate mental status for recent change.
- Is the weakness of arms or legs of recent onset?
- Describe the type and location of pain.
- Evaluate hemodynamic status.

THE ECG (See Chapters 1 and 2)

Evaluate the ECG for the following factors:

- Heart rate. A slow (fewer than 50 beats/min) or high (100 beats/min or more) rate indicates increased risk.
- Presence or absence of ectopic beats or abnormal rhythms.
- ST segment deviation score (the sum of the ST segment elevation and depression by all 12 leads). The higher the score, the larger the area at risk.
- Determine the site of occlusion in the coronary artery, which also indicates the size of the area at risk.

- The QRS width and presence of intraventricular conduction defects.
- Presence of high-risk anterior wall MI (occlusion before the first septal and first diagonal branch of the LAD), as indicated by:
  ST elevation: leads V_1 (more than 2 mm), V_2, V_3, aVR, aVL
  ST depression: leads II, III, aVF
- For medium- and low-risk LAD coronary artery occlusion locations, see Chapter 1.
- Presence of high-risk inferior wall MI. In addition to the usual findings in the inferior leads, high risk is indicated by ST segment elevation of 1 mm or more in lead V_4R, which identifies patients with an occlusion high in the RCA.
- Transmit the ECG to the physician at the base hospital. Thereafter, the decision is made for rapid percutaneous coronary intervention, initiation of thrombolytic therapy, or further evaluation in the hospital.

USEFULNESS OF LEAD V_4R IN ACUTE INFERIOR MI

Lead V_4R has the following four important roles in the risk assessment and management of patients with acute MI:

1. Identification of patients with a large inferior MI
2. Determination of whether RV MI has occurred
3. Identification of patients who are at high risk for developing AV block
4. Identification of the location of the coronary artery occlusion

SIGNIFICANCE OF BUNDLE BRANCH BLOCK IN ACUTE ANTERIOR MI

In acute anterior wall MI, acquired (new) bundle branch block is an ominous finding, preferably requiring rapid percutaneous coronary intervention. This information must therefore be transmitted to the base hospital. Paramedics should be able to recognize these conditions. The ECG signs of bundle branch block with and without MI are discussed in Chapter 1.

Thrombolytic Therapy

The value of thrombolytic therapy is highly time dependent; it is most beneficial when administered within 1 to 4 hours of the onset of pain, the earlier the better. These benefits are proportionally reduced the later the treatment occurs. These facts place the focus of prehospital management of patients with acute MI on rapid identification and treatment, possibly including thrombolytic therapy. Once the decision is made in favor of a program for prehospital thrombolytic therapy, certain requirements and procedures should be met, including a physician-directed plan for a quick, effective response.

INITIATION OF PREHOSPITAL THROMBOLYTIC POLICY

The following three facts should be considered when deciding to initiate a prehospital thrombolytic policy and should emphasize the importance of correct ECG analysis (with or without computer assistance) and ongoing contact with the hospital-based physician.

1. Only a limited number of patients with chest pain in the prehospital setting actually have acute MI.[5]
2. Accurate screening of patients for thrombolytic therapy in the prehospital setting requires correct interpretation of the ECG and the absence of contraindications.
3. Mistakenly administering thrombolytic therapy to noncandidates may have important medical and legal implications.

EVALUATION OF THE PATIENT FOR THROMBOLYTIC THERAPY IN THE FIELD

When thrombolytic therapy is initiated in the field, the following evaluation of the patient is quickly carried out:

- Patients with chest pain or tightness, acute epigastric distress, or other symptoms of acute MI are placed on an established protocol.
- Any contraindications to thrombolysis are noted.
- The patient's status and ECG are transmitted to the emergency department for physician guidance.

WHEN REPERFUSION THERAPY IS INDICATED

When reperfusion therapy is indicated, the physician will advise regarding the preferred mode: a rapid intracoronary intervention or thrombolytic therapy. As discussed in Chapter 1, both the size of the area at risk and the distance between the patient and the hospital where a percutaneous intervention can be performed play a role in decision making.

RESPONSE AT THE BASE HOSPITAL

Cardiac monitoring should be continuous and a physician should see the patient within the first few minutes of arrival. Delays of any kind should not be permitted in the admission and evaluation of these patients.

High-risk patients. High-risk patients are promptly identified from the 13-lead ECG (12 standard leads plus lead V_4R) and the clinical assessment.

For patients who are in cardiogenic shock, have a large acute MI, or have a contraindication to thrombolytic therapy, the first choice of reperfusion therapy is primary angioplasty with stenting of the culprit coronary artery.

Rural areas. In rural areas where hospitals do not have special cardiac facilities or physicians trained in emergency cardiac care, a protocol should be established for telephone communication with a nearby well-equipped medical center. Protocols for initiating thrombolytic therapy in patients from rural hospitals before transferring them to metropolitan centers have been shown to be safe and effective.

CAUSES FOR DELAY

The American College of Cardiology/American Heart Association special task force advises that in the critical setting of acute MI no unnecessary delays in initiating treatment should occur, such as those consumed by administrative procedures (e.g., establishing insurance coverage and prolonged efforts to consult with the patient's private physician). Such delays "must not be allowed to occur" and are "inappropriate."[1]

Other delays also occur. For example, patients with chest pain sometimes wait their turn in busy emergency departments. Once admitted, additional delay may occur while a cardiologist is located for decision making about therapy. Sometimes therapy is not initiated until the patient is transferred to the cardiac care unit. The sum of these delays reduces the potential benefit of early reperfusion. Evaluation of these delays by emergency department directors and hospital administrators is the first step in eliminating them. The goal is to start the intravenous thrombolytic treatment in the proper candidate within 30 minutes of the onset of chest pain or to proceed to primary angioplasty within 60 minutes of arrival in the emergency department.

CANDIDATES FOR THROMBOLYSIS

To be considered a candidate for thrombolytic therapy, the patient should have a qualifying 12-lead ECG and the following characteristics:

- Be oriented and cooperative
- Have had chest discomfort for 20 minutes or more but fewer than 24 hours
- Have a systolic blood pressure of more than 80 mm Hg but less than 200 mm Hg
- Have a systolic blood pressure difference of less than 30 mm Hg and diastolic blood pressure of less than 20 mm Hg between the right and left arm

ABSOLUTE CONTRAINDICATIONS FOR THROMBOLYSIS

When the contraindications for thrombolysis are absolute, other reperfusion strategies are considered, such as percutaneous transluminal coronary angioplasty or coronary artery bypass surgery. The following are absolute contraindications for thrombolysis:

- Altered consciousness
- Active internal bleeding
- Suspected aortic dissection or pericarditis
- Recent head trauma
- Known spinal cord or cerebral arteriovenous malformation or tumor
- Known previous hemorrhagic cerebrovascular accident
- Intracranial or intraspinal surgery within 2 months
- Trauma or surgery within 2 weeks that could result in bleeding into a closed space
- Persistent blood pressure greater than 200/120 mm Hg
- Pregnancy
- Previous allergy to streptokinase product (other thrombolytic agents may be used)

RELATIVELY MAJOR CONTRAINDICATIONS (INDIVIDUAL EVALUATION OF RISK VERSUS BENEFIT)

The following conditions are relatively major contraindications for thrombolytic therapy:

- Active peptic ulcer disease (recent)
- Gastrointestinal or genitourinary hemorrhage
- History of ischemic or embolic cerebrovascular accident
- Current use of oral anticoagulants with therapeutic international normalized ratio
- Known bleeding disorder
- Major trauma or surgery within past 2 weeks
- History of chronic uncontrolled hypertension (diastolic blood pressure greater than 100 mm Hg, treated or untreated)
- Subclavian or internal jugular venous cannulation or puncture of central noncompressible vessel
- Prolonged, traumatic cardiopulmonary resuscitation
- Unwitnessed syncope or fall with potential central nervous system trauma

When these contraindications have paramount importance, such as very recent trauma, surgery, or active peptic ulcer disease with recent bleeding, they become absolute contraindications when weighed against a less than life-threatening and evolving acute MI.

RELATIVELY MINOR CONTRAINDICATIONS

The relatively minor contraindications for thrombolytic therapy are diabetic retinopathy and endocarditis.

Cardiopulmonary resuscitation was originally considered a contraindication for thrombolytic therapy, but increasing evidence shows that thrombolytic therapy may be beneficial for patients undergoing cardiopulmonary resuscitation for circulatory arrest.[6-8]

Unstable Angina with ST Segment Depression or Negative T Waves

In the presence of unstable angina with ST segment depression or negative T waves, use the following procedures:

1. Take a history and perform a physical examination.
2. Obtain a 12-lead ECG and transmit it to the base hospital.
3. Evaluate the ECG for signs of critical proximal LAD coronary artery stenosis and count the number of leads showing ST segment deviation to recognize left main and three-vessel disease. Both situations are indications for rapid cardiac catheterization and revascularization therapy. Especially at risk are patients showing these ECG findings in the presence of low blood pressure and an elevated troponin value.
4. Transmit findings to the base hospital.

RECOGNITION OF CRITICAL PROXIMAL LAD CORONARY ARTERY STENOSIS
(See Chapter 2)

- Unstable angina
- No pathologic precordial Q waves
- ST segment isoelectric or minimally elevated (1 mm), concave or straight
- Symmetric T-wave inversion, which may begin with very slight negativity at the terminal part of the T wave in leads V_1 to V_3

This ECG is typically recorded when patient is *without pain.* In contrast, the ECG changes of left main stem and three-vessel disease are typically present *during pain,* whereas those of critical proximal LAD stenosis usually develop *after* the chest pain has subsided.

RECOGNITION OF LEFT MAIN STEM AND THREE-VESSEL DISEASE

- Unstable angina
- ST elevation in leads aVR and V_1 during pain
- ST depression in eight or more leads during pain

Conscious Patient with a Tachycardia

When the patient is conscious with a rapid heart rate:

1. Record a 12-lead ECG and transmit it to the base hospital.
2. Obtain vital signs and evaluate neck veins for cannon A waves and changing loudness of the first heart sound (AV dissociation) or the frog sign (SVT).
3. Determine if the patient has a narrow (less than 0.12 seconds) or a broad (0.12 seconds or more) QRS tachycardia.

NARROW QRS TACHYCARDIA (See Chapter 4)
Physical Signs

Pulse: Regular in regular SVT.
Blood pressure: Constant in regular SVT.
First heart sound: Constant in regular SVT. Pulse, blood pressure, and loudness of the first heart sound vary in atrial fibrillation and atrial flutter with changing AV conduction.
Neck veins: Flutter waves are visible in atrial flutter. In AV nodal reentry and circus movement tachycardia, regular pulsation in the jugular veins is noted.

Effect of Carotid Sinus Massage

Carotid sinus massage is an essential skill for clinicians (see Chapter 4). The gag reflex is an excellent vagal maneuver and substitute for carotid sinus massage, which is usually performed by the physician. Carotid sinus massage has the following effects:

Sinus tachycardia: Gradual and temporary, slowing heart rate.
Atrial tachycardia: Cessation or temporary slowing (AV block) of tachycardia or no effect.
Atrial flutter: Temporary slowing (AV block), conversion to atrial fibrillation, or no effect.
Atrial fibrillation: Temporary slowing (AV block) or no effect.
AV nodal reentry tachycardia: Cessation of tachycardia or no effect.
Circus movement tachycardia by an accessory AV pathway: Cessation of tachycardia or no effect.

BROAD QRS TACHYCARDIA (See Chapter 5)

If broad QRS tachycardia is present, proceed as follows:
- Remain calm.
- Determine if lead V_1 is positive or negative and apply morphologic rules to differentiate SVT from VT (see Chapter 5).
- Systematically evaluate the 12-lead ECG and examine the patient for physical signs of AV dissociation (a sign of VT).
- If in doubt, *do not give verapamil;* give procainamide.

Physical Signs of AV Dissociation

AV dissociation is present in VT in approximately 50% of cases. Thus the following physical signs of AV dissociation during a broad QRS tachycardia are helpful in the differential diagnosis:

Blood pressure: Beat-to-beat changes in systolic blood pressure.
First heart sound: Varying loudness of the first heart sound.
Neck veins: Irregular cannon A waves in the jugular venous pulse.

ECG in Lead V_1–Positive Broad QRS (RBBB-Like) Tachycardia

- SVT is most likely with a triphasic pattern in lead V_1 (rSR′).
- VT is most likely with a monophasic or biphasic pattern in lead V_1.
- The "rabbit ear clue" is also an indication of VT (two peaks in lead V_1 with the left peak being taller).
- When lead V_1 is not diagnostic, examine lead V_6.
- A triphasic pattern (qRS) in lead V_6 suggests SVT, whereas a deep S (R/S ratio of less than one) or QS indicates VT.
- Left axis deviation in the frontal plane suggests VT.

ECG in Lead V_1–Negative Broad QRS (LBBB-Like) Tachycardia

The following findings in leads V_1, V_2, and V_6 are highly predictive of VT:

- A broad R wave of 0.03 seconds or more in lead V_1 or V_2.
- A notched or slurred downstroke on the S or QS wave in lead V_1 or V_2.
- A distance of 0.06 seconds or more from the onset of the ventricular complex to the nadir of the QS or S in lead V_1 or V_2.
- A Q wave in lead V_6 strongly suggests VT, but *only* if the complex is mainly negative in lead V_1.
- In SVT with LBBB aberration, if an r wave is present it is narrow and sharp in lead V_1 and/or lead V_2, and the S wave has a clean, swift downstroke (see Chapter 5). If the recording from lead V_1 looks like VT, it is treated as VT; if the recording from lead V_1 looks like SVT, check leads V_2 and V_6 before deciding.
- Right-axis deviation suggests VT.

Other Helpful ECG Clues

■ QRS width more than 0.14 seconds favors VT (except in the case of digitalis toxicity or in the presence of drugs that slow intraventricular conduction).

■ Fusion beats, capture beats, and precordial concordance (all precordial leads showing either a completely positive or negative QRS complex) also favor a diagnosis of VT.

TREATMENT
VT

1. Administer intravenous procainamide 10 mg/kg body weight over a 5-minute period or intravenous lidocaine 1 mg/kg body weight if an acute MI is suspected.
2. If unsuccessful, cardiovert.
3. Obtain a history regarding frequency of tachycardia episodes and symptoms during an attack of tachycardia.

SVT with Aberration

In patients with SVT with aberration, transmit the 12-lead ECG to the base hospital. The following procedure may be ordered:

■ Apply vagal stimulation.
■ Administer adenosine as a 6-mg bolus (12 mg may be repeated twice) or intravenous verapamil 10 mg over a 3-minute period. If unsuccessful:
■ Administer intravenous procainamide 10 mg/kg body weight over a 5-minute period. If unsuccessful:
■ Cardiovert.

If in Doubt

■ Do *not* give verapamil.
■ On advice of the physician, give intravenous procainamide 10 mg/kg body weight over a 5-minute period.

Broad and Irregular Rhythm

1. Transmit the 12-lead ECG to the base hospital.
2. Do *not* give digitalis or verapamil.
3. On advice of the physician, give intravenous procainamide 10 mg/kg body weight over a 5-minute period. If unsuccessful:
4. Cardiovert (see Appendix B).

Torsades de Pointes

1. Transmit the 12-lead ECG to the base hospital. The patient's history will usually implicate class IA or III drugs.
2. Maintain continuous monitoring.
3. Establish an intravenous line; the physician may advise magnesium administration, which is advocated even when magnesium levels are normal. Give MgCl or $MgSO_4$ as a 1- to 2-g bolus over a 5-minute period, followed by an infusion, 1 to 2 g/hr for 4 to 6 hours.
4. If intravenous magnesium is unsuccessful, advise the physician because cardiac pacing may be necessary on arrival at the hospital.

Possible Digitalis Intoxication

1. Transmit the 12-lead ECG to the base hospital.
2. Protect the patient from stress (catecholamines may exacerbate the arrhythmia).
3. Do not use vagal maneuvers.
4. Establish an intravenous line and transport without delay.
5. Continue monitoring.
6. A temporary pacemaker or digitalis antibodies may be indicated on arrival at the hospital.

A Conscious Patient in Bradycardia

1. Record a 12-lead ECG and transmit it to the base hospital.
2. Take a history and do a physical examination.
3. Evaluate the ECG for MI, arrhythmia, PR interval, and QRS axis and width. The PR interval and QRS axis and width help evaluate for AV and intraventricular block.
4. Determine type of arrhythmia and note:
   ■ Regularity (suggests sinus bradycardia or heart block).
   ■ Abrupt pauses or group beating. Abrupt pauses in the atrial rhythm or group beating suggests SA block or sick sinus syndrome; abrupt pauses or group beating in the ventricular rhythm suggests AV block.
5. Treatment is governed by the cause of the bradycardia:
   ■ *If sinus bradycardia,* give no treatment unless hypotension or hypoperfusion is present; if so, administer atropine 0.04 mg/kg body weight.
   ■ *If SA block or sinus arrest,* give no treatment unless hypotension develops; if so, give atropine.
   ■ *If sick sinus syndrome,* advise the physician because a pacemaker may be indicated on arrival at the hospital.
   ■ *If complete AV block with narrow QRS,* give no treatment unless hypotension or hypoperfusion is present; if so, give atropine and advise the physician because a pacemaker may be indicated on arrival at the hospital.
   ■ *If complete AV block with broad QRS,* with or without hypotension, a temporary pacemaker may be indicated.

Unconscious Patient

UNCONSCIOUS PATIENT IN TACHYCARDIA

1. Cardiovert, then transmit the 12-lead ECG to the base hospital.
2. Obtain vital signs and a history from the family if possible; advise the physician regarding medications being taken by the patient.
3. Establish an intravenous line.

UNCONSCIOUS PATIENT IN BRADYCARDIA

1. Record a 12-lead ECG and transmit it to the base hospital.
2. Take a history and perform a physical examination.
3. Give intravenous atropine 0.04 mg/kg body weight.
4. Advise physician of results because temporary pacing may be necessary if atropine is unsuccessful.

Emergency Cardioversion

Cardioversion is performed promptly with minimal premedication in patients who have tachycardia, discernible R and T waves, and a deteriorating hemodynamic status. This status would include those with the following conditions:

- Atrial flutter or atrial fibrillation with conduction over an accessory pathway that does not respond to procainamide or ajmaline (in Europe) or is associated with hemodynamic instability
- SVT that does not respond to vagal maneuvers or antiarrhythmic therapy, is not caused by digitalis intoxication, and is associated with hemodynamic instability
- VT refractory to antiarrhythmic drug therapy and associated with hemodynamic instability

ENERGY SETTINGS FOR DEFIBRILLATION AND CARDIOVERSION OF UNCONSCIOUS PATIENTS

VT (synchronized cardioversion): 10 J is usually adequate; 100 J is almost always successful.

SVT (synchronized cardioversion): 10 J is frequently effective; 100 J is almost always successful.

Ventricular fibrillation (defibrillation): Initially 200 J; if unsuccessful, follow immediately by 350 J. (For children weighing 2.5 to 50 kg, use 2 J/kg.)

AUTOMATIC EXTERNAL DEFIBRILLATOR

The automatic external defibrillator is a combination of an ECG monitor and a defibrillator powered by long-life batteries. It contains sophisticated rhythm-detection algorithms capable of detecting ventricular fibrillation or VT with high specificity and sensitivity and responding appropriately by automatically charging itself and alerting the rescuer to stand clear and push the defibrillator button.[9-11]

Further information on the automatic external defibrillator can be found in Appendix B.

PRECORDIAL THUMP

If administered at the onset of ventricular fibrillation or rapid hypotensive VT, the precordial thump can sometimes return the heart to a normal sinus rhythm.

REFERENCES

1. Antman EM, Anbe DT, Armstrong PW, et al: ACC/AHA guidelines for the management of patients with ST-elevation myocardial infarction—executive summary: a report of the American College of Cardiology/American Heart Association Task Force on Practice Guidelines (Writing Committee to Revise the 1999 Guidelines for the Management of Patients With Acute Myocardial Infarction), *Circulation* 110:588-636, 2004.
2. Goldberg RJ, Garwitz JH, Gore JM: Duration of, and temporal trends (1994-1997) in, prehospital delay in patients with acute myocardial infarction: the second National Registry of Myocardial Infarction, *Arch Intern Med* 159:2142-7, 1999.
3. Hurst JW, Logue RB: Angina pectoris: words patients use and overlooked precipitating events, *Heart Dis Stroke* 2:89-96, 1993.
4. Karagounis L, Ipsen SK, Jessop MR, et al: Impact of field-transmitted electrocardiography on time to in-hospital thrombolytic therapy in acute myocardial infarction, *Am J Cardiol* 66:686-91, 1990.
5. Weaver WD, Cerqueira M, Hallstrom AP, et al: Pre-hospital-initiated vs hospital-initiated thrombolytic therapy: the myocardial infarction triage and intervention trial, *JAMA* 270:1211-6, 1993.
6. Van Campen LC, Van Leeuwen GR, Verheugt FW: Safety and efficacy of thrombolysis for acute myocardial infarction in patients with prolonged out-of-hospital cardiopulmonary resuscitation, *Am J Cardiol* 69:953-5, 1994.
7. Bottiger BW, Bode C, Kern S, et al: Efficacy and safety of thrombolytic therapy after initially unsuccessful cardiopulmonary resuscitation: a prospective clinical trial, *Lancet* 357:1583-5, 2001.
8. Abu-Laban RB, Christenson JM, Innes GD, et al: Tissue plasminogen activator in cardiac arrest with pulseless electrical activity, *N Engl J Med* 346:1522-8, 2002.
9. Weisfeldt ML, Kerber RE, McGoldrick RP et al: Public access defibrillation: a statement for health care professionals from the American Heart Association Task Force on the automatic defibrillator, *Circulation* 92:2763-72, 1995.
10. Marenco JP, Wang PJ, Link MS, et al: Improving survival from sudden cardiac arrest: the role of the automated external defibrillator, *JAMA* 285:1193-200, 2001.
11. Myerburg RJ, Fenster J, Velez M, et al: Impact of community-wide police car deployment of automated external defibrillators on survival from out-of-hospital cardiac arrest, *Circulation* 106:1058-64, 2002.

Determining the Axis of the ECG Components

The ECG consists of components such as the P wave and the QRS complex, representing depolarization of the atria and ventricles, and the ST-T segment, reflecting repolarization of the ventricles.

The spatial orientation of the current flow during these parts of the ECG results in the configuration of the P wave, the QRS complex, the ST segment, and the T wave. The mean current flow of these components can be expressed as the frontal and horizontal axis of the P wave, the QRS complex, the ST segment, and the T wave.

Many factors determine the direction of the axis of the different parts of the ECG, such as the position of the heart in the chest, the site of impulse formation in the heart, and the direction of impulse propagation in the atria and ventricles, plus factors such as dilation, hypertrophy, and scarring of the cardiac chambers.

Examining the direction of the axis is important during both depolarization and repolarization.

As stated in Chapter 1, in acute cardiac ischemia the ST segment deviation points in the direction of the ischemic area and is quite helpful in determining the site and size of the area at risk and the location of the coronary occlusion.

The T wave also has a certain spatial direction that may be concordant or discordant with the axis of the QRS complex, providing diagnostic implications.

HISTORIC BACKGROUND

More than a century ago, Willem Einthoven introduced the three bipolar leads that define Einthoven's triangle (Figure A-1). The triangle is composed of leads I, II, and III. Lead I is across the arms (shoulders), with the negative electrode on the right arm (shoulder) and the positive electrode on the left arm (shoulder). Lead II has the negative electrode on the right arm (shoulder) and the positive electrode on the left leg. Lead III has the negative electrode on the left arm (shoulder) and the positive electrode on the left leg.

The unipolar limb leads (aVR, aVL, aVF) are formed by a positive electrode at each point of Einthoven's triangle with the zero reference point in the center of the electrical field of the heart. This reference point is created by the sum of the electrical potentials from the three bipolar leads.

The lead axes of the three unipolar and three bipolar limb leads are illustrated in Figure A-2. These six limb leads provide information about the direction of the axis in the frontal plane.

THE HEXAXIAL FIGURE

The hexaxial figure helps estimate the frontal plane axis in degrees. This figure is drawn by shifting the axis of the six limb leads so they all pass through the center of the electrical field of the heart (Figure A-3).

DETERMINING THE AXIS

When the mean current of the P wave, the QRS, the ST segment, or the T wave is perpendicular to the axis of a lead, an equiphasic deflection is produced. When this current is parallel to the axis of the lead, the resulting ECG complex is either the most positive or

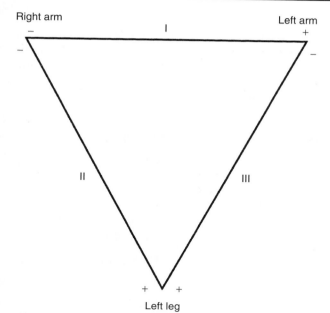

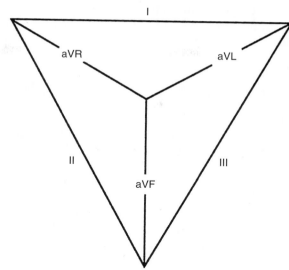

Figure A-1 Einthoven's triangle consists of the three bipolar limb leads I, II, and III. Lead I represents the electrical potential difference between the arms, and leads II and III represent the potential difference between the arms and the left leg.

Figure A-2 The six limb leads consist of Einthoven's triangle plus the three unipolar leads. The unipolar limb leads are achieved by placing a positive electrode on each arm (aVR and aVL) and one on the left leg (aVF). There is an electrical potential between this positive electrode and a reference point at the center of Einthoven's triangle.

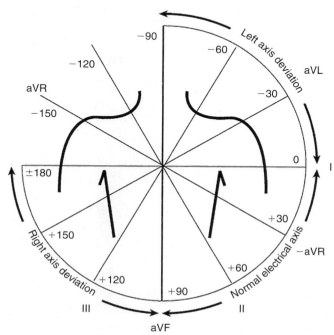

Figure A-3 The hexaxial figure. All lead axes are drawn through the center of the electrical field of the heart; each lead axis has a 30-degree angle with its neighboring lead axis.

the most negative deflection depending on whether current flows toward the positive or the negative electrode.

Frontal Plane Axis

Therefore, to determine the frontal plane axis, the following two steps must be taken:

1. Find the equiphasic deflection (as much positive as negative forces) in the six frontal leads; the mean current of the heart is perpendicular to this lead axis. If no equiphasic deflection is present in any of the six limb leads, select the one that is smallest (i.e., almost equiphasic).
2. To discover in which direction the current is traveling, look for the lead in which the QRS complex has an axis parallel to the current flow. For example, if the equiphasic deflection were in lead aVL (Figure A-4), the mean current would be perpendicular to the axis of lead aVL and parallel to the axis of lead II. Thus if lead II is positive, the frontal plane axis is normal.

Horizontal Plane Axis

Similarly, the axis can be determined in the horizontal plane by using lead I and the precordial leads. The horizontal plane axis helps determine the spread of atrial and ventricular depolarization in the horizontal plane and is of special importance for localizing abnormal impulse formation or conduction in the atrium or ventricle.

NORMAL FINDINGS DURING SINUS RHYTHM

The following features are present in the frontal plane:

■ The P-wave axis varies from +10 to +80 degrees.
■ The QRS axis varies from 0 to +90 degrees.
■ The T-wave axis varies from +10 to +80 degrees.

An axis to the left or the right of these values (left-axis or right-axis deviation) should be considered abnormal.

CLINICAL USE OF AXIS DETERMINATION
P Wave

The P-wave axis provides information about the direction of atrial activation. For example, a negative P wave in lead I during an SVT indicates that atrial activation

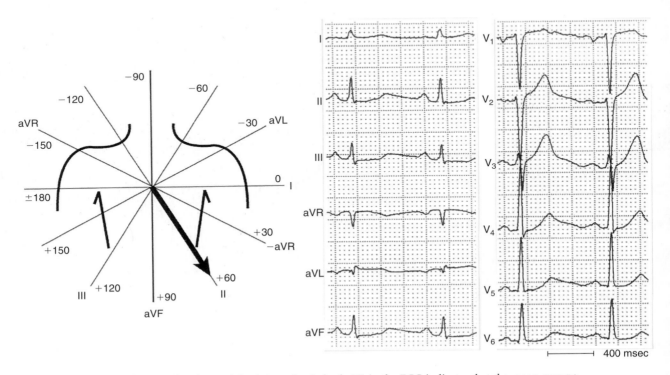

Figure A-4   *Right,* The equiphasic complex in lead aVL in the ECG indicates that the mean current is perpendicular to the axis of lead II. Lead II reveals which way the current is flowing because the axis of lead II is parallel with the current flow. *Left,* The direction of the axis is shown in the hexaxial figure.

starts in the left atrium, as it would in left atrial tachycardia or when a left-sided accessory pathway is being used as the retrograde arm of a reentry circuit.

When atrial activation starts low in the atrium close to the intraatrial septum—such as in AV nodal tachycardia, low atrial tachycardia, tachycardias by a posteroseptal accessory pathway as the retrograde arm in the reentry circuit, or ventriculoatrial conduction during VT—the P wave will be negative in leads II, aVF, and III and positive in leads aVR and aVL. Examples of P-wave axis determination and its use in determining the direction of atrial activation are given in Chapter 4.

The QRS Complex

Emergency situations in which the QRS axis is altered include the following:

- The appearance of conduction disturbances in acute MI, such as the development of left-axis deviation in a patient with an acute anterior MI. This situation indicates an interruption of conduction in the left anterior fascicle and means that the patient has a very proximal occlusion in the LAD. This situation calls for an immediate intracoronary reopening of the vessel (Figure A-5).
- Acute pulmonary embolism in which sudden dilation of the RV leads to a shift in the frontal plane QRS axis to the right (see Chapter 9).
- Wide QRS tachycardia in which an abnormal axis supports a diagnosis of VT. An axis to the left of −30 degrees is highly suggestive of a VT in an RBBB-shaped QRS in lead V_1. In lead V_1, an LBBB-shaped QRS complex with right-axis deviation of more than +90 degrees is diagnostic of VT (Figures A-6 and A-7).

ST Segment Axis

As discussed in Chapter 1, in acute cardiac ischemia the ST segment deviation points in the direction of the area of maximal ischemia and allows identification of the location of that area in the anterior, posterior, inferior, and lateral part of the LV and in the RV by adding right precordial leads, as well as the culprit coronary artery and the location of the occlusion in that artery. As shown in Chapter 1, both the frontal and the horizontal plane leads must be analyzed to determine that information. For example, the ST deviation axis in the horizontal plane points toward the precordial leads V_1 to V_3, indicating anterior wall MI, but the exact location of the occlusion in the LAD comes from the analysis of the ST deviation axis in the frontal leads (Figure A-8).

SUMMARY

Axis determination of the different components of the ECG is an essential step in diagnosing the type and site of origin of cardiac arrhythmias, localizing conduction disturbances, and localizing the site and size of ischemia in coronary artery disease.

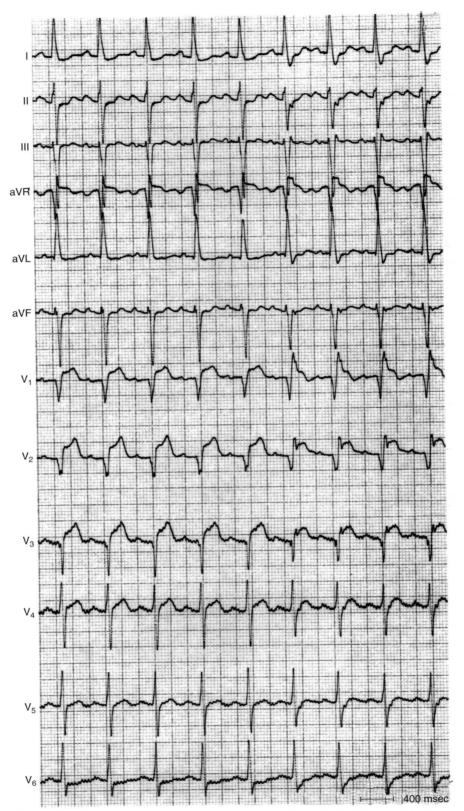

Figure A-5 An acute anterior wall MI showing left-axis deviation in the *left* part of the figure, indicating left anterior hemiblock. This pattern suddenly changes to RBBB in the *right* part of the figure. These changes indicate an occlusion in the LAD proximal to the first septal branch.

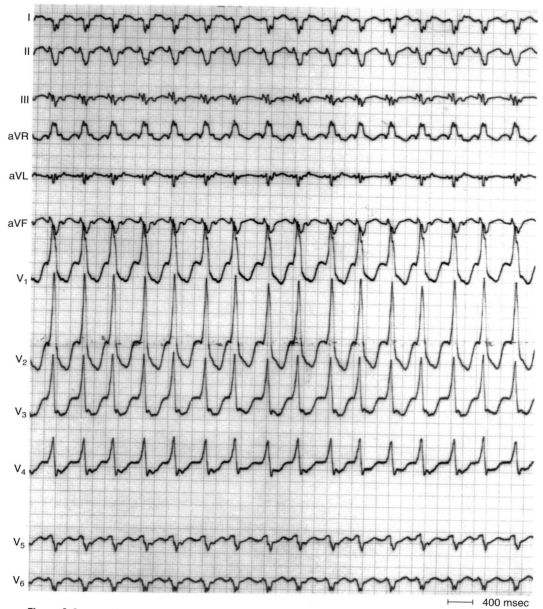

Figure A-6 A wide QRS tachycardia with an RBBB-like configuration in lead V_1. Left-axis deviation supports a ventricular origin of the arrhythmia. In addition, other findings indicate the arrhythmia is a VT.

⊢——⊣ 400 msec

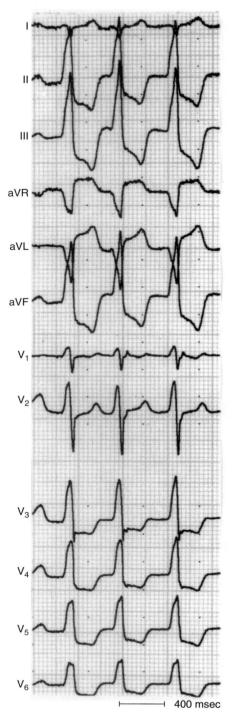

Figure A-7   Wide QRS tachycardia with an LBBB-like configuration in lead V_1. Right-axis deviation in the frontal plane indicates a ventricular origin of the tachycardia in the outflow tract of the RV.

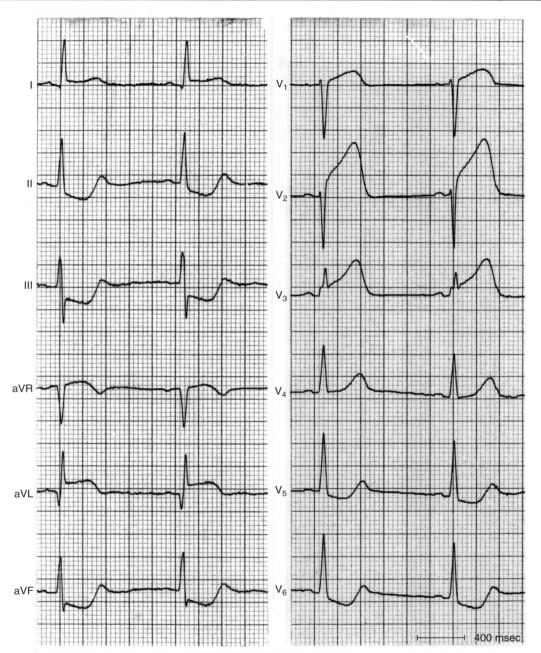

Figure A-8   A patient with an acute anterior wall MI. The ST deviation vector in the horizontal plane indicates ischemia on the anterior wall of the heart, but the ST deviation vector in the frontal plane pointing to the base of the heart indicates that the occlusion is located in the LAD coronary artery proximal to the first septal branch.

B

Electrical Treatment of Arrhythmias and the Automated External Defibrillator in Out-of-Hospital Resuscitation

EMERGENCY CARDIOVERSION

Cardioversion is the electrical conversion of an atrial or ventricular arrhythmia to a normal sinus rhythm by the delivery of a direct current shock to the heart synchronized to discharge with the QRS complex. Biphasic defibrillators are currently used after studies demonstrated a higher defibrillation efficacy with lower energies, resulting in less cardiac damage and fewer skin burns.[1-3]

During tachycardia, the electrical current from the defibrillator depolarizes the heart and interrupts the arrhythmia; during fibrillation, the current reduces the amount of excitable myocardium so that fibrillation cannot be perpetuated. Synchronization of the electrical discharge with the QRS complex (cardioversion) is necessary to avoid delivering a depolarizing current during the vulnerable period when the heart is more susceptible to ventricular fibrillation. The vulnerable period is an interval that begins and ends with the T wave but is at its peak for approximately 30 msec just before the apex of the T wave. At this point, the current required to elicit ventricular fibrillation is at its lowest. Additionally, in the ischemic heart the stimulus required to cause fibrillation is much less than it is in the normal heart.

Cardioversion is performed promptly with minimal premedication in patients who have tachycardia and discernible R and T waves and a deteriorating hemodynamic status. These patients include those with the following conditions:

- Atrial flutter or atrial fibrillation with conduction over an accessory pathway that does not respond to procainamide or ajmaline (in Europe) or is associated with hemodynamic instability
- SVT that does not respond to vagal maneuvers or antiarrhythmic therapy, is not caused by digitalis intoxication, and is associated with hemodynamic instability
- VT refractory to antiarrhythmic drug therapy and associated with hemodynamic instability

Cardioversion for Patients with Implanted Pacemakers

Patients with implanted pacing systems needing emergency cardioversion or defibrillation require special attention to avoid endocardial burns and increased fibrosis at the electrode-endocardial interface. Energy can be shunted to the myocardium by way of the pacing electrode, causing endocardial burns and an increase in the stimulation threshold; this in turn results in a loss of capture.[4]

DEFIBRILLATION

Defibrillation is nonsynchronized cardioversion and is used when QRS complexes and T waves are not distinguishable, as in ventricular fibrillation. Early defibrillation is the most useful measure in resuscitation; the earlier it is initiated, the better the chance of success. Even if the rhythm appears to be asystole, it may still respond to defibrillation because, depending on the recorded ECG lead, both fine and coarse ventricular fibrillation may mimic asystole. The coarse fibrillation waves of ventricular fibrillation may actually produce zero electrical vectors, resulting in a relatively straight line.[5]

RISKS

Risks associated with cardioversion and defibrillation include the following:

- Postcardioversion tachyarrhythmias (VT or ventricular fibrillation)
- Bradyarrhythmias or asystole
- Embolism (systemic or pulmonary)
- Myocardial injury
- Ventricular dysfunction
- Pulmonary edema
- Hypotension

ENERGY SETTINGS FOR DEFIBRILLATION AND CARDIOVERSION OF UNCONSCIOUS PATIENTS

VT: 10 J is usually adequate; 100 J is almost always effective.

SVT: 10 J is usually adequate; 100 J is almost always effective.

Ventricular fibrillation: Initially 200 J; if unsuccessful, follow immediately with 350 J. (For children weighing 2.5 to 50 kg, use 2 J/kg.)

EMERGENCY PACING

Emergency pacing is rarely needed during cardiopulmonary resuscitation. Ventricular fibrillation is treated with defibrillation and drugs. Electromechanical dissociation is frequently based on inadequate coronary perfusion or myocardial rupture with pericardial tamponade and does not respond to pacing. In bradyasystolic cardiac arrest, apart from airway establishment with effective ventilation and institution of chest compression and drugs (epinephrine, atropine), emergency pacing may be required.

USE OF THE AUTOMATED EXTERNAL DEFIBRILLATOR IN OUT-OF-HOSPITAL RESUSCITATION

In the Western world, one fifth of all deaths occur suddenly and unexpectedly, with ventricular fibrillation being a frequent mechanism.[6] Both in the United States and Europe sudden death occurs approximately 300,000 times per year.[7] Most of these people cannot be identified as being at high risk for this event. In fact, half of them have no history of cardiac disease.[8]

Time Factor

Following cardiac arrest, normal cardiac rhythm must be restored within 5 to 6 minutes to ensure survival without neurologic damage. Essential, therefore, in the chain of survival is the rapid recognition of cardiac arrest and the rapid initiation of cardiac resuscitation with restoration of the normal heart rhythm. An important step in the restoration of normal heart rhythm in out-of-hospital cardiac arrest is the automated external defibrillator (AED).

Simplicity of the Automated External Defibrillator

The AED is a combination of an ECG monitor and a defibrillator powered by long-life batteries. It contains a rhythm-detection algorithm capable of detecting ventricular fibrillation with high specificity and sensitivity and responding appropriately by automatically charging itself and alerting the rescuer to stand clear and push the defibrillator button. Most units give verbally recorded instructions. The simplicity, portability (4 to 7 lbs), and built-in safety of the device allow its use by nonprofessional rescuers, a practice that is rapidly growing worldwide.[9-11] Many airlines, large airports, large businesses, casinos, and stadiums have installed AEDs.[12]

The Nonshockable Rhythm

Early defibrillation is life saving for those in ventricular fibrillation. However, the sudden collapse of an individual may be caused by asystole or pulseless electrical activity, a so-called nonshockable rhythm. In that situation, the AED is of no help.

Survival Rate

Although the process of dying can be delayed by early cardiopulmonary resuscitation, its effectiveness disappears within minutes and, for those in ventricular fibrillation, only defibrillation returns the patient to an organized rhythm.[13] Ideally, the interval between collapse and defibrillation should not exceed 5 to 6 minutes,[14] necessitating that an AED be near the victim and a bystander be capable of responding with speed and comprehension. The survival rate is almost 100% if patients are immediately defibrillated, a feat not possible with the AED because 40% of circulatory arrests are unwitnessed and the system has built-in delays (locating and retrieving the AED, setting it up, and pausing for the ECG diagnosis and automated instructions).[6] The survival rate decreases to 14% to 40% when the resuscitation attempt is started after 4 to 5 minutes. When normal cardiac rhythm is restored after 10 minutes, 95% die even with cardiopulmonary resuscitation.[14]

Legal Restrictions

Most countries have removed legal restrictions by expanding their "Good Samaritan" laws to include the use of AEDs.

Procedure

The AED must be used within minutes after the onset of cardiac arrest. The following procedure should be used:

1. The first rescuer on the scene should call for help, check for pulse and respirations, and, if finding none, provide cardiopulmonary resuscitation.
2. When the AED arrives, quickly apply the electrode pads, one over the apex of the heart and the other over its base.
3. Push the "on" button. The device will take a moment to analyze. Wait for the machine to give the order to either defibrillate or not defibrillate.
4. If ventricular fibrillation is detected the rescuer will be told by the machine to stand clear and push the defibrillator button. After the shock is delivered, the AED will then recycle and repeat the process of ECG evaluation and instructions.
5. If ventricular fibrillation is again detected, the device will instruct the rescuer to deliver another shock. If the AED detects asystole, it will prompt the rescuer to check the airway and begin cardiopulmonary resuscitation.

The Future

Although the presence of AEDs has resulted in improved survival from sudden cardiac arrest, the actual number successfully resuscitated is typically less than 5%.[10] Even with a much wider density of AED placement, the ability to save people from cardiac arrest will likely be disappointing because of the many weak links in the chain of survival (Box B-1). To reach the essential goal of restoration of normal cardiac rhythm within a very short time, the following facts must be considered:

1. The interval between collapse and call for help should be as short as possible. This situation requires a bystander who quickly overcomes the paralysis that occurs when witnessing cardiac arrest. Even with a bystander trained in cardiopulmonary resuscitation, confirmation of circulatory arrest easily takes 1 minute.
2. Prompt external chest compression at a rate of 90 to 100 beats/min is essential in the resuscitation effort. There is growing concern about having thoracic compression interrupted by mouth-to-mouth breathing. This leads to interruption of cerebral and coronary perfusion. As recently pointed out by

---

BOX B-1

Weak Links in the Chain of Survival

- No witness
- The time interval from collapse to start of resuscitation
- Absence of a trained bystander
- Dispatch time
- First responder and advanced life support not rapidly available
- Absence of information about the exact time of collapse and the subsequent steps during the resuscitation effort
- Interruption of chest compression with mouth-to-mouth breathing

---

Ewy,[15] both the fibrillatory heart and the brain can maintain vitality better by continuous chest compression.

3. An average of 2.5 minutes expires after the call comes in for trained responders to be sent to the scene. The dispatch time could be shortened by having a special telephone number other than 911 in the United States and 112 in Europe that is exclusively used for cardiac emergencies.[11]
4. Time between collapse and defibrillation can also be shortened by having a dense network of AEDs and "cardiac arrest watchers" (those who can be summoned when cardiac arrest occurs) in the community.

A major breakthrough in improving results of cardiac resuscitation requires the development of a device specifically geared toward minimizing the time between collapse and the resuscitation effort.[16] By continuous registration of vital signs such as cardiac rhythm or arterial pulsations, such a device would promptly recognize circulatory arrest. This device would reduce the time spent to arrive at the correct diagnosis by giving an audible alarm to attract bystanders, especially when no witnesses are present. The location of the victim would then be transmitted to the nearest site of an AED in the community and to emergency medical services, resulting in a marked reduction in time required for diagnosis and dispatch. The device should also have a clock that allows for precise identification of the time of collapse and subsequent intervention, providing information essential for decision making regarding the patient.

Weisfeldt and Becker,[17] in their three-phase, time-sensitive model, indicated that optimal treatment of cardiac arrest might be phase specific. Their model is as follows:

Electrical phase: In this phase, which lasts approximately 4 minutes, early defibrillation is required.

Circulatory phase: In the next phase (4 to 10 minutes after cardiac arrest), oxygen delivery should precede attempts to restore normal rhythm by defibrillation.

Metabolic phase: In the last phase (starting approximately 10 minutes after cardiac arrest), the value of interventions to improve postischemic ventricular recovery should be investigated, such as controlled reperfusion after treatment with apoptosis inhibitors and external cooling.

Wearing the device would also indicate that the person wants to be resuscitated, a question that cannot be answered with anonymous victims. A reliable device, one able to continuously register artifact-free vital signs, probably requires intracutaneous or subcutaneous sensors. Vital signs should be transmitted to a wearable receiver able to analyze them and sound an alarm in case of circulatory arrest and to transmit the location of the victim.

As shown in Figure B-1, the development of such a device may speed up the chain of survival, resulting in a marked reduction of sudden death outside the hospital.

It might also allow more phase-specific therapies, according to time elapsed after cardiac arrest. If the overall success rate of a resuscitation attempt after a cardiac arrest could be raised from 5% to 25%, an additional 70,000 lives would be saved per year, both in the United States and Europe.

REFERENCES

1. Augostini RS, Tchou PJ, Love C, et al: Multicenter trial of a biphasic external defibrillation waveform, *PACE* 22(4 part II):827, 1999.
2. Faddy SC, Powell J, Craig JC: Biphasic and monophasic shocks for transthoracic defibrillation: a meta analysis of randomized controlled trials, *Resuscitation* 58:9-16, 2003.
3. Walcott GP, Killingsworth CR, Ideker RE: Do clinically relevant transthoracic defibrillation energies cause myocardial damage and dysfunction? *Resuscitation* 59:59-70, 2003.
4. Gould L, Patel S, Gomes GI, et al: Pacemaker failure following external defibrillation, *PACE* 4:575-7, 1981.
5. Weaver WK, Cobb LA, Dennis D, et al: Amplitude of ventricular fibrillation waveform and outcome after cardiac arrest, *Ann Intern Med* 102:53-5, 1985.
6. De Vreede-Swagemakers JJ, Gorgels AP, Dubois-Arbouw WJ, et al: Out-of-hospital arrest in the 1990s: a population based study in

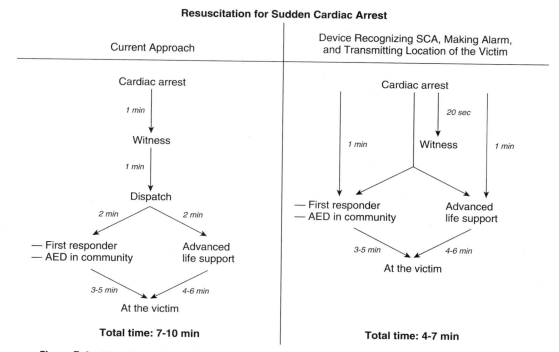

Resuscitation for Sudden Cardiac Arrest

Figure B-1 Time intervals during a currently "ideal" approach to resuscitation compared with the use of a monitoring device that recognizes cardiac arrest, sounds an alarm, and transmits the location of the victim directly to the first responder. *SCA,* Sudden cardiac arrest.

the Maastricht area on incidence, characteristics and survival, *J Am Coll Cardiol* 30:1500-5, 1997.

7. Priori SG, Aliot E, Blomstrom-Lundqvist C, et al: Task force on sudden cardiac death of the European Society of Cardiology, *Eur Heart J* 22:1374-1450, 2001.

8. Zipes DP, Wellens HJJ: Sudden cardiac death, *Circulation* 106:28-36, 2002.

9. Weisfeldt ML, Kerber RE, McGoldrick RP, et al: Public access defibrillation: a statement for healthcare professionals from the American Heart Association task force on the automatic external defibrillator, *Circulation* 92:2763-72, 1995.

10. Marenco JP, Wang PJ, Link MS, et al: Improving survival from sudden cardiac arrest: the role of the automated external defibrillator, *JAMA* 285:1193-200, 2001.

11. Myerburg RJ, Fenster J, Velez M, et al: Impact of community-wide police car deployment of automated external defibrillators on survival of out-of-hospital cardiac arrest, *Circulation* 106:1058-64, 2002.

12. Weaver WD, Peberdy MA: Defibrillators in public places—one step closer to home, *N Engl J Med* 347:1223-4, 2002.

13. Cummins RO: Emergency medical services and sudden cardiac arrest: the "chain of survival" concept, *Ann Rev Public Health* 14:313-29, 1993.

14. Holmberg M, Holmberg S, Herlitz J, for the Swedish Cardiac Arrest Registry: Factors modifying the effect of bystander cardiopulmonary resuscitation on survival in out-of-hospital cardiac arrest patients in Sweden, *Eur Heart J* 22:511-9, 2001.

15. Ewy GA: Cardiocerebral resuscitation. The new cardiopulmonary resuscitation, *Circulation* 111:2134-42, 2005.

16. Wellens HJJ, Gorgels AP, De Munter H: Cardiac arrest outside of a hospital. How can we improve results of resuscitation? *Circulation* 107:1948-50, 2003.

17. Weisfeldt ML, Becker LB: Resuscitation after cardiac arrest: a time-sensitive model, *JAMA* 288:3035-8, 2002.

APPENDIX C

Emergency Drugs

TABLE C-1	Intravenous Dosage (Adult) of Drugs Commonly Used During Bradycardia, Tachycardia, or Following Cardiac Resuscitation*
Drug	**Dosage**
Adenosine (Adenocard)	6-12 mg
Atropine	0.5-1.0 mg
Bretylium (Bretylol)	2-5 mg/kg
Calcium chloride	500 mg or 6.8 mEq (5 ml of 10% solution)
Digoxin (Lanoxin)	0.125-0.5 mg
Ephedrine	5-10 mg
Epinephrine (Adrenalin)	0.5-1.0 mg
Ibutilide	1 mg in a 10-minute period when body weight is ≥60 kg; 0.01 mg/kg when body weight is <60 kg
Lidocaine (Xylocaine)	1-1.5 mg/kg body weight
MgCl or MgSO$_4$	1-2 g (5-10 ml of 20% solution)
Nitroglycerin (Tridil)	200-400 µg
Phenytoin (Dilantin)	100-250 mg intravenously at 50 mg/min†
Procainamide (Pronestyl)	10 mg/kg per minute to 1000 mg
Propranolol (Inderal)	1-2 mg
Sodium bicarbonate	1 mEq/kg; 50-75 ml of 8.4% solution
Verapamil (Isoptin, Calan)	5-10 mg in 2- to 3-minute period

*Usually mixed in 5-10 ml 5% dextrose in water or normal saline.
†Use 0.22- to 0.45-µm filter.

TABLE C-2	Infusion Mixtures for Drugs Used During Bradycardia, Tachycardia, or Following Cardiopulmonary Resuscitation

| | | | Usual Dose | |
Drug	Dose*		Per Milliliter	Per Minute†
Amiodarone (Cordarone)	5 mg/kg body weight in 250 ml 5% glucose in 20-120/min			
Bretylium (Bretylol)	1000 mg		4 mg	1-2 mg
Dobutamine (Dobutrex)	500 mg		2 mg	5-15 µg/kg
Dopamine (Intropin)	200 mg		800 µg	2.5-20 µg/kg‡
Epinephrine (Adrenalin)	1 mg		4 µg	1-8 µg
Isoproterenol (Isuprel)	8 µg		1-8 µg	2 mg
Lidocaine (Xylocaine)	1000 mg		4 mg	1-4 mg
$MgSO_4$	4 g		16 mg	16 mg
Nitroglycerin (Tridil, Nitrostat, Nitro-Bid, Nitrocine, Nitrol)	50 mg		200 µg	25-1000 µg
Nitroprusside (Nipride, Nitropress)	50 mg		200 µg	10-500 µg
Norepinephrine (Levophed)	4 mg		16 µg	1-8 µg
Phenytoin (Dilantin)	500 mg		2 mg	200-300 µg
Procainamide (Pronestyl)	1000 mg		4 mg	1-4 mg

*Concentration per 250 ml 5% dextrose in water.

†Usually started at a low dose and titrated to desired action. If high doses are used, use higher concentration (×2, ×4) to limit volume of infusion.

‡Low dose: 2.5 to 5 µg/kg per minute. High dose (predominant alpha action): 5 to 20 µg/kg per minute. For high-dose infusion, use a more concentrated solution.

BOX C-1

Dosage of Drugs Used Intravenously to Treat Circus Movement Tachycardia by an Accessory Pathway

- Adenosine 6 mg; if unsuccessful, 12 mg (may repeat)
- Verapamil 10 mg over a 3-minute period
- Ajmaline 1 mg/kg over a 3-minute period
- Procainamide 10 mg/kg over a 5-minute period
- Diltiazem hydrochloride 0.25 mg/kg

BOX C-2

Dosage of Drugs Used Intravenously to Treat Atrial Fibrillation by an Accessory Pathway

- Procainamide 10 mg/kg over a 5-minute period
- Ajmaline 1 mg/kg over a 3-minute period
- Disopyramide 1.5 to 2 mg/kg over a 5-minute period

D

Mechanisms of Aberrant Ventricular Conduction

Aberrant ventricular conduction is a widening of the QRS caused by delay or block in a bundle branch or intramyocardial conduction. Following are the four different causes:

1. Sudden marked shortening of the ventricular cycle length (phase 3 aberration)
2. Retrograde invasion into one of the bundle branches (concealed retrograde conduction)
3. Marked lengthening of the ventricular cycle length (phase 4 aberration)
4. A modest shortening of the ventricular cycle length (acceleration-dependent block)

Delay or block in the right bundle branch is the most common cause of short cycle length aberration because that bundle usually has the longest refractory period.[1-3] LBBB aberration accounts for approximately one third of cases with aberrant ventricular conduction.

PHASE 3 ABERRATION

Functional or physiologic phase 3 aberration (bundle branch block) may occur in normal fibers if the impulse is premature enough to reach the cell when the membrane has not fully repolarized and is therefore refractory. This form of aberration is commonly observed after a conducted APB and at the beginning of an SVT.

Phase 3 aberration occurs following a long-short cycle sequence because the refractory period of the beat following the long cycle is prolonged. Figure D-1 shows that different degrees of RBBB are present, depending on the prematurity of the APB. Figure D-2 shows left bundle branch aberration in a patient with an SVT when a long-short sequence occurs at the initiation of the tachycardia.

CONCEALED RETROGRADE INVASION IN THE BUNDLE BRANCH

Retrograde concealed conduction into one of the bundle branches is a common mechanism of aberration during SVT.[4] Although the mechanism at the onset of PSVT may be phase 3 aberration, the sustaining mechanism is often concealed retrograde conduction up one of the bundle branches.[5] Figure D-3 is a schematic drawing of how, during sinus rhythm, LBBB aberration can be initiated by an APB. The initial mechanism of bundle branch block is phase 3 block in the left bundle. Perpetuation of LBBB during SVT is, however, caused by continuing retrograde invasion into the left bundle branch. As shown, the critical time relations required for continuing retrograde invasion into the left bundle branch are disturbed by an induced VPB. Examples of concealed retrograde invasion causing bundle branch block during SVT are

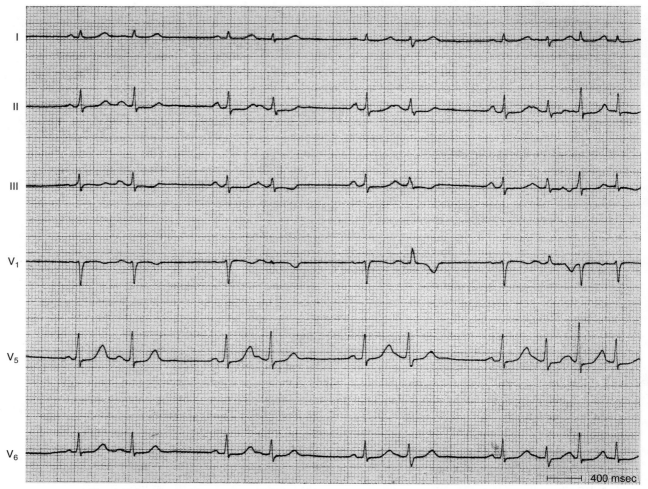

Figure D-1 Phase 3 aberration. Depending on the prematurity of the APB, the QRS complex shows different degrees of aberrant conduction in the right bundle branch.

given in Figures D-4 and D-5. In both instances, a VPB disrupts the critical time relations required for retrograde invasion into the bundle branch.

PHASE 4 ABERRATION

Phase 4 aberration is bundle branch block or hemiblock that occurs only following a critical lengthening of the cardiac cycle. Conduction velocity is optimal in fibers with a transmembrane potential of −90 mV, and it becomes slower when the membrane potential becomes less negative. During a long pause, the fibers of the His-Purkinje system spontaneously depolarize (become less and less negative), possibly blocking the impulse that terminates the pause in one of the bundle branches. This

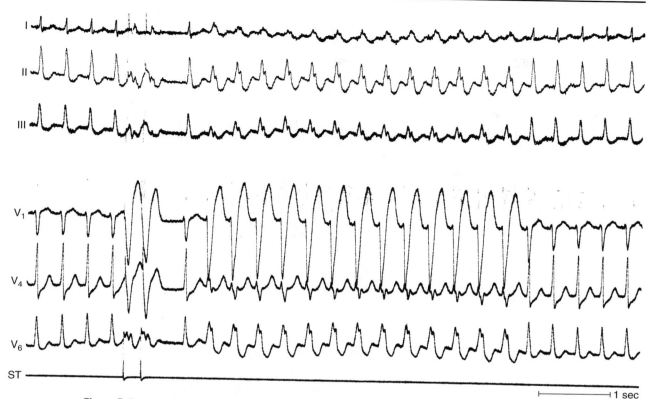

Figure D-2 Example of phase 3 aberration in the left bundle branch on shortening the ventricular cycle length at the initiation of an SVT. Note that rate-related shortening of the refractory period of the left bundle branch leads to disappearance of LBBB after 13 tachycardia QRS complexes.

shift in threshold membrane potential to a less negative level and a change in membrane responsiveness are seldom seen in normal hearts.

Figure D-6 illustrates phase 4 LBBB aberration in a patient with atrial fibrillation. During a long cycle the membrane potential of the left bundle branch has become less and less negative, so that local delay or block takes place for the descending impulse in the left bundle branch.

ACCELERATION-DEPENDENT BLOCK

As shown in Figure D-7, RBBB occurs when the sinus cycle shortens to values less than 1000 msec. This condition is obviously not phase 3 block because such an interval is much longer than the refractory period of the bundle branch. It points to poor conduction in the bundle branch and is a forerunner to complete block in that bundle branch.

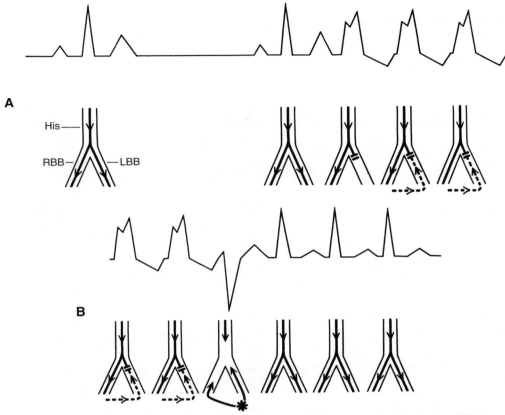

Figure D-3   Initiation, maintenance, and termination of left aberrant conduction during SVT. **A,** The first beat of the SVT is unable to pass the left bundle branch because of phase 3 block. That impulse conducted over the right bundle branch travels through the interventricular septum to invade the left bundle branch in a retrograde direction. The frequency of the SVT is such that all following impulses coming from above reach the left bundle branch when the structure has been made refractory by retrograde invasion from the preceding beat. Persistent left aberrant conduction results. **B,** If the excitation pattern described in **A** is disturbed, as shown here by a fortuitously timed VPB, the left bundle branch is no longer refractory when the next supraventricular impulse arrives. Now nonaberrant conduction takes place at the same frequency of the SVT.

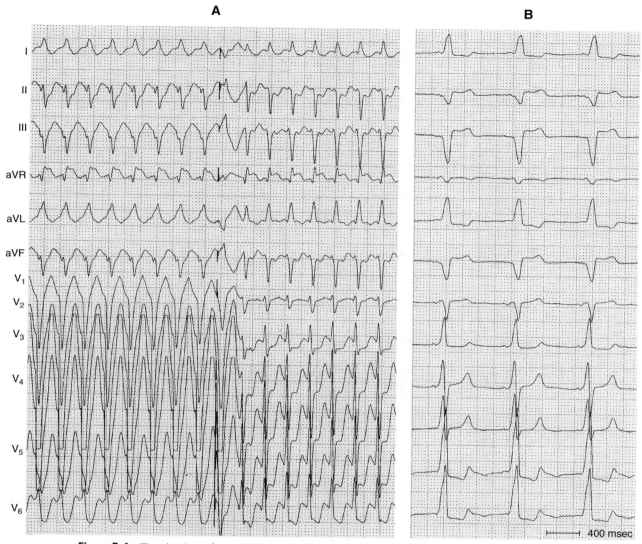

Figure D-4   Termination of concealed retrograde invasion into the left bundle branch by an induced VPB. See Figure D-3 for details. The tachycardia was a circus movement tachycardia (**A**) in a patient with a posteroseptal accessory pathway (**B**).

A

B

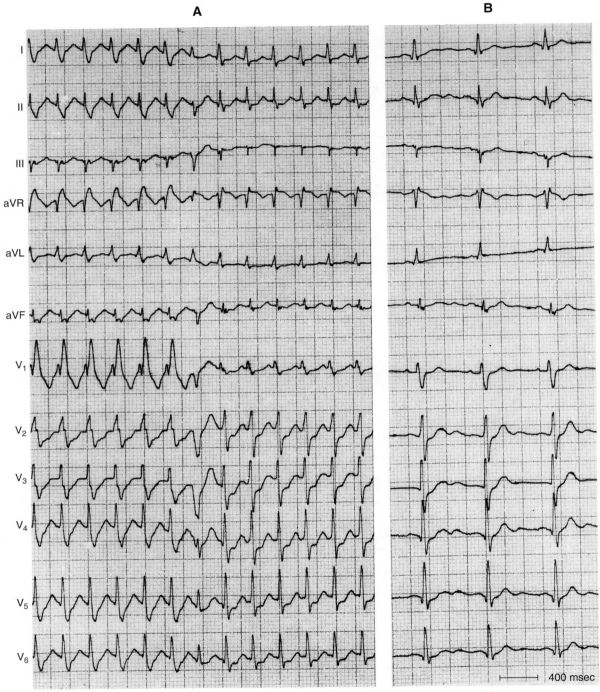

Figure D-5   Termination of concealed retrograde invasion into the right bundle branch by a spontaneously occurring VPB. The tachycardia was a circus movement tachycardia (**A**) in a patient with a concealed posteroseptal accessory pathway (**B**).

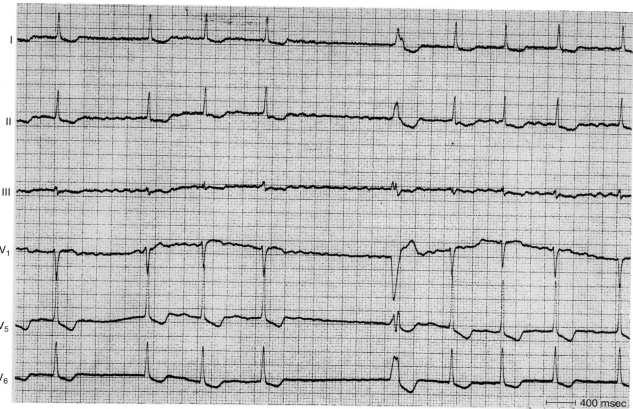

Figure D-6 Phase 4 aberration. In this patient with atrial fibrillation, the QRS after a long pause (1800 msec) shows LBBB caused by phase 4 block in the left bundle branch.

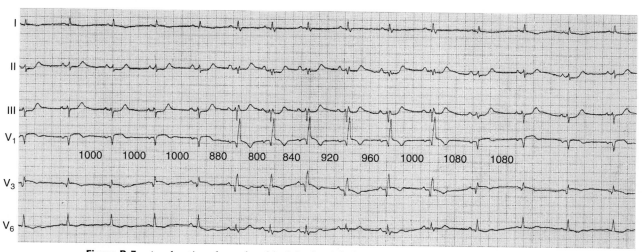

Figure D-7 Acceleration-dependent block in the right bundle branch. As shown, RBBB occurs when the sinus rate rises above 60 beats/min. This patient has an old anteroseptal MI.

REFERENCES

1. Lewis R: Paroxysmal tachycardia, the result of ectopic impulse formation, *Heart* 1:262-9, 1919.
2. Couax FJL, Ashman R: Auricular fibrillation with aberration simulating ventricular paroxysmal tachycardia, *Am Heart J* 34:366-72, 1957.
3. Moe GK, Mendez C, Han J: Aberrant AV impulse propagation in the dog heart: a study of functional bundle branch block, *Circ Res* 16:261-9, 1965.
4. Wellens HJJ, Ross DL, Farre J, et al: Functional bundle branch block during supraventricular tachycardia in man: observations on mechanisms and their incidence. In Zipes D, Jalife J, editors: *Cardiac electrophysiology and arrhythmias*, New York, 1985, Grune & Stratton, pp. 435-41.
5. Wellens HJJ, Durrer D: Supraventricular tachycardia with left aberrant conduction due to retrograde invasion into the left bundle branch, *Circulation* 38:474-9, 1968.

Index

Major discussions are boldface.
Page numbers followed by *f* indicate figures; *t,* tables; *b,* boxes.

Emergency Decisions in Acute ST Segment Elevation MI

1. Ascertain the time from onset of pain.
2. Determine the site, size, and severity of cardiac ischemia and the location of the occlusion in the coronary artery by analyzing the amount and direction of the ST segment deviation vector.
3. In inferoposterior MI, record lead V_4R.
4. Look for conduction disturbances—sinoatrial, AV nodal, and sub–AV nodal—and the presence of bundle branch block.
5. Decide on the necessity and type of reperfusion attempt (primary percutaneous coronary intervention or fibrinolysis).

The ECG in Anterior Wall MI

LAD OCCLUSION PROXIMAL TO FIRST SEPTAL AND FIRST DIAGONAL BRANCH

Apart from ST elevation in the precordial leads V_1 to V_4, the frontal ST vector points toward the base of the heart.

- ST elevation in aVR, aVL, and V_1
- ST depression in II, III, aVF, V_5, and V_6
- Acquired right bundle branch block (qR in lead V_1) with or without hemiblock indicates a proximal LAD occlusion.

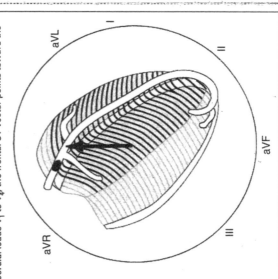

The ECG in Anterior Wall MI

LAD OCCLUSION BETWEEN THE FIRST SEPTAL AND FIRST DIAGONAL BRANCH

Apart from ST elevation in precordial leads V_2 to V_5, the frontal ST vector points toward aVL and away from III.

- ST elevation in I and aVL
- ST depression in III
- ST isoelectric in II

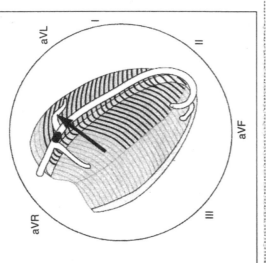

The ECG in Anterior Wall MI

LAD OCCLUSION DISTAL TO THE FIRST DIAGONAL OR INTERMEDIATE BRANCH BUT PROXIMAL TO THE FIRST SEPTAL BRANCH

Apart from ST elevation in precordial leads V_1 to V_5, the frontal ST deviation vector is directed rightward and inferiorly.

- ST elevation in aVR and III
- ST depression in I and aVL

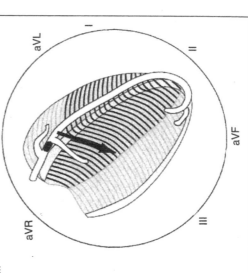

The ECG in Inferoposterior MI

Right coronary artery MI

Circumflex coronary artery MI

RCA occlusion: Frontal ST deviation vector points to III, resulting in ST elevation in III > II

CX occlusion: Frontal ST deviation vector points to II, resulting in ST elevation in II > III

over

Emergency Response to Non–ST Elevation MI and Unstable Angina

RECOGNITION OF EXTENT AND SEVERITY OF CORONARY ARTERY DISEASE DURING CHEST PAIN

1. Count the number of leads with ST segment deviation and determine the total ST deviation score (ST segment deviation in more than eight leads suggests left main or three-vessel disease).
2. Look for ST segment elevation in leads aVR and V_1, which suggests left main or three-vessel disease.
3. Determine the troponin value.
4. Decide on early invasive versus noninvasive management.

RECOGNITION OF A CRITICAL NARROWING IN THE LAD IN UNSTABLE ANGINA

1. Determine the troponin level. There will be little or no elevation in ischemia because of critical narrowing in the LAD.
2. Be alert to the three ECG signs of critical narrowing in the LAD when the patient is without pain. When these signs are present, an early invasive diagnostic (and possible therapeutic) approach is suggested.
   - Little or no ST elevation
   - No loss of R-wave progression in precordial leads
   - Terminal T-wave negativity progressing to deep symmetrical T-wave inversion in the precordial leads (usually most prominent in V_2 and V_3) after the chest pain has subsided

The ECG in Anterior Wall MI

DISTAL LAD OCCLUSION

Apart from ST elevation in V_2 to V_6, a frontal ST deviation vector points in an apical direction.

- ST elevation in the inferior leads with lead II greater than lead III

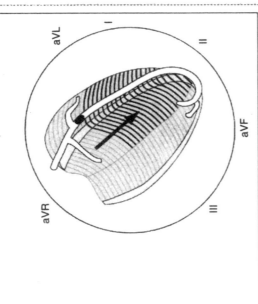

The ECG in Left Main Occlusion

The combination of acute ischemia in the LAD and CX region results in a frontal ST deviation vector pointing toward aVR and a horizontal ST deviation vector directed away from the posterior wall.

over

Proximal RCA: V_4R: ST elevation with positive T wave

Distal RCA: V_4R: ST isoelectric with positive T wave

CX occlusion: V_4R: ST isoelectric or depressed with negative T wave

LV posterior involvement: Horizontal ST deviation vector points to the posterior wall, resulting in ST depression in the anterior precordial leads

LV lateral involvement: Horizontal ST deviation vector points to the lateral wall

- Low lateral: ST elevation in V_5 and V_6
- High lateral: ST elevation in I and aVL

Isolated RV infarction: Horizontal ST deviation vector points to the anterior (right ventricular!) wall, leading to ST elevation in leads V_4R to V_4, and sometimes even V_5 and V_6.

- ST elevation in aVR and V_1
- ST depression in I, II, and aVF and V_2 to V_6

Emergency Approach to Regular Narrow QRS Tachycardia

1. Obtain a 12-lead ECG.
2. Assess the hemodynamic situation.

IF HEMODYNAMICALLY UNSTABLE
1. Cardiovert.
2. Obtain a history.
3. Record postconversion ECG.
4. Using a systematic approach, examine and compare precardioversion and postcardioversion ECGs to determine the type of SVT.

IF HEMODYNAMICALLY STABLE
1. Look for the frog sign in the jugular pulse.
2. Perform vagal stimulation. If unsuccessful:
3. Give adenosine 6 mg as a rapid IV bolus; if unsuccessful, follow after 3 minutes with 12 mg IV. If unavailable:
4. Give verapamil 10 mg IV over 5 to 10 minutes; reduce to 5 mg if the patient is taking a beta-blocker or is hypotensive. If hypotensive. If unsuccessful:
5. Give procainamide 10 mg/kg body weight over 5 minutes. If unsuccessful:
6. Perform electrical cardioversion.
7. Obtain a history.
8. Record a postconversion ECG.
9. Using a systematic approach, examine and compare preconversion and postconversion ECGs to determine the type of SVT.

Emergency Approach to SA Conduction Abnormalities

1. Record a 12-lead ECG.
2. If hypotension, dizziness, and presyncope are absent, no immediate treatment is required.
3. Evaluate the ECG for:
   - MI
   - Mechanism of bradycardia; look for:
     P-wave regularity (indicates a regular sinus or atrial rhythm)
     Abrupt pauses or group beating during sinus rhythm (suggests SA block)
4. In case of sinus bradycardia, give no treatment unless hypotension is present; then give IV atropine 0.04 mg/kg body weight.
5. In case of SA block or sinus arrest, give no treatment unless hypotension is present or the rhythm is digitalis induced (stop the drug).
6. If the diagnosis is sick sinus syndrome, treatment depends on symptoms (dizziness, presyncope, congestive heart failure).

Emergency Approach to Wide QRS Tachycardia

Do not panic when confronted with wide QRS tachycardia. Obtain a 12-lead ECG.

IF HEMODYNAMICALLY UNSTABLE
1. Cardiovert.
2. Obtain a history.
3. Examine precardioversion and postcardioversion ECGs to determine the etiology of the arrhythmia.

IF HEMODYNAMICALLY STABLE
1. Examine the patient for clinical signs of AV dissociation.
2. Systematically evaluate the 12-lead ECG.
3. Obtain a history.

IF VT
1. Give procainamide 10 mg/kg body weight IV over 5 minutes unless the tachycardia is ischemia related; then give lidocaine. If unsuccessful:
2. Cardiovert.
3. Examine the ECG during the VT and the ECG during sinus rhythm to determine the etiology of the tachycardia.

over

Emergency Approach to AV Block

1. Record a 12-lead ECG.
2. Evaluate the ECG for presence of MI.
3. When MI is excluded, determine the site of AV block using noninvasive methods.

IN ACUTE INFERIOR WALL MI
- *High-grade AV nodal block* indicates the need for early reperfusion. Resolution of the block indicates successful reperfusion.
- *AV conduction problems* are transient and usually do not require a pacemaker. The patient should be observed.
- If *complete AV block develops*, the escape pacemaker is usually a dependable AV junctional rhythm not requiring a pacemaker. The patient should be observed.
- Insert a *temporary ventricular or dual-chamber pacemaker* in cases of pump failure or cardiogenic shock or when both *frequent ventricular ectopic activity* and *high-degree AV nodal block* occur.
- *The need for permanent* pacing is very rare and is indicated only when symptomatic second- or third-degree AV nodal block is present and persists for more than 2 weeks after MI.

TYPE II AV BLOCK (MOBITZ II AV BLOCK)
- Evaluate for anterior MI.
- Determine the likely site of AV block by measuring the PR interval and the effect of exercise, carotid sinus pressure, and atropine on AV conduction.

over

SVT WITH ABERRATION

1. Perform vagal stimulation. If unsuccessful:
2. Give adenosine 6 mg by rapid IV bolus; if unsuccessful follow after 3 minutes with a 12 mg IV bolus. If unavailable:
3. Give verapamil 10 mg IV over 5 to 10 minutes; reduce to 5 mg if the patient is taking a beta-blocker or is hypotensive. If unsuccessful:
4. Give procainamide 10 mg/kg body weight IV over 5 minutes. If unsuccessful:
5. Cardiovert.
6. Examine SVT and postconversion ECGs to determine mechanism.

IF IN DOUBT

- Do not give verapamil; give IV procainamide.

IF WIDE QRS AND IRREGULAR

- Do not give digitalis or verapamil.
- Give IV procainamide unless torsades de pointes is present (see Chapter 7).

- A temporary pacemaker is required when type II AV block is associated with syncope. In patients with chronic fibrotic disease of the conduction system, this is followed by a permanent pacemaker.

TWO-TO-ONE AV BLOCK

- Determine the level of AV block by measuring the PR interval.
- Although the block may become complete in acute inferior wall MI, a pacemaker is usually not necessary because of a dependable junctional escape mechanism.
- A *temporary pacemaker* may be indicated in acute anterior wall MI if the QRS is broad and the patient is symptomatic (syncope or hemodynamic deterioration).

COMPLETE AV BLOCK (THIRD-DEGREE AV BLOCK)

- The insertion of a pacemaker is usually required when associated with a broad QRS.
- No immediate treatment is necessary when the QRS is narrow. Determine the cause of the block and then make a judgment regarding the necessity of pacemaker insertion.
- Complete AV block in acute anterior MI requires temporary pacing. A permanent pacemaker usually is not needed if the patient survives the acute stage of MI.

PAROXYSMAL AV BLOCK

- A pacemaker is indicated because of the unreliability of the escape mechanism and the risk of sudden death.

Emergency Approach to Potassium-Related Emergencies

ECG RECOGNITION OF SEVERE OR PROGRESSIVE HYPERKALEMIA

- Slow heart rate
- P-wave widening with low voltage, followed by loss of P wave
- Broad QRS
- Frequently, left axis deviation
- Loss of ST segment (S wave merges with T wave)
- Tall, tented T waves
- Normal or shortened QTc interval

TREATMENT

1. Give calcium gluconate (10%) 10 to 30 ml IV over 1 to 5 minutes with constant ECG monitoring.
2. Administer 10 units of insulin in 500 ml 10% glucose IV in 30 minutes.
3. Add salbutamol 5 μg/kg body weight in 15 ml glucose 5% IV in 15 minutes.
4. Add sodium bicarbonate (2 to 3 ampules) to 1 L of 5% dextrose in 0.9% saline solution.
5. Administer cation exchange resins (sodium polystyrene sulfonate) by retention enema; this may be repeated until potassium levels are within safe limits. Oral doses of 20 g are given 3 or 4 times a day together with 20 ml of 70% sorbitol solution.
6. In the event of renal failure, institute hemodialysis or peritoneal dialysis with one of the treatments above.

over

Emergency Approach to Acute Pulmonary Embolism

EXAMINE THE ECG FOR

- Rhythm disturbances
- A shift in the axis to the right in comparison with the ECG prior to the acute event (need not be outside the normal range of +90 to −30 degrees)
- Appearance of an RBBB pattern
- Pseudoinfarction patterns

IF SUDDEN CHANGES OCCUR IN THE ECG SUGGESTING PULMONARY EMBOLISM,

CALL FOR

- Emergency echocardiogram
- Arterial oxygen saturation and
- D-Dimer measurement

THERAPY

- Oxygen
- Analgesics
- Full-dose heparin
- Thrombolytic therapy

PREVENTION

Avoid Venous Stasis

- Early mobilization and ambulation when possible
- External compression of the legs for patients on complete bed rest

over

Digitalis-Induced Emergencies

SYSTEMATIC DIAGNOSTIC APPROACH

1. Obtain periodic 12-lead ECGs on all patients in your care who are taking digitalis.
2. Question the patient regarding noncardiac symptoms of digitalis toxicity and concomitant medication that may interact with digitalis.
3. Know the ECG signs of digitalis-induced arrhythmias.
4. Look specifically for bradycardia, tachycardia, inappropriate regularity (such as in atrial fibrillation or flutter), or group beating.

EMERGENCY MANAGEMENT

1. Stop digitalis administration.
2. Prescribe bed rest (no sympathetic stimulation!).
3. Initiate continuous ECG monitoring.
4. If hemodynamically unstable, administer phenytoin unless digitalis antibodies are available.
5. Insert a ventricular pacemaker:
   - In symptomatic bradycardia
   - During treatment with phenytoin because suppression of the tachycardia may be followed by asystole
6. Evaluate kidney function and correct potassium and magnesium deficits.

AVOID

- Sympathetic stimulation (stress, anxiety, exercise, sympathomimetic drugs)
- Carotid sinus massage
- Fast or sudden cessation of ventricular pacing

Emergency Treatment of Drug-Induced Arrhythmic Emergencies

TORSADES DE POINTES

1. Stop the offending drug.
2. Establish continuous ECG monitoring.
3. Give magnesium as MgCl or MgSO₄, 1 to 2 g IV bolus over 5 minutes; infusion: 1 to 2 g/hr for 4 to 6 hours. If unsuccessful:
4. Increase heart rate with isoproterenol or by pacing.

SUSTAINED (INCESSANT) MONOMORPHIC VT

1. Stop the offending drug.
2. In case of hemodynamic compromise, give inotropic support with isoproterenol or epinephrine. This will also counteract slowing in conduction velocity induced by class IA or class IC drugs.
3. If VT persists and is poorly tolerated, pace the atrium at the rate of the VT. Use an AV interval that will provide maximal contribution of atrial contraction to ventricular filling.

DRUG-INDUCED BRADYCARDIA

1. Stop the offending drug.
2. Give atropine or start temporary transvenous pacing in case of (a) Adams-Stokes attacks, (b) a low ventricular rate leading to hypotension, and/or (c) bradycardia-dependent ventricular arrhythmias.

over

ECG RECOGNITION OF SEVERE HYPOKALEMIA (SERUM LEVEL <2.5 mEq/L)

- ST depression
- Decrease in T-wave amplitude
- Increase in U-wave amplitude
- QT prolongation

TREATMENT

1. Give potassium chloride IV not to exceed 40 mEq/L at an infusion rate not to exceed 20 mEq/hr (approximately 200 to 250 mEq/day).
2. Give oral potassium chloride.

Anticoagulants

- If heart failure is present or the patient is on long-term bed rest

Emergency Approach to Hypothermia

ECG RECOGNITION

- Slow heart rate
- Widened P waves
- Widened QRS
- Osborn waves
- Prolonged QT

TREATMENT

1. Gradually rewarm the patient in cases of exposure to a cold environment.
2. Identify the cause and treat accordingly. The hypothermia may be caused by nonenvironmental conditions.

Emergency Approach to Monogenic Arrhythmic Diseases

When the patient presents with a broad QRS tachycardia, either monomorphic or polymorphic VT, or ventricular fibrillation:

IF HEMODYNAMICALLY UNSTABLE

1. Cardiovert.
2. Obtain a history.
3. Examine the preconversion and postconversion ECGs to determine possibility and type of monogenic disease.

IF HEMODYNAMICALLY STABLE

1. Evaluate the 12-lead ECG.
2. In case of long QT with torsades de pointes (see card on Emergency Treatment of Drug-Induced Arrhythmic Emergencies), a beta-blocking agent may be added. If unsuccessful:
   - Cardiovert.
   - Obtain a history.
   - Examine the preconversion and postconversion ECGs to determine possibility and type of monogenic disease.
   - Discuss the value of a genetic evaluation of the family.